369 0123793

Clinical Judgment and Communication in Nurse Practitioner Practice

Clinical Judgment and Communication in Nurse Practitioner Practice

Susan K. Chase, APRN, BC, FNP, EdD

Associate Professor
Christine E. Lynn College of Nursing
Florida Atlantic University
Boca Raton, Florida

F. A. DAVIS COMPANY • Philadelphia

F. A. Davis Company
1915 Arch Street
Philadelphia, PA 19103
www.fadavis.com

Printed in the United States of America

Last digit indicates print number: 10 9 8 7 6 5 4 3 2 1

Acquisitions Editor: Joanne P. DaCunha, RN, MSN
Developmental Editor: Rose Foltz
Production Editor: Jessica Howie Martin
Cover Designer: Joan Wendt, Design Manager

As new scientific information becomes available through basic and clinical research, recommended treatments and drug therapies undergo changes. The author and publisher have done everything possible to make this book accurate, up to date, and in accord with accepted standards at the time of publication. The author, editors, and publisher are not responsible for errors or omissions or for consequences from application of the book, and make no warranty, expressed or implied, in regard to the contents of the book. Any practice described in this book should be applied by the reader in accordance with professional standards of care used in regard to the unique circumstances that may apply in each situation. The reader is advised always to check product information (package inserts) for changes and new information regarding dose and contraindications before administering any drug. Caution is especially urged when using new or infrequently ordered drugs.

Library of Congress Cataloging-in-Publication Data

Chase, Susan K.
  Clinical judgment and communication in nurse practitioner
practice / Susan K. Chase. — 1st ed.
    p. ; cm.
  Includes bibliographical references and index.
  ISBN 0-8036-0797-0 (pbk. : alk. paper)
    1. Nurse practitioners. 2. Clinical competence. 3. Nurse and
patient.   I. Title.
  [DNLM: 1. Nurse Practitioners. 2. Nursing Process. 3. Decision Making. 4. Nurse-Patient Relations.   WY 128 C487c
2004]
  RT82.8.C485 2004
  610.73′06′92—dc22

                                        2003026077

This book is dedicated to the nurses
who have been my students over the years
and who have taught me so much through
their presence, and to the patients who open
their lives to us in the unique relationship that
exists between nurse practitioner and patient
as together we work to support their health.

Preface

This book is designed to be useful throughout a nurse practitioner student's education. It supplements the typical health assessment course by illustrating how to approach relationship building and history taking. It bridges the gap between data gathering, which is the main focus of health assessment courses, and diagnostic reasoning, which is required in clinical management courses. It supplements primary-care management textbooks, which in many programs include medical textbooks, by providing strategies that include nursing diagnoses and interventions. It supports clinical-management courses by providing support for high-quality documentation and by addressing issues both within nursing itself and between the nurse and other professionals. Finally, it considers the philosophical and ethical grounding for how we relate to patients as nurse practitioners. In this way, it can be useful to advanced practitioners already in the field. Throughout the chapters, where appropriate, Words of Wisdom is included as a feature that offers the perspectives of actual nurse practitioners as they reflect on their practice. Clinical judgment is more than application of a step-by-step process. It requires the consideration of the meaning of an encounter. Words of Wisdom point out these relationships. Rules of Thumb, another feature, offers shortcuts to reasoning that develop in a particular practice area and serve as supports to clinical judgment in the field.

The model for care presented here is not the type of care that student nurse practitioners can deliver in their early months of practice. It is held out here, however, as a model so that, after mastering the technical skills of history taking, physical examination, and treatment planning, the nurse practitioner will be able to grow into a model of care that is emancipatory for both nurse practitioner and patient. Students can observe their preceptors for the humanistic and holistic care that is described here. They can begin to assemble their experience narratives so that they can continue to grow in their practice. Becoming a nurse practitioner is an exciting adventure. Faculty members, fellow students, and preceptors are available to help the novice nurse practitioner develop the type of relationship-centered care described in this book.

Susan K. Chase

Acknowledgments

I want to thank the many people who have supported me through the process of envisioning and completing this book. Joanne DaCunha and Rose Foltz from F. A. Davis have been consistent supports. My contributing authors, Robin Whittemore and Pamela Grace, delivered their wonderful chapters without prompting. Fellow faculty members Carol Lynn Mandle, Patricia Tabloski, Laurel Eisenhauer, Barbara Brush, and Margaret Murphy helped me shape my teaching. Many friends have supported me during the process, including Jean D'Meza Leuner, who helped me shape an early conception of this book; Lynne Dunphy, who shared her research interview data; and Kristin Parent, Carolyn Hayes, Connie Phillips, Ken and Nancy Krienke, Patti Kinzer, Marcene Powell, and Roberta Kaplow, who were tremendous personal supports. My dean at Boston College, Barbara Hazard Munro, supported me in my attendance of the post-doctoral nurse practitioner program at the University of Wisconsin at Oshkosh. My teachers' words and philosophy are interspersed throughout this book. These teachers include Roxanna Huebscher, Nancy Elsberry, Mary Barker, and my preceptor Laura Frankenstein. My fellow nurse practitioners at the Massachusetts General Hospital, Brenda Smith and Catherine Grams, and physicians Richard Wiklund and Annetta Murphy were great colleagues and partners. Finally, I want to thank my parents, Nyla and Orville Krienke, for their support and pride in all that I do; and my sons, Peter and Andrew, whose generous sharing of my time and attention have supported my career and, more importantly, my life.

SKC

Contributors

Pamela J. Grace, APRN, BC, PhD
Adult Nurse Practitioner
Assistant Professor, William F. Connell School of Nursing
Boston College
Boston, Massachusetts

Robin Whittemore, RN, PhD
Assistant Professor
School of Nursing
University of Connecticut
Storrs, Connecticut

Reviewers

Sherri Beck, RN, MSN, ANP, GNP
Nurse Practitioner
Aspen Medical Associates
Teaneck, New Jersey

Linda Caldwell, RN, CS, DNSc
Chairperson
Curry College
Milton, Massachusetts

Nancy Campbell-Heider, RN, PhD
Associate Professor/FNP
SUNY at Buffalo
Buffalo, New York

Evelyn L. Cesaroti, FNP-C, GNP-C, PhD
Assistant Professor
Arizona State University
Phoenix, Arizona

Judith A. Conedera, RN, MSN
Assistant Professor
Purdue University, Calumet
Hammond, Indiana

Sherri Davidson, RN, MSN, CCRN, CS, ACNP
Acute Care Nurse Practitioner
Hillcrest Baptist Medical Center
Waco, Texas

Roger A. Green, ARNP, FNP, CS, MSN
Adjunct Faculty, Family Nurse Practitioner Program
The University of Tampa
Tampa, Florida

Sandra M. Handley, RN, CS, FNP, PhD
Family Nurse Practitioner, School-based Clinic
Instructor, FNP Program
University of Missouri–Kansas City
Kansas City, Missouri

Diane S. Harper, MS, CANP
Assistant Professor
Molloy College
Rockville Center, New York

Mary D. Knudtson, RN, MSN, FNP, PNP
Assistant Clinical Professor
Director, FNP Program
University of California–Irvine
Irvine, California

Denise L. McKinney, RN, CPNP, MS
Pediatric Nurse Practitioner
Pediatric Associates
Ellicott City, Maryland

Karen Koozer Olson, PhD, FNP-CS
Professor, Graduate Program Director
and FNP Student Health Center
Texas A&M University
Corpus Christi, Texas

Mary Carol Galichia Pomatto, RN, MS, ARNP, EdD
Assistant to the President and Professor
Pittsburg State University
Pittsburg, Kansas

Jacqueline Rhoads, RN, CCRN-ACNP-CS, PhD
Professor, FNP Program
Louisiana State University
New Orleans, Louisiana

Denise Robinson, RN, FNP, PhD
Professor and Director, MSN Program
Northern Kentucky University
Highland Heights, Kentucky

Cynthia K. Russell, RN, CS, PhD
Assistant Professor and Adult Nurse Practitioner
University of Tennessee–Memphis
College of Nursing
Memphis, Tennessee

Judith Schilling, CRNP, PhD
Director, MSN FNP Program
Edinboro University
Department of Nursing
Edinboro, Pennsylvania

Leane Schimke, RN, MSN, FNP
Family Nurse Practitioner
New Holland Family Health Center
New Holland, Pennsylvania

Mary M. Sullivan, RN, MSN
Clinical Specialist, Nurse Practitioner
University of California, San Francisco
San Francisco, California

Linda M. Tenofsky, RN, CS, PhD
Professor
Curry College
Milton, Massachusetts

Contents

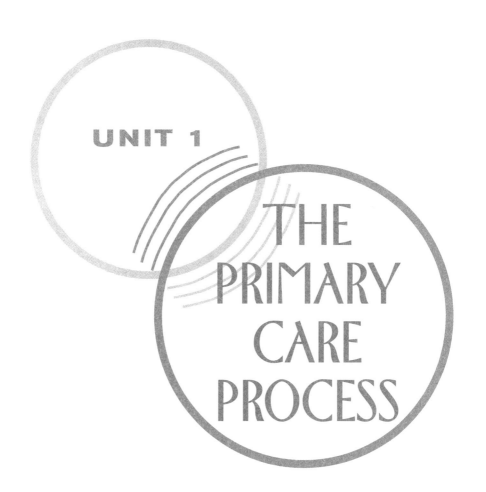

UNIT 1

THE PRIMARY CARE PROCESS

CHAPTER 1

Nurse Practitioners and Relationship-Centered Care

)) UNIQUENESS OF NURSE PRACTITIONER PRACTICE

Since the inception of the nurse practitioner role, its practitioners have demonstrated that they deliver safe and effective care (Brown & Grimes, 1995; Mundinger et al., 2000). When compared with primary medical caregivers, nurse practitioners have been shown to deliver care that provides patient outcomes that are at least equivalent. Nurse practitioners also provide care with which patients are highly satisfied (Matas, Brown, & Holman, 1996).

This book is about the processes used by nurse practitioners in delivering that care. It supplements knowledge from pathophysiology, treatment options for various diseases, health promotion strategies, and physical assessment skills by providing the links that the nurse practitioner must make among all these areas when dealing individually with patients and their families. The clinical judgment process brings together the basic knowledge of disease within the context of a patient's life so that the nurse practitioner can create a unique view of the patient's experience and devise an appropriate health management plan. The process of bringing together general knowledge of health and illness with personal knowledge of the patient's story is called clinical judgment (Crabtree, 2000).

Nurse practitioner practice is different from the practice of nurses who work in staff nurse roles in acute, long-term, or community-based settings because nurse practitioners are responsible for developing a full treatment plan, including nursing and medical measures. Clinical judgment by nurse practitioners involves making decisions about ordering diagnostic tests and prescribing medications. It also differs from medical primary care because nurse practitioners function within a nursing model, even in a primary care setting. The range of problems or life issues is broader than a medical diagnosis list. This means that the nursing database is broader and richer than the standard medical database. The nurse practitioner is expert in providing teaching and counseling to patients that helps patients develop self-care skills. Nurses function from a holistic model that involves more than physical illness: they are concerned with a body-mind-spirit view of each patient's life situation. These unique features not only distinguish nurse practitioner practice from other nursing and primary care practices, but also render the clinical judgment process more complex.

Nurses experienced in acute care will find that they are challenged to learn both new content areas and new approaches to patient care. Primary care has been defined by the Institute of Medicine (IOM) as "the provision of integrated, accessible, health care services by clinicians who are accountable for addressing a large majority of personal health care needs, developing a sustained partnership with patients, and practicing in the context of family and community" (IOM, cited in Donaldson & Vanselow, 1996, p. 114). The process of developing relationships over time that takes into account the family and the community is the basis for primary care by nurse practitioners.

⟩⟩ MUTUALITY IN NURSE PRACTITIONER-PATIENT RELATIONSHIP

The nurse practitioner-patient relationship involves more than treatment of disease. The nurse practitioner's goal is to become a partner in health management with patients and families. Nurse practitioners establish a relationship with patients and family members that respects the patient's knowledge, skills, and values. This respect invites patients to be open and honest about their health concerns and struggles. This, in turn, provides a fuller picture of the patient's situation and allows the nurse practitioner to make accurate diagnoses and to fashion an individualized management plan. Even within the constraints of busy office practices, the nursing model that values time and personal attention helps patients to feel that they are being heard and not rushed. This feeling results in increased patient satisfaction (Chase, 2001).

In a concept analysis of mutuality, Henson (1997) differentiates mutuality from autonomy, in which decisions are made in isolation by a patient, and paternalism, in which decisions are made solely by the health-care provider. Mutuality implies a relationship that is collaborative, reciprocal, negotiated, and participatory. Consequences of mutuality are:

◎ An increased sense of control for both provider and patient
◎ An increase in self-care by the patient
◎ An increase in accountability by the provider
◎ An initial investment of time and energy, with a concomitant increase in efficiency of care delivery
◎ A new creativity in reaching alternative care strategies
◎ An increase in empowerment for the patient
◎ Positive growth for both patient and provider

Patients come to a health-care appointment because of some health concern, but they also come expecting to be heard and attended to. It has been argued that during the health-care encounter, "an important component of healing, apart from the effect of any technology applied, derives from the relationship between the healer and the patient" (Matthews, Suchman, & Branch, 1993, p. 973). Several explanations for the power of this relationship have been proposed (Bensing, Schreurs, & DeRijk, 1996; Keller & Carroll, 1994). These explanations include an enhanced placebo effect when the patient has confidence in the care provider, the relief of being able to share one's burdens with another, and the general social support provided by a personal relationship. Each visit is prompted by two needs: a need to obtain a diagnosis and treatment for a health concern and a need to be understood and accepted as a person.

A model for how the nurse practitioner and patient work together in a clinical encounter is presented in Figure 1–1. Clinical judgment is a process that occurs in a dialogue between patient and provider. Open communication about what the encounter is meant to accomplish will improve both effectiveness and satisfaction for both parties. The model includes patient

Figure 1–1
PATIENT-NURSE PRACTITIONER LINKAGES

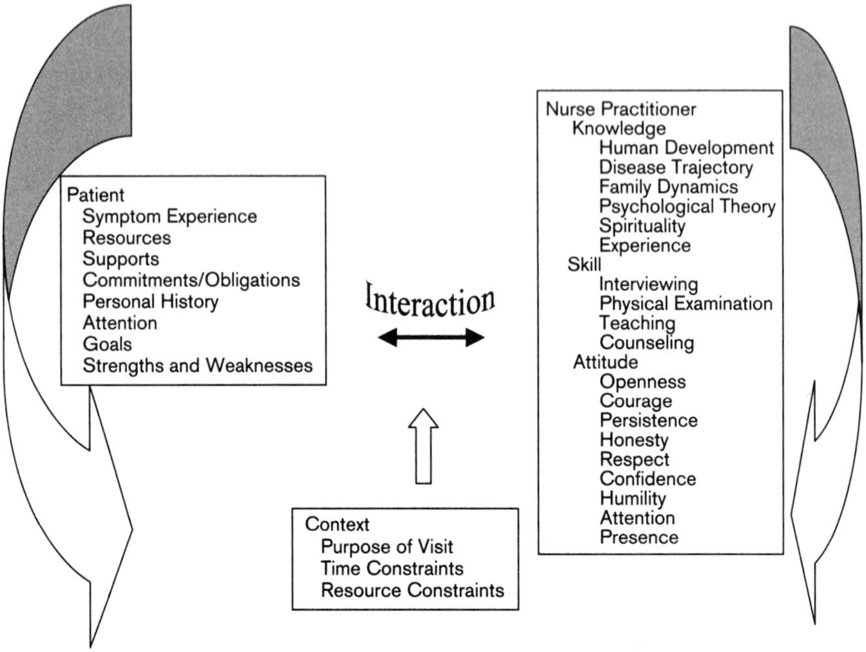

Nurse Practitioner
  Knowledge
    Human Development
    Disease Trajectory
    Family Dynamics
    Psychological Theory
    Spirituality
    Experience
  Skill
    Interviewing
    Physical Examination
    Teaching
    Counseling
  Attitude
    Openness
    Courage
    Persistence
    Honesty
    Respect
    Confidence
    Humility
    Attention
    Presence

Patient
  Symptom Experience
  Resources
  Supports
  Commitments/Obligations
  Personal History
  Attention
  Goals
  Strengths and Weaknesses

Interaction

Context
  Purpose of Visit
  Time Constraints
  Resource Constraints

factors, nurse practitioner factors, and contextual factors, all of which have an influence on the clinical judgment process.

Patient Factors Influencing Clinical Judgment

The patient brings his or her experience of symptoms and his or her attempts to manage them. Symptoms can have a variety of meanings to patients, from minor annoyances to potential threats to life or vitality. Symptoms also affect patients differently when they are part of a long-term pattern of chronic illness as compared to a new problem. Each patient has unique resources in terms of economic support, family or other social supports, and previous experience in dealing with health problems. Each patient is also balancing a unique set of commitments and obligations, such as work, child care, or elder care, that determine the amount of energy that he or she will be able to devote to lifestyle change or even to rest. Each person has a personal history of successes, failures, hopes, and dreams that shape how he or she responds to the stress of an illness situation. Patients vary in how much attention they pay to their symptoms. They also present with varying cognitive and reasoning skills that they can use in self-management of their condition. Finally, individual patients and families have unique values and goals as to how they choose to live their lives. Patients bring a unique set of strengths and weaknesses to the health situation. It is important to understand these strengths and weaknesses when devising a treatment plan that will maximize health.

Nurse Practitioner Factors Influencing Clinical Judgment

Just as each patient and family brings uniqueness to the nurse practitioner-patient encounter, the nurse practitioner brings his or her own uniqueness to the situation. Nurse practitioner knowledge, although it meets a basic standard for certification, varies widely from one person to another. Nurse practitioners may have various experiences in caring for patients in a wide range of settings. Some nurse practitioners have experience in caring for diabetic patients in other settings that can be used in primary care settings. Others have extensive experience in working with children and understand how to form linkages that have healing power by applying their knowledge of developmental issues and individual temperament. The types of knowledge that nurse practitioners use in their practice include disease and pathophysiology, human and family development, knowledge of stress and its effects, and general concepts of how humans make sense and meaning of their experience. Nurse practitioners are cognizant of their own experiences as humans interacting with an environment that makes demands and provides supports. Each brings a specific set of skills in data collection, diagnostic reasoning, teaching, counseling, and treatment delivery that forms a major part of the clinical encounter. Over a lifetime, nurse practitioners also have developed a set of their own personal and professional values and goals that become part of every human encounter.

The values that assist the development of clinical judgment include openness to humans and their expression of distress, courage in facing difficult situations, persistence in diagnostic reasoning, and staying with patients as they develop new health management skills. This is founded in respect for other people, whether they are the patient or other members of the practice setting. In order to deal with the complexities of primary care, the nurse practitioner needs confidence in his or her own abilities tempered by humility in recognizing the limits of knowledge and skill. Ultimately, offering human presence in the clinical judgment phase or the treatment phase of the nurse practitioner-patient relationship is life affirming for both patient and nurse practitioner.

Contextual Factors Influencing Clinical Judgment

Finally, the context of the encounter partly determines what will occur. Context includes both the environment of care and the purpose or goal of the encounter. A busy primary care office shapes the visit in one way. A nursing home visit brings a unique set of opportunities and constraints to the encounter. A college health setting or homeless shelter provides a different set of values and perspectives that influence the nurse practitioner-patient interaction. All these factors that are at play in every nurse practitioner-patient encounter shape the uniqueness of the nurse practitioner-patient relationship. A patient may perceive that the purpose of a visit is to solve what he or she perceives to be a simple problem. In order to include health-promoting activities, the nurse practitioner must negotiate the purpose of the visit to meet the patient's needs as he or she perceives them, as well as to inform the patient about other potential benefits that could be obtained through health promotion.

Holistic Relationships

All nurse practitioners must deal with family issues as part of the relationship-centered care that they provide. Patients' relationships with other people, primarily their own families, provide a backdrop for the relationship with the nurse practitioner. Knowledge of these relationships can shed light on the patient's style of life and provide information about social support that may affect treatment regimens. A study of family practice in direct observation of 4454 office visits in 138 family practice offices showed that there are two styles of operating with a family focus. The first style places family as the context of care of an individual patient. The second model treats the family itself as the unit of care (Medalie, Zyzanski, Langa, & Stange, 1998). Nurse practitioners are able to operate most broadly within the second model. This supports choosing interventions such as teaching the family together about food choices. Nurse practitioners must be aware that an individual patient's definition of family may be different from the traditional nuclear family. Family can mean any significant ongoing relationships that provide mutual support.

A model of primary care that promotes holistic care has been described by Dacher (1995). He asserts that the holistic model expands to include psychological, spiritual, community, and environmental concerns. The relationship formed between provider and patient becomes a focus of healing. The relationship with the holistic practitioner is one of partnership. The advantage of this model is that the responsibility for outcome does not rest solely on the professional. Patients are empowered to increase their self-care ability.

Recently patients have gained access to information and treatment guidelines from the popular press, the Worldwide Web, or support groups. As a result, the purpose for the primary care visit is changing. It is no longer solely designed to obtain a diagnosis and prescription, but is expanding to establish a partnership that supports patient self-management. Patients come to nurse practitioners for relationship and individual attention, not for decontextualized medical management.

⟩⟩ NURSING MODEL OF PRACTICE

Nurse practitioners perform in both the nursing and medical domains. The medical domain contains diagnosis and treatment of diseases. The nursing domain contains consideration of individual and family responses to actual or potential threats to health. The nursing domain also involves helping patients cope with disease processes that might be occurring. The nurse practitioner anticipates human distress and works on the level of what an illness experience means to the patient.

Too many nurse practitioner students are entranced by entering the medical realm and seem to leave their nursing values behind. When they do so, they leave the patient vulnerable. Barbara Bates, the author of the classic physical examination text, commented, "by expanding into medicine, nurse practitioners will need more than ever before, to increase their consciousness of what nursing is all about. The values of nursing must not get lost in the dominant medical culture. If they do, nurse practitioners justly risk the epithet of junior doctor" (1990, p. 139). Dunphy and Winland-Brown's model described as the "Circle of Caring" (1998) confronts this issue. This model combines components of traditional biomedicine and traditional holistic nursing practice. It synthesizes the problem-solving approaches of these two domains.

When nurses become nurse practitioners, they do not need to leave their nursing practice model. Rather, as they gain a medical domain of practice skills, they learn new diagnostic reasoning skills and new treatment options for specific medical problems. These new skills are additions to the nursing framework. They do not replace the nursing basis for practice. Nurse practitioners have been proven to be effective and efficient care providers for patients with acute and chronic health problems (Brown & Grimes, 1995). Their effectiveness stems from their holistic view of patients and their health problems (Courtney & Rice, 1997).

Although much of this textbook provides a framework for managing medical problems, all that the nurse has learned in caring for patients still applies. A nurse practitioner's approach to patient problems is often very individualized and therefor less easy to summarize in a textbook. Nevertheless, the nursing model supports and nurtures the nurse practitioner's practice and values a holistic view of patients.

Nursing models as taught in Concept or Theory courses in nurse practitioner programs might be chosen for application to practice. General nursing models, such as Orem's Self Care model or Roy's Adaptation model, provide a way of understanding patient problems and nursing's contribution to care. Specific models focus the nurse's attention in specific ways. For example, in a rehabilitation context, Orem's Self Care model works particularly well in helping both nurse and patient understand the role of patient self-care and nursing support. Roy's model, with its emphasis on the adaptation process, might be appropriate for use in a chronic illness situation. By choosing an explicit model, nurses are guided in collecting data about functional status or responses to health/illness concerns. Even if an explicit nurse theorist is not chosen as a model, nursing models support collecting data from such broad perspectives as the Functional Health Model (Gordon, 1994). By collecting data about varying aspects of the patient's life, the nurse practitioner is able to understand health and illness concerns from a wider perspective than that of a list of medical diagnoses. This understanding allows the nurse practitioner to be more efficient in meeting the true concerns of the patient. See Chapter 3 for a fuller discussion of Functional Health Pattern Assessment.

For example, a 46-year-old man was being evaluated for chest pain with a cardiac catheterization, which found no blockages of any coronary arteries. An in-depth history, taken by a nurse practitioner student after the cardiac catheterization, revealed that he also suffered from irritable bowel syndrome, stomach ulcers, and asthma. Furthermore, her interview revealed that he was unhappy in his work life. If this patient had been initially evaluated by a nurse practitioner, the broad range of his concerns could have been addressed and perhaps the expensive cardiac catheterization might have been avoided. Nurse practitioners have many tools such as the functional health pattern assessment, several depression indexes, and life stress indexes to use in assessing patients. The nursing model allows creative and flexible evaluation and management of patient concerns. Box 1–1 is a sample dialogue between the student nurse practitioner (SNP) and the patient (PT) in this case. Throughout assessment, diagnosis, and treatment, the nurse practitioner brings an authentic presence, which is in itself humanizing and healing.

Nursing has claimed concern for caring as the essence of its practice.

Box 1–1 Sample Student Nurse Practitioner Encounter

SNP: Mr. B., my name is Jane Martin. I am a nurse practitioner student, and I am here to explore your health problems. I will discuss what we talk about with my preceptor, Miss Jenkins. She will then come in, and together we will work out a plan for your care. I understand that you have been having chest pain. Can you tell me about your pain?

PT: Well, it has been bothering me more and more lately.

SNP: When did you first notice it?

PT: I guess 2 months ago.

SNP: Were you doing anything in particular at the time?

PT: I guess I had just had a big dinner with clients from my work. It's hard to remember.

SNP: And how long did the pain last?

PT: Oh, I guess for an hour or so.

SNP: Can you point on your body to where you felt the pain?

PT: Right here (indicating upper abdomen, lower sternum).

SNP: Did it stay in that place or move?

PT: I guess it stayed there.

SNP: How often does the pain come back? And does it come at any particular time?

PT: Well, I guess I get it twice a week or so. I get it at night a lot. I also notice that it feels better to eat something, so I've been eating more. I guess I put on a few pounds.

SNP: When you have your pain, do you notice anything else about how you feel?

PT: What do you mean?

SNP: Well, do you feel sweaty or nauseated or dizzy or short of breath?

PT: Oh, well, I guess my stomach gets upset, but I don't think I get short of breath. I do have asthma, but that hasn't bothered me much lately, and I know what that feels like.

SNP: What do you do to relieve the pain?

PT: Mostly try to ignore it, but it's been getting worse.

SNP: Have you called your doctor or any other provider because of this pain?

PT: Well, I have new insurance, so I called a guy on the list they gave me and he said to go to the emergency room, and that's how I ended up here.

SNP: And before that, when did you last see a health-care provider?

(Continued)

Box 1–1 Sample Student Nurse
Practitioner Encounter *(Continued)*

PT: Oh, maybe 2 or 3 years. I'm awful busy at work.

SNP: Have you had your cholesterol checked or had a stress test for your heart?

PT: Well, they did one just before this last test, but not before that.

SNP: So to summarize this, you've been having pain for 2 to 3 months, often at night. You have some stomach pain that is better when you eat something. The pain seems to be centered in your lower chest or upper abdomen, and your new physician asked you to come here for an evaluation. You have never had a cardiac examination before. Does that sound right?

PT: Yeah, I think you've got it.

SNP: OK, let me ask a few more general questions about your health.

PT: OK, shoot.

SNP: How would you describe your health?

PT: Fairly good until this.

SNP: What do you do to stay healthy?

PT: Try to eat right, but that's hard with my work. I have to take clients out to dinner a lot. And I've been traveling more. I used to use asthma inhalers, but I haven't needed them for a while and don't even know where they are.

SNP: Has work been stressful for you?

PT: Yeah, but it goes with the territory.

SNP: What do you do to relieve stress?

PT: Have a drink, watch some TV.

SNP: Are you married?

PT: No. I've been divorced for 3 years.

SNP: Do you have friends or a roommate who are part of your life?

PT: Yeah, I've got my buddies I watch football with, although my travel has interfered with that lately. My parents live nearby and my ex-wife and my teenage daughter live in the next town. I see my daughter a few times a month. She's hard to catch these days.

SNP: Are you sexually active?

PT: Not since I broke up with my girlfriend 6 months ago.

SNP: What would you say is important to you in life?

PT: Gee, that's a tough one. I guess providing for my daughter, doing well at my work.

SNP: OK, now let me ask you some more basic questions. What did you have to eat yesterday?

PT: Well, I had some coffee and a Danish at the conference I attended for breakfast. Then I grabbed a sandwich and a Coke for lunch. I guess I had

(Continued)

> ### *Box 1–1 Sample Student Nurse*
> ### *Practitioner Encounter (Continued)*
>
> some French fries, too. Not so good, huh? Then for dinner, I had a salad, a steak, and a potato. I had a couple glasses of wine, too.
>
> **SNP:** Do you have any trouble with your bowels or bladder?
>
> **PT:** Well, I've had a lot of loose stools and cramping lately. Seems like I'm either constipated or I'm running to the bathroom.
>
> **SNP:** Is that a new problem?
>
> **PT:** I guess I've had it on and off, but it seems worse now.
>
> **SNP:** How much alcohol do you drink in a week?
>
> **PT:** Oh, I guess 7 to 10 drinks in a week.
>
> **SNP:** Do you smoke or have you ever smoked?
>
> **PT:** I quit 10 years ago. Before that I smoked for 15 years, about 2 packs a day.
>
> **SNP:** Do you take any medications?
>
> **PT:** None.
>
> **SNP:** Are you allergic to anything?
>
> **PT:** Not that I know of.
>
> **SNP:** Let me just review the form you filled out when you came in about your previous illnesses and surgeries. I see that you list asthma and that you had your tonsils out when you were a child. Is there anything else you'd like to tell me?
>
> **PT:** No. I think you know more about me than my best friend!
>
> **SNP:** Well, thank you for telling me so much about yourself. I will do a physical examination on you now and then I am going to go out and get my preceptor to come back to review my findings and discuss your plan of care.
>
> In the physical examination, Jane noted pink skin with no diaphoresis. The patient had full visual fields by confrontation, intact extraocular movements, and good visual and hearing acuity. He had no thyroid enlargement. The mucous membranes of the mouth and nose were pink with no exudates. Chest auscultation revealed normal breath sounds with no wheezes. His heart sounds were normal S_1 and S_2 with no murmurs, rubs, or gallops. His abdominal examination revealed hyperactive bowel sounds but no areas of tenderness or masses. He had a groin dressing in place over the cardiac catheterization site with no sign of hematoma. His pulses were present and equal in the radial, dorsalis pedis, and popliteal spaces. The femoral pulse was present on the right but not palpable on the left because of the dressing. He had deep tendon reflexes in a normal pattern and equal muscle strength and range of motion bilaterally.
>
> *(Continued)*

Box 1—1 Sample Student Nurse Practitioner Encounter *(Continued)*

When the student and preceptor returned, the preceptor clarified some data on the bowel complaints and history, performed a physical examination focusing on the chest and abdomen, and reviewed the CBC and blood chemistry studies already obtained. She ordered thyroid function tests (because hyperthyroidism can cause increased frequency of stools) and a fecal occult blood test and suggested that the patient avoid dairy products for 2 weeks to rule out lactose intolerance. She also recommended a gradual increase in regular exercise as a stress reducer. She scheduled a return appointment in 2 weeks to evaluate symptoms and go over test results. She explained that the cardiac catheterization test had not shown evidence of coronary heart disease, but that it was important to evaluate and interpret the symptoms he was experiencing. The student nurse practitioner was able to establish a beginning relationship with this new patient, and his return appointment was scheduled for a day when the student would be scheduled in the clinic.

Nurse practitioners function in an advanced-practice role, but also retain their nursing function and role as nurses. This core of knowing what it is to be a nurse provides a framework for practice that is rich and human. Nurses are not primarily concerned with disease, but with the person who is experiencing the illness. Being person centered rather than disease centered provides a basis for forging authentic relationships with patients. The value of the authentic relationship is that patients are more likely to be open and honest with the nurse practitioner, who is then better able to understand the patient's condition.

Quinn describes a practice goal of nurse practitioners as supporting healing. She defines healing as a process that moves a person toward wholeness. Healing is different from curing. It is the tendency of any living thing to evolve to its intended purpose. Healing involves wholeness and organization, which lead to actualization and transcendence (Quinn, 1989, 1997). A healing relationship changes both the patient and the nurse (Doona, Haggerty, & Chase, 1997). According to Quinn, healing:

- ◎ Increases coherence of the whole system
- ◎ Decreases chaos or disorder in the whole
- ◎ Maximizes free energy in the whole

◎ Maximizes freedom, autonomy, and choice in the whole
◎ Increases the capacity for creative unfolding of the whole (Quinn, 1997, p. 3)

Mutuality in care between the patient and the nurse practitioner requires more than an open attitude on the part of the nurse. The nurse practitioner must be skilled in assembling data and arriving at true understanding of the patient's condition in both a medical and a personal sense. The processes used by the nurse practitioner and the influences on this process in the clinical setting are the subjects of this book.

CLINICAL JUDGMENT PROCESS USED IN NURSE PRACTITIONER PRACTICE

Essential to high-quality clinical judgment is the ability of the nurse practitioner to form a link between patients' life experiences, their problems, and the full range of diagnostic and therapeutic choices available to achieve a range of possible outcomes. The nurse practitioner must be expert at eliciting the true patient story and in recognizing patterns presented in the data. This assists in arriving at an appropriate diagnostic statement. Accurate diagnosis is essential for developing an effective therapeutic plan. This book will focus on applying the results of research into diagnostic reasoning and clinical judgment to the processes used by the advanced-practice nurse in forming clinical judgments. It will include examples of care situations throughout to assist the nurse practitioner student in applying concepts of clinical judgment.

The Patient-Nurse Practitioner Model is based on research in diagnostic reasoning and the particulars of the primary care encounter. Johnson (1993) described the discourse between patient and nurse as containing four phases:

1. Establishing the agenda for the encounter
2. Eliciting information from the patient, which includes being alert to cues
3. Conducting the physical examination, which includes attending to comfort level as well as preparing and informing the patient
4. Developing a plan of care, using a teachable moment

Teaching in this case is not content centered but patient centered, based on understanding the perspective of the patient. Finally, the nurse practitioner personalizes solutions based on knowing the patient. The unique basis for the work of the nurse practitioner is the personal relationship between himself or herself and the patient. The process continues with increasing refinement and individualization as the nurse practitioner increases in "knowing" the patient. Although this is not addressed by Johnson, the process continues through evaluation of the plan and forging the next steps of the relationship or terminating it in a way that is supportive to the patient.

Experienced nurse practitioners eventually transcend the step-by-step process of data collection, diagnostic hypothesis evaluation, and selection of a treatment plan and begin to practice intuitively. Exemplary cases stored in memory guide management decisions and assist the nurse practitioner in delivering seamless, efficient care (Brykczynski, 1989, 1999). Students will need to follow a systematic approach to develop memory systems for their developing case experience.

From the patient's point of view, the purpose of some visits to nurse practitioners might be to solve a physical problem. But the nurse practitioner goes beyond problem solving, keeping in mind that every visit is an opportunity for disease prevention, screening for high-risk problems, and health promotion. The patient must know that his or her initial concerns are taken seriously and not ignored, but the nurse practitioner can establish a tone that attends to body, mind, and spirit in every visit. Diagnostic reasoning to solve problems, promote health, and screen for disease or illness requires a sensitivity to complex stories, contextual factors, and a sense of probability and uncertainty. The mental tasks of eliciting and sorting through large amounts of data, clustering those data elements into meaningful patterns, connecting patterns to reasonable diagnostic statements, and selecting appropriate interventions require the highest order of cognitive processes. These mental functions distinguish the professional and are the reason why patients seek our services. The range of problems in the scope of practice of nurse practitioners distinguishes this practice from those of registered nurses, physicians, and other health professionals. The human element of caring by the nurse practitioner helps to elicit rich data and establish the trust necessary to encourage patients to adjust their short- or long-range living patterns. The next chapter deals in depth with the processes used in diagnostic reasoning.

⟩⟩ LEARNING TO BE A NURSE PRACTITIONER

Learning the nurse practitioner role is a challenge for many nurses experienced in acute, long-term, or community-based care. Primary care is a unique specialty with problems and concerns that are different from acute-care problems. Many students come to nurse practitioner programs with extensive experience in acute or critical-care nursing. They are committed to learning an expanded mode of nursing practice, but may be overwhelmed with the bulk of new material that must be mastered. Even students who have primary-care or community-health experience find that the issues faced in primary care are different from those in their previous practice, requiring development of new knowledge and skills. Going from the nursing role to the nurse practitioner role is a complex process. Entering primary care is entering a new world with a different set of problems to be solved, different kinds of constraints on choices, and a different culture of care. Entering this world with sensitivity to its differences can reduce anxiety for new nurse practitioner students and can explain other reactions to the setting that might arise, such as a feeling of overwhelming responsibility (Rubin, 1995).

Types of Problems

The types of problems addressed in primary care are different from those encountered in acute or critical-care settings. Upper respiratory infections, common abdominal complaints, skin rashes, and vaginal discharges are problems not often dealt with in acute-care settings. Even chronic conditions present differently in primary care. Hypertension, congestive heart failure, arthritis, and diabetes present with day-to-day management problems that are different from the crises that acute-care nurses encounter in tertiary-care settings. The sense of responsibility for clinical judgment accuracy is new in the nurse practitioner role. Patients with psychosocial problems such as anxiety and depression frequently present with vague, nonspecific complaints.

Pace and Focus of Care

The pace of care is also different in primary care. Nurses who are seeking refuge from busy acute-care duties will be surprised by the mental fatigue that comes from diagnosing and treating up to 20 different patients or families in a day. The sheer variety of possible problems faced in a day's time is exciting and interesting, but it is also challenging. The office visit allows for focused attention with an individual patient, but the former staff nurse will realize that an organized approach to obtaining and processing information is necessary because the patient will not be available to fill in missing pieces of information at the end of the day. On the other hand, the relationship with a growing family or the treatment of patients with chronic conditions will continue over many years. This long-term relationship is very rewarding to both the nurse practitioner and the patient and family.

Primary care includes more than problem solving and symptom management. It involves screening for problems as yet undetected as well as health promotion and disease and injury prevention at every opportunity. Teaching patients of all ages about how their bodies work, risk reduction, or treatment options helps patients assume more responsibility for their own wellness.

Increased Autonomy and Uncertainty

Primary care and the increased autonomy that nurse practitioners enjoy also bring an increase in uncertainty. Patient problems are not already labeled when the nurse practitioner sees the patient. Many different conditions present in similar ways. Laboratory test results must be evaluated for their reliability and validity. Once a diagnosis is made, multiple treatment approaches are available even for simple problems. Furthermore, patients do not always carry out recommended treatment plans. Many problems require lifelong lifestyle adjustment. At the end of the day, the nurse practitioner may have nagging doubts about the decisions that were made on many levels. For new nurse practitioners, preceptors and new employers are available to support the development of confidence in diagnostic and treatment planning, but even experienced nurse practitioners describe learning to live with the "not knowing" of primary care. Uncertainty in clinical judgment is one of the factors that leads to unnecessary testing and higher costs of health care (Kassirer, 1989). Intellectual honesty and humility are important aspects of thoughtful practice and should be cultivated. This must be balanced with confidence based on experience, which also serves to increase the effectiveness of the nurse practitioner.

Tasks to Be Performed

The tasks of primary care are also quite different for nurse practitioners. Multiple tasks need to be accomplished. These include data collection, diagnostic and treatment decision making, arranging consultation visits and continuity of care, and teaching to support patient and family self-management. Staff nurses who are accustomed to changing dressings or providing treatments themselves will need to learn to work through others, most especially the patient. The goals of primary care are prevention of illness, screening for signs of illness that might not yet be detectable, treatment of minor, self-limiting ill health conditions, and maintenance of function in the face of illnesses that cannot be cured. This level of responsibility is different from that of the staff nurse, who collects data for a team that decides on diagnoses and plans and carries out interventions as a member of a team.

Primary-Care Relationships

Nurse practitioner students are frequently surprised that the nature of the relationship between nurse practitioner and patient is different from the relationship between nurse and patient to which they are accustomed. The primary care relationship is different in several aspects. First, the time-limited nature of the nurse practitioner-patient encounter is different from that of the hospital-based staff nurse relationship. Because the nurse cannot expect to have 8 or 12 hours in which to get to know the patient, there is pressure to collect all necessary information in a shortened time frame. After the encounter, the patient returns home and may not see the nurse practitioner again for weeks or months, if ever. This time difference can create a kind of distance between the nurse practitioner and the patient that the new practitioner must learn to deal with. On the other hand, the boundaries of inpatient admissions are dropped. Telephone follow-up and return visits over time are common. The nurse practitioner-patient relationship deepens because of these long-term connections.

◉) SUMMARY

Nurse practitioners provide essential services in maintaining and improving health for patients in a variety of settings. The role of nurse practitioner incorporates much of what is considered traditional medicine while maintaining a nursing model for care. The unique contributions of nurse practitioners in providing holistic care are based on understanding the patient's life situation. Learning the knowledge and skill essential to nurse practitioner practice for the nurse involves increasing knowledge about recognition of disease states and health patterns and increased knowledge about treatment modalities not available to registered nurses. Further, the nurse practitioner role provides a way of relating to the patient in the context of family and community that offers humanistic care. This care enhances the quality of life for patients, families, and nurses alike. This book is about learning the clinical judgment processes that support such care.

REFERENCES

Bates, B. (1990). Twelve paradoxes: A message for nurse practitioners. *Journal of the American Academy of Nurse Practitioners, 2*(4), 136–139.

Bensing, J., Schreurs, K., & De Rijk, A. (1996). The role of the general practitioner's affective behaviour in medical encounters. *Psychology and Health, 11*, 825–838.

Brown, S. A., & Grimes, D. E. (1995). A meta-analysis of nurse practitioners and nurse midwives in primary care. *Nursing Research, 44*, 332–339.

Brykczynski, K. A. (1989). An interpretive study describing the clinical judgment of nurse practitioners. *Scholarly Inquiry for Nursing Practice, 3*(2), 75–104.

Brykczynski, K. A. (1999). Reflection on clinical judgment of nurse practitioners. *Scholarly Inquiry for Nursing Practice, 13*(2), 175–184.

Chase, S. K. (2001). The art of diagnosis and treatment. In L. M. Dunphy & J. E. Winland-Brown (Eds.). *Primary care: The art and science of advanced practice nursing* (pp. 85–104). Philadelphia: F. A. Davis.

Crabtree, K. (Ed.). (2000). Teaching clinical decision making in advanced nursing practice. Washington, D.C.: National Organization of Nurse Practitioner Faculties.

Courtney, R., & Rice, C. (1997). Investigation of nurse practitioner-patient interactions: Using the nurse practitioner rating form. *Nurse Practitioner, 22*(2), 46–65.

Dacher, E. S. (1995). Reinventing primary care. *Alternative Therapies, 1*(5), 29–34.

Donaldson, M. S., & Vanselow, N. (1996). The nature of primary care, *The Journal of Family Practice, 42*, 113–116.

Doona, M. E., Haggerty, L. A., & Chase, S. K. (1997). Nursing presence: An existential exploration of the concept. *Scholarly Inquiry for Nursing Practice, 11*, 3–16.

Dunphy, L. M., & Winland-Brown, J. E. (1998). The Circle of Caring: A transformative model of advanced practice nursing. *Clinical Excellence for Nurse Practitioners, 2*, 241–247.

Gordon, M. (1994). *Nursing diagnosis: Process and application* (3rd ed.). St. Louis: Mosby.

Henson, R. H. (1997). Analysis of the concept of mutuality. *Image: Journal of Nursing Scholarship, 29*(1), 77–81.

Johnson, R. (1993). Nurse practitioner-patient discourse: Uncovering the voice of nursing in primary care practice. *Scholarly Inquiry for Nursing Practice, 7*, 143–157.

Kassirer, J. P. (1989). Our stubborn quest for diagnostic certainty: A cause of excessive testing. *New England Journal of Medicine, 320*, 1489–1491.

Keller, V. F., & Carroll, J. G. (1994). A new model for physician-patient communication. *Patient Education and Counseling, 23*, 131–140.

Matas, K. E., Brown, N. C., & Holman, E. J. (1996). Measuring outcomes in nursing centers: Otitis media as a sample case. *Nurse Practitioner, 21*(6), 116–125.

Matthews, D. A., Suchman, A. L., & Branch, W. T. (1993). Making "connections": The therapeutic potential of patient-client relationships. *Annals of Internal Medicine, 118*, 973–977.

Medalie, J. H., Zyzanski, S. J., Langa, D., & Stange, K. C. (1998). The family in family practice: Is it a reality? *The Journal of Family Practice, 46*, 390–396.

Mundinger, M. O., Kane, R. L., Lenz, E. R., Totten, A. M., Tsai, W., Cleary, P. D., Friedewald, W. T., Siu, A. L., & Shelanski, M. L. (2000). Primary care outcomes in patients treated by nurse practitioners or physicians. *Journal of the American Medical Association, 283*(1), 59–68.

Quinn, J. F. (1997). Healing: a model for an integrative health care system. *Advanced Practice Nursing Quarterly, 3*(1), 1–7.

Quinn, J. (1989). On healing, wholeness and the haelan effect. *Nursing and Health Care, 10*, 553–556.

Rubin, R. H. (1995). Differences between inpatient and outpatient medicine. In R. Rubin (Ed.). *Primary care* (pp. 5–7). Philadelphia: W. B. Saunders.

The Process of Clinical Judgment

Every patient encounter involves at least two people, the patient and the nurse practitioner, and good clinical work requires communication from both of them. The focus of this chapter, however, is on the cognitive processes of the nurse practitioner. It examines the kinds of thinking involved in deciding what data to collect, how to cluster the data into something meaningful, how to decide what is going on with the patient, how to decide what plan to implement, and how to follow up with the patient. All these decisions occur in the mind of the nurse practitioner while he or she is carrying on a conversation, performing a physical examination, and often, documenting the encounter. This is a complex cognitive process, and a focused look at it can help the new nurse practitioner avoid common errors and increase the speed at which the new skills of being a nurse practitioner can be acquired.

All nurses are taught the nursing process as part of basic nursing education (Carnevali & Thomas, 1993), and in some ways the basic steps used by the nurse practitioner are similar to those in basic nursing. In other ways, however, the difference in the judgment that nurse practitioners make is what separates them from basic nurses. For example, nurse practitioners are responsible for selecting from among a much wider scope of diagnostic possibilities and treatment options than basic nurses. The biggest difference, however, lies in the responsibility for independent practice carried by the nurse practitioner, and therefore the quality of the clinical thinking is a focus for both new and experienced nurse practitioners.

)) MODELS OF DIAGNOSTIC REASONING

Two major schools of thought describe how practitioners of any kind use their minds to arrive at a diagnosis. Sufficient evidence exists supporting both views, and it is likely that nurse practitioners will find useful elements in both models that can help them learn and improve diagnostic reasoning. The two major areas are information processing and intuitive models. A third model, decision analysis, is useful under certain circumstances, but is less likely to be used in everyday practice.

Information Processing

Information processing ideas first arose from cognitive psychologists who had discovered a new tool that they could use to explore reasoning processes (Newell & Simon, 1972; Shaw, Newell, & Simon, 1958). That tool was the computer, and we can see many examples of describing the brain as a computer in projects that use information processing as a model. Certainly the human brain is more than a computer, but in many ways we can understand the human brain by seeing how it is similar.

Memory

Information processing models account for the memory and processing capacities of the human system. Early research on the human mind showed that there are two kinds of memory, long term and short term

(Baddeley, 1999). Clinical judgment makes extensive use of various types of memory. By understanding the forms and types of memory, the nurse practitioner can maximize memory capacity, which will assist in the clinical judgment process.

Long-Term Memory

Long-term memory has a large capacity and stores information in several different ways. The first way is called *semantic memory*. This form contains facts as well as concepts and language. Knowledge from books or journal articles is stored as factual data. These facts are retrievable from long-term memory when needed for processing or matching patterns.

Episodic memory is the way in which we remember experiences that we have had. For example, patients are remembered as cases. Some authors have called these exemplar cases when describing powerful experiences that teach us something, but even routine cases are stored in episodic memory. It is frequently the narrative or story of the case that we remember. Language is involved as we recount the narrative of a situation that has a beginning, middle, and end, although language has its limits as we try to describe the richness of the case or vignette. Episodic memory helps the clinician to develop possible causal relationships (Tulving, 1972); that is, to understand and remember cause and effect relationships evident in daily practice.

A different kind of memory involves sensory data. Remembering the sound of a heart murmur or the feel of skin when a person is in shock are examples of *sensory memory*. Sensory memory is useful in pattern matching and does not require language to be available. Another kind of memory, called *production memory*, involves remembering "how to do" something. For example, we remember how to drive after we are experienced in such a way that we do not need to consciously remember how much pressure to apply to the gas pedal. In clinical practice, we remember how to perform a phlebotomy in doing it, not in abstract thought about it. We find the vein through the "feel" of it and learn the act as a production sequence.

Clinical judgment requires the use of all these kinds of memory. The capacity of our long-term memories is huge, and things that are stored in long-term memory are stored for a lifetime. Even patients with dementia can remember experiences from their childhoods.

Short-Term Memory

Another large category of memory, which differs from long-term memory but is essential to consider in describing the clinical judgment process, is *short-term* or *working memory*. If long-term memory is likened to the hard drive of a computer, short-term memory is more like random access memory (RAM) or processing capacity. When the computer is turned off, anything held only in RAM is lost. The information-processing model describes the use of short-term or working memory as being quite limited in comparison with long-term memory. Short-term memory has been described as being limited to "the magic number seven, plus or minus two" (Miller, 1956). It may seem hard to realize that our processing memory can hold only seven bits of information. It seems that we have so much more on our minds. The fleeting nature of short-term memory accounts for how easily we may forget the name of a person to whom we were just introduced or something we just heard when distracted immediately after hearing it. Working memory is the space where all the information needed to form judgments and decide on actions takes place.

How do busy clinicians maximize the limited capacity of short-term memory? Research has shown that we expand our memory limitation by "chunking" information together so that, rather than remembering every discrete reading of vital signs as a separate piece of information, we cluster the data into "vital signs," which are remembered as one piece of information (Larkin, McDermott, Simon & Simon, 1980). This frees up short-term memory capacity to bring together additional information. Increasing the efficiency and accuracy of reasoning by using this limited space is a key feature of learning to perform good clinical judgments.

Other Types of Memory

A newer model of human memory that has been proposed is the neural network. This means that a cue or an idea is related by means of a rich network of connections with many other ideas and experiences. These connections are more complex than the simple associational models previously described and help account for the human mind's ability to respond to novel conditions in reasonable ways (Baxt, 1991).

The process of evaluating information and building an appropriate understanding of the patient's clinical problems requires efficient use of all our different types of memory and processing capacities. How do these processes come together? First, long-term memory information is easier to access if it is stored in recognizable and retrievable ways. One common way of organizing the information in our brains is by thinking in terms of body systems. For example, in most cases, chest pain involves cardiovascular, pulmonary, musculoskeletal, or digestive systems. We can use body systems to pull out information that is related to the problem under consideration and to generate possible diagnoses.

Research has shown that frequent retrieval of information makes it more accessible (Waldorp, 1987). It works similarly to computer systems that identify your favorite programs or recent documents to make them easier to access. Retrieval of memory allows us to build a list of possible diagnoses, to evaluate the meaning of various symptoms and signs, and to develop treatment approaches for our patients. Production memory is involved as we remember the sequence of history taking and physical examination. This frees up more processing capacity when our sequence of steps becomes more automatic. Sensory memory is used as we collect objective data and compare it with what we know about potential problems. Episodic memory is involved as we match features of the patient's story with other experiences we have had. This can trigger both diagnostic and treatment solutions. Semantic memory is used as we recall terminology to document our findings and plan. We also use semantic memory to recall relationships between cues and conditions or groups of medications that might treat a condition.

Problems with memory can occur at several levels. Facts stored in long-term memory can be difficult to retrieve. For example, a nurse practitioner who is trying to describe a certain kind of skin rash distribution that he or she has read about in a book must be able to access the word for it when writing in the patient record. Memories can be distorted when we misinterpret facts and store them incorrectly. An exciting or vivid case can be more easily recalled and have more importance in our memory than a common or simple case. Recency is a principle that states that information recently retrieved will be more likely to be retrieved again. A rare case will be less likely to be recalled.

The hypothetico-deductive method uses the strategy of generating a list of hypotheses based on a few pieces of information obtained early on. When each new piece of data is collected, the relative likelihood of each hypothesis is re-evaluated. The clinician proceeds until he or she is sufficiently confident that one hypothesis about the patient's problem can be selected. Computer expert systems can simulate this kind of thinking and can make use of epidemiological and statistical data to recalculate relative probabilities. Working through cases and comparing diagnostic decisions with computer-generated decisions can help students gain skill in diagnostic reasoning (Lange et al., 1997).

In actuality, although the information processing model is a useful starting point, the human brain functions differently from the computer. Humans are able to sense patterns of data and to include emotional responses to experiences with other human beings. In advanced-practice nursing, the ability to empathize with a patient, to be available personally, and to be invested with the patient in maximizing health make the human decision maker much richer in function than any computer or protocol system. The nurse practitioner and patient can together develop approaches and solutions that are individualized and creative. If protocols were enough for effective management, the Internet or some other computer system would be sufficient to provide health care for anyone with access. Patients come to a health-care provider for more than a diagnosis; they come for a human connection. The human aspect of the nurse-patient relationship adds rather than detracts from diagnostic accuracy.

Intuition

Several researchers noted that there were limitations in the research approaches used to develop the information processing models of clinical judgment. First of all, most studies used simulated case situations and relied on the clinician's report about mental processes that are used without conscious thought in actual practice (Elstein, Shulman & Sprafka, 1978). When observational studies of real situations conducted by experienced clinicians were done, it was noted that many times steps in the process were seemingly skipped, that the clinician just "knew" what the patient's problem was after collecting only a few pieces of data, and that the clinicians arrived at problem solution strategies almost immediately.

Staff nurses with years of experience can recount times when their intuition told them what was going to occur with the patient before any of the objective signs were present. This happens with nurse practitioners as well. A different model for studying clinical processes was proposed that used naturalistic inquiry such as phenomenology or ethnography and that tried to describe actual practice situations, not simulated cases. This approach will be discussed as the intuitive practice model.

Intuitive research programs were conducted mostly with expert practitioners. Benner (1984), in her work with multiple levels of nurses, showed that processes used by expert nurses differed from those used by novices. She argued that intuitive practice required years of experience in the particular specialty before intuitive judgments could be made. What is meant by intuition? Authors have described intuition as knowing without needing to use conscious processes (Benner & Tanner, 1987; Rew & Barrows, 1987). Rew (1988) describes three aspects of intuition: an immediate reception of the knowledge of the situation; perception of the wholeness of the situation; and knowledge that is gained without a conscious, deliberative process. Benner, Tanner, and Chesla describe intuition as "a judgment without a rationale, a direct apprehension and response without recourse to calculative rationality" (1996, p. 8). A grasping of the "big picture" in a situation before all the data elements can be assembled or a gut reaction to a clinical situation is often associated with intuition.

The beginning nurse practitioner cannot exert intuitive judgments in the new role without gaining experience first. However, the new nurse practitioner can bring to the clinical situation the years of experience gained in multiple clinical and life situations. Even if grasp of a situation is perceived as an intuition, the novice or expert nurse practitioner is required to collect data to confirm or disconfirm the intuitive judgment. Intuition can lead a clinician to certain understandings but is not sufficient to justify a treatment course without the collection of confirming data. For this reason, nurse practitioner students need to be familiar with both intuitive and information processing models.

Several features of the intuitive model described by Benner, Tanner, and Chesla (1996) in critical-care practice have direct transference to primary-care practice. First is an overall sense of a goal. This distinguishes intuitive practice from the problem-solving mode of practice. There are times when nurse practitioners are called on to be with patients in ways that go beyond the immediate solving of a particular problem. This often occurs at times when a patient is making a major life transition. The goal might be symptom management or improved communication.

A second feature of intuitive practice concerns knowing the particulars of the individual patient's situation. This often involves coming to know the patient over time and to know the type of responses this patient typically has. For example, if a patient of the type known as a "minimizer" (one who tends to downplay symptoms or concerns) calls with a complaint and "sounds worried," the nurse practitioner would know to pay particular attention to the complaint. The nurse practitioner would respond differently to a patient who is frequently made anxious by simple symptoms. This relates to research on knowing the patient that has been carried out in other practice arenas (Jenny & Logan, 1992; Tanner, Benner, Chesla, & Gordon, 1993).

A third aspect of intuitive practice is that the context matters, as does the nurse's emotional response. Experienced nurse practitioners recognize a nagging fear when hearing certain complexes of complaints, such as unexplained weight loss, unexplained fatigue, and night sweats. The alarm that the nurse feels is not coming from the patient. The patient may not know enough to feel alarmed, but the meaning of the complex of symptoms in a previously well person spells danger, and the nurse recognizes the pattern.

A fourth feature of intuitive practice is that recognizing patterns supports intuition. Patterns are learned over years of experience. Nurses frequently relate the telling of one story by comparing it with a similar story and by remembering how that story turned out. This pattern recognition is different in character from the pattern of symptoms described in information processing that can be clustered by an expert system on a computer. The pattern takes into account many aspects of the patient situation that a computer model might not be sensitive to. Patterns include how the person finds meaning in his or her world and lives in it.

Finally, intuitive practice is sensitive to the narrative. In an interview study (Dunphy, 1999) in which nurse practitioners described a case in which they knew they had made a difference, the nurse practitioners could not help but resort to telling the story in rich detail. The narrative is a way of remembering patterns, of being able to bring them to bear in a new patient situation. New nurse practitioners and students can learn much from the narrative accounts of experienced nurse practitioners. Students can use time with preceptors to prompt them to tell practice narratives related to the patients they are currently seeing. They can also develop skill in intuitive practice by recording narratives of their own practice.

A study of nurse practitioner judgment that included direct observation of patient management revealed that experienced nurse practitioners were able to attach meaning to subtle cues. The interpretation of cues is an important feature of expert clinical judgment. Before any specific hypotheses were evaluated, the nurse practitioner attended to a response in herself that indicated that "there was a little voice in the back of my head that said 'something else is going on here' " (Brykczynski, 1989, p. 84). Nurse practitioners describe gut feelings, those physical responses to fear or threat that the patient's symptoms might indicate. Intellectual flags indicate that there is a puzzle yet to be solved.

Nurse practitioners also describe a sixth sense, a way of listening below the surface. One nurse practitioner described the case of a man who complained of narcolepsy. His anxiety was palpable despite previous negative workups. The nurse practitioner stayed with the patient to determine what was causing his problem. Other providers whom he had contacted over the previous year had failed to pursue his complaints. Eventually it was determined that he had an inoperable glioma. The nurse, by weighing the cues and attending to her own impressions, was led to pursue the diagnostic challenge that his case presented.

Decision Analysis

Another approach to clinical judgment that has been promoted in the past is decision analysis (Corcoran, 1986). This model proposes that a probability model will assist decision makers in making the "best" decisions

(Nicoll, Pignone, & Detmer, 2000). It uses mathematical probabilities of various likely outcomes if different approaches are tried. Table 2–1 represents a decision analysis of empirical treatment for suspected streptococcal pharyngitis with and without conducting a strep antigen test. The model allows considering relative "costs" of the various approaches as well as the likely response of the problem to the various options. (This model is based on Bayes' theorem, a model for decision making presented more than 200 years ago.) Although it is based on the idea of relative certainties, which may appeal to diagnosticians bothered by the uncertainty of clinical judgment, this method is time consuming and not well suited to daily practice demands. It could be useful for cases that do not respond to obvious treatment decisions, and it offers a way for the patient to specify preferences for treatment.

Table 2–1 illustrates that for a patient with a presentation of sore throat, fever and lymphadenopathy, the nurse practitioner knows that the likelihood of streptococcal pharyngitis is 60 percent. There are three management options:

1. Treat empirically with antibiotics.
2. Treat with comfort measures only and wait to see if the condition progresses.
3. Perform a Quick Strep test on everyone and treat patients with positive results with antibiotics.

Decision analysis allows examination of each of the decision options. The first, treating all patients has financial costs, exposes some patients to antibiotic side effects unnecessarily (40%), and increases the likelihood of antibiotic resistance in the pool of bacteria present in the community. The second option saves money, but exposes some patients to untreated streptococcal infection (60%), which can have serious sequelae such as glomerulonephritis and rheumatic heart valve disease. The third option costs the most and increases the proportion of appropriate care (84%), but does not completely eliminate unnecessary treatment (4%) or failure to treat actual disease in some patients (12%).

The point of this exercise is to show the limits of decision analysis in real-world situations. Nurse practitioners make management decisions with a respect for the uncertainty of diagnostic decisions even when using laboratory tests. Factors such as the likelihood of the patient to contact providers if the condition does not improve, availability of laboratory tests, availability of treatment, and underlying susceptibility to side effects or complications affect management decisions in individual cases. Decision

TABLE 2-1

Decision Analysis: Sore Throat, Fever, Lymphadenopathy*

Decision	Patient Status	Test[†]	Cost	Risk	Outcome
Option 1: Treat with antibiotics	60% with disease	No	Antibiotics	Side effects	Appropriate care
	40% with no disease	No	Antibiotics	Side effects	Unnecessary care
Option 2: Treat with comfort measures only	60% with disease	No	None	Complications Untreated disease	Disease persists
	40% with no disease	No	None	None	Appropriate care
Option 3: Test and treat positives	60% with disease	Test positive (48%)	Test Antibiotics	Side effects	Appropriate care
		Test negative (12%)	Test	Complications Untreated disease	Disease persists
	40% with no disease	Test positive (4%)	Test Antibiotics	Side effects	Unnecessary care
		Test negative (36%)	Test	None	Appropriate care

*The likelihood of streptococcal pharyngitis, given the symptoms, is 60%.
[†]Sensitivity of the Quick Strep test is 80%. Specificity is 90%.

analysis is a good exercise to evaluate decision processes, but it does not relieve the nurse practitioner from the burden of making decisions for individual patients.

◎》 PHASES OF CLINICAL JUDGMENT

Hypothesis Generation

The goal of the clinical encounter is to select accurately from a range of diagnostic possibilities a label that best fits the patient's signs and symptoms. Essential features of diagnostic reasoning using an information-processing model include generating hypotheses and then narrowing the range of diagnostic possibilities early in the encounter. Figure 2–1 illustrates the process used in primary care when a patient seeks help for a new problem. The figure represents the cognitive process of the nurse practitioner as well as the part that the patient plays in assisting the judgment process.

Figure 2–1

CLINICAL JUDGMENT IN PRIMARY CARE

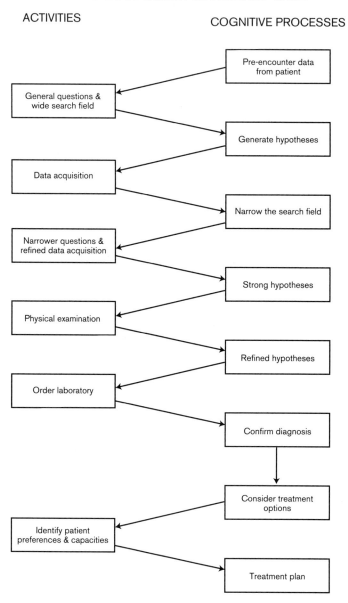

Even before meeting the patient, the nurse practitioner can obtain baseline or pre-encounter data from most office systems. Data such as age and gender already focus the range of diagnostic possibilities. A 65-year-old woman is unlikely to be pregnant. A 65-year-old man is likely to have benign prostatic hypertrophy. Back pain could indicate muscle strain, herniated lumbar disc, vertebral fracture, sciatica, dissecting aortic aneurysm, cholecystitis, pyelonephritis, or drug-seeking behavior. When meeting the patient for the first time, the nurse practitioner observes the general distress of the patient, his or her level of self-care, and posture and mobility restrictions.

One rule of thumb or heuristic to use in generating diagnostic hypotheses is to work from the "outside in." For example, chest pain could be caused by angina, esophagitis, or other problems. A systematic way to generate hypotheses is to start at the skin. Could the pain be the first symptom of herpes zoster? The distribution of the pain would be a clue leading in this direction. Below the skin are fascia, muscles, and bones. Muscle strain or inflammation such as costochondritis might elicit point tenderness or pain on movement. Below the ribcage are lung tissue and pleurae. Pain on inspiration or pleuritic pain could indicate pleurisy or pulmonary embolus. Concomitant fever might corroborate a diagnosis of pneumonia. Within the mediastinum is the esophagus. Pain associated with meals or stomach emptiness could indicate esophagitis, gastritis, or referred cholecystitis. Also found in the mediastinum are the great vessels. A history of tearing, burning pain could indicate aneurysm. Finally, pain associated with activity, accompanied by diaphoreses or nausea, or radiating to the shoulder or jaw could be coronary in origin. This method of generating hypotheses helps the inexperienced clinician to generate a wide range of possible diagnostic hypotheses and can help to prevent premature closure on one diagnostic label.

Experienced clinicians keep their antennae raised for the most serious conditions. Abdominal pain could be from gas, but if it is from a ruptured ectopic pregnancy, a dissecting abdominal aortic aneurysm, or a ruptured appendix, immediate surgical consultation is necessary. The clinician must collect and document data that rule out the presence of a serious condition.

Data Collection

The nurse practitioner starts taking the history of an illness by asking questions that elicit the story of the illness from the patient's point of view. (Chapter 3 discusses assessment in greater depth.) The nurse practitioner starts with broad general questions to allow the patient to tell his or her point of view most clearly. Each piece of data helps the nurse practitioner to judge the likelihood of each of the competing hypotheses or to raise new hypotheses. The nurse practitioner asks increasingly specific questions in order to eliminate some hypotheses and to support others.

After the full history taking, the nurse practitioner begins the physical examination with the intention of distinguishing the most likely hypotheses. While focusing on the problem identified by the patient, the nurse practitioner maintains openness to other cues that indicate related problems or new problems that need attention during this or another visit.

Students are taught in physical assessment or health assessment courses to collect a wide range of data. These courses focus on learning history-taking techniques and organizational approaches as well as new psychomotor skills in physical assessment. Too often the seeming goal of data collection is presented as "Collection of Data," and students are surprised when they enter the clinical practice arena that the "full history and physical" is seldom done and that time pressure forces them to omit steps of the data collection process. The solution to this bewilderment is for the student to realize that the purpose of data collection is to arrive at a clinical judgment. Collecting data without engaging in critical thinking about what data are appropriate to collect is not advanced–practice-level thought. Chapter 3 provides details on data collection, but students must keep in mind that even data collection requires clinical judgment because there are many options to consider in collecting data. Is a mini-mental status examination indicated? Is a full neurosensory examination useful in determining the patient's problem or health risk?

A research study of nurse practitioners based on a simulated case showed that participants used several approaches to data collection. The first, called "symptom driven," confined data collection to information related to the specific problem. A second approach was termed "extended physical" and included focused data collection, but added other body systems for data collection consideration. The final approach was termed "comprehensive care" and looked broadly at the person's health situation. It used the symptom as an opportunity to discuss health. The study further showed that participants developed potential hypothesis lists early and collected data related to active hypotheses. Inexperienced nurse practitioners generated longer hypothesis lists (White, Nativio, Kobert, & Engberg, 1992).

For experienced clinicians, data acquisition in history taking and physical examination is most effective if it is hypothesis driven. That is, the information that is selected and gathered is related to the list of possible diagnoses. For common problems, the data collection approach becomes routinized and therefore takes less active processing space in short-term memory. In contrast, novices tend to use a shotgun approach and ask a little bit about everything that might be possible, not considering which diagnoses are likely.

Hypothesis-driven data collection means that the nurse practitioner specifically seeks and records data that would confirm or disconfirm a specific hypothesis being evaluated. It is not enough to note only data that fit with one possible problem. Competing hypotheses must be ruled out by seeking disconfirming data. In doing this, the clinician must be open to changing the priority list of hypotheses based on new information. For example, rhinitis might present like a viral infection, but if, when asked whether this has happened before, the patient says, "Yes, I had the same thing 2 weeks ago," this decreases the likelihood of viral illness and increases the likelihood of allergy. An approach to data collection that is completely symptom driven, however, can result in leaving out important concepts. The nurse practitioner should have an agenda for the visit that includes the patient's agenda but that expands the visit to provide health promotion.

As the patient encounter proceeds, the clinician raises diagnostic possibilities or hypotheses and constantly evaluates the hypotheses in light of new data. Early hypothesis generation has been found to be related to accuracy of diagnostic reasoning for nurses and physicians. If the hypothesis list does not contain the accurate diagnosis early on, the search process takes longer or wrong answers are selected (Tanner, Padrick, Westfal & Putzier, 1987). Clinicians need to be realistic in evaluating possible diagnostic hypotheses. Even experienced clinicians can be fooled into selecting a label they commonly see. For example, an active pediatric nurse practitioner who has seen many patients with viral upper respiratory infections might fail to recognize signs of bacterial sinusitis.

After the physical examination, confirmatory or screening laboratory tests are ordered. By focusing diagnostic testing on the specific hypotheses being considered, the nurse practitioner saves the health-care system from paying for unnecessary testing and saves the patient from inconvenience and risk (Flagler, 2000).

Hypothesis Evaluation

In addition to this hypothetico-deductive example, clinicians also make use of rich pattern matching in recognizing clusters of findings. Data are clustered together into meaningful chunks that explain and account for the different elements of the history. Clinicians are alert to any data bits that do not fit the pattern of what is expected. This can be seen as an analytic process, but clinicians often report that they are alert to the feeling in themselves that "Something is just not right here." This experience is similar to that described using intuitive models of reasoning. This can indicate that the problem is more serious than it initially appeared or that there are data bits that are not yet accounted for. Diagnosticians are persistent in trying to fit the pieces of data into a coherent picture. One must be on guard not to ignore the discrepant data pieces that exist. Research has shown that we see what we expect to see in many cases, so nurse practitioners must remain open to the patient situation in order to continue seeing all the data that are present.

Problem Identification

Problem identification by the nurse practitioner involves more than simple medical diagnosis labeling. The theoretical background that supports nurse practitioner practice is a nursing model. Although there are many nursing models to choose from, all include a holistic view of body, mind, and spirit. There is always more going on in a person's life than a medical diagnosis label. The nurse and patient together decide how wide and deep the focus of an encounter will go. The experience of a simple infectious disease exists in the context of the person's immune system integrity and the perceived stresses and meaning in the person's life. All these issues may become part of the picture of the person's condition that the nurse practitioner develops.

Every encounter with a nurse practitioner becomes an opportunity for health screening and health promotion. Deciding on how to conceive of the problems presented by the patient is the basis for the richness of nurse practitioner practice. Patients recognize when their whole person is being addressed. An engagement in life decision making assists patients who must make serious lifestyle adjustment to prevent or minimize the effects of disease. The nurse practitioner-patient relationship serves as the basis for this kind of support, and the nurse must consider including more than "hypertension" as part of the problem list. That problem list might include situational stressors, social isolation, obesity, or sedentary lifestyle. Prescribing drugs to control hypertension is never enough to treat it effectively. Furthermore, patients benefit from the understanding and care provided by the nurse practitioner. This way of thinking of problems and planning is discussed further in Chapter 4.

Diagnoses are frequently interrelated. Obesity, hypertension, hyperlipidemia, and type 2 diabetes frequently occur together. When evaluating competing hypotheses, cluster related problems together. The lifestyle recommendations are the same for all these conditions, but the medication approach might differ. When considering nursing diagnoses, the nurse practitioner may find that many occur together. The expert tries to approach the core diagnosis, which, if managed, will ameliorate all the others. For instance, ineffective coping with stress can result in altered sleep patterns, constipation, difficulty concentrating, and interpersonal tension. If the underlying problem is dealt with, the other problems might not need direct intervention. If the nurse practitioner focuses only on the superficial problem level, the problems may remain.

Treatment Decision Making

Often the diagnostic hypotheses are so strong that they do not need specific testing, or they need to allow empirical treatment to begin before the diagnostic test results are returned. Treatment considerations are as much a part of clinical judgment as diagnostic judgments. Again, the patient and family should be included as sources of important information to guide treatment decision making. Because most conditions can be treated in a number of different ways, the patient's preferences and abilities for management choices are considered. This is sometimes confusing to the new nurse practitioner student. For example, if the patient is unable to manage medication that is divided into three daily doses, a form of the medication that is given once daily might be preferable, even if it is more expensive. The patient may need medication, special diet, exercise, or rest. Patients should always be instructed in comfort measures and self-care to support healing and recovery as well as the more medical aspects of the treatment plan. Health promotion should be included in every visit. When the patient has an acute upper respiratory infection, it might be easier to stop smoking. An illness experience often gives the patient new focus on choosing healthy lifestyle patterns.

Following a rigid protocol is characteristic of beginner practice. Bryczynski (1989) showed that nurse practitioners frequently use an efficiency in managing conditions known as a "set." Others have referred to this clustering as a "script." An example of this is the management of a newly diagnosed diabetic patient. The cognitive load associated with the elements of beginning care for a diabetic is large. By tying a set of responses together, the nurse practitioner increases the reliability of his or her response to the patient and maintains working memory space for individualizing the approach. A set can be thought of as a "chunk" related to actions, not data elements. The nurse practitioner then evaluates the patient's responses to the plan and has certain expectations about how the patient might respond if the plan is well designed. This is an element of follow-up described previously.

As practitioners gain experience, they become more innovative and creative in how they choose treatment plans. Furthermore, as they gain experience, they trust their own judgments better and are more willing to begin a treatment plan before diagnostic certainty, which is elusive at best, can be achieved. In all kinds of practice, from acute to primary care, there are times when the patient's response to initial treatment approaches is the only way to confirm a diagnostic hypothesis. This book does not argue that beginners should engage in "shooting from the hip." However, beginners should know, when they see a preceptor presumably "jumping" to a treatment decision, that the decision comes only after long years of experience and a realistic sense of confidence in clinical judgment abilities.

When the diagnosis list is settled, there might still be some uncertainty. A treatment plan is discussed with the patient in light of mutually shared goals. Honest conversation about ability and willingness to follow treatment recommendations will result in more realistic plans. Part of the treatment plan always includes a plan for follow-up. Patients should always know when to return for a visit and under what circumstances they should telephone. If possible, written instructions should be provided to help patients adjust to complicated treatment directions.

Follow-Up Visit Reasoning

The clinical judgment process used in follow-up visits with patients is illustrated in Figure 2–2. Here the focus is on evaluating the effectiveness of the entire clinical process. If the patient is not responding at all to the plan, one must consider that the wrong diagnosis was made. A re-examination of symptoms and history can shift the hypothesis list into new areas and a new plan for diagnostic testing and treatment can be initiated. A partial response can indicate a less than optimal treatment plan or difficulty that the patient might be having in following the plan. This reopens consideration of the treatment plan. Finally, good response assists in confirming the diagnosis and plan, although the possibility exists that the condition is resolving itself regardless of the treatment initiated. In any case, the visit provides a deepening relationship with the patient as the nurse practitioner listens to new concerns or satisfactions with care. The visit can set the course for further treatment and for new health promotion activities.

Clinical judgment is always an informed guess. Clinicians learn to be open with patients about how they should be responding to treatment and

Figure 2–2

EVALUATION OF PATIENT OUTCOMES

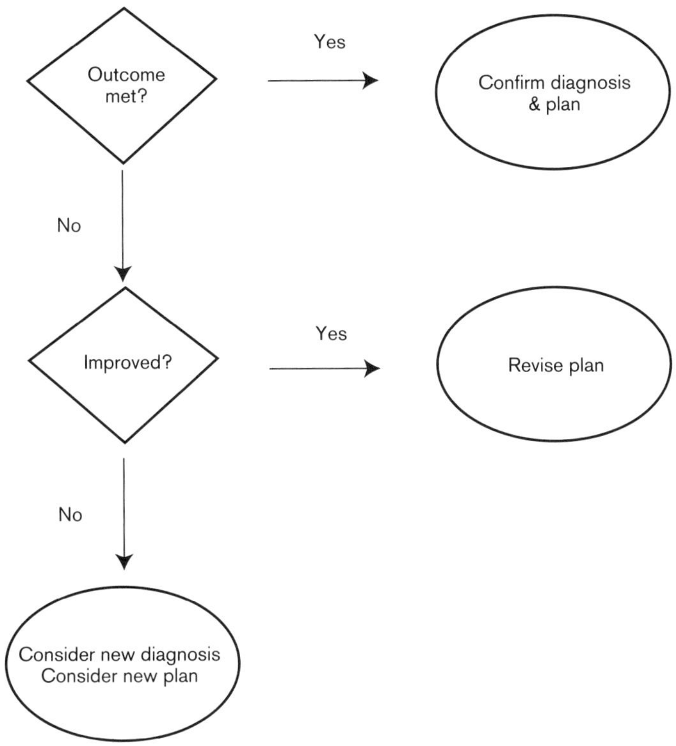

what they should do if their condition worsens or they do not respond to the treatment. Patients should also know when they should plan to return to the clinic, either for a follow-up on the current problem or for the next healthy visit. If there is any concern about how a patient will do at home, the nurse practitioner can telephone the next day to check on progress.

Health Promotion Reasoning

Some patient appointments are not related to specific problems. Annual physicals, school health examinations, and pre-employment physicals are examples of situations in which the nurse practitioner sees patients who have no identified problems. In this case, clinical judgment is also required. Figure 2–3 represents the steps in the process of a health promotion visit. Patients are encouraged to share any health concerns or questions that they might have. Their general health patterns are elicited using a format such as the functional health pattern assessment (Gordon, 1994). This helps to determine life patterns and values. The nurse practitioner asks focused questions about health risks that are significant for the type of patient being seen. In deciding which questions to ask, one considers

Figure 2–3

HEALTH PROMOTION REASONING

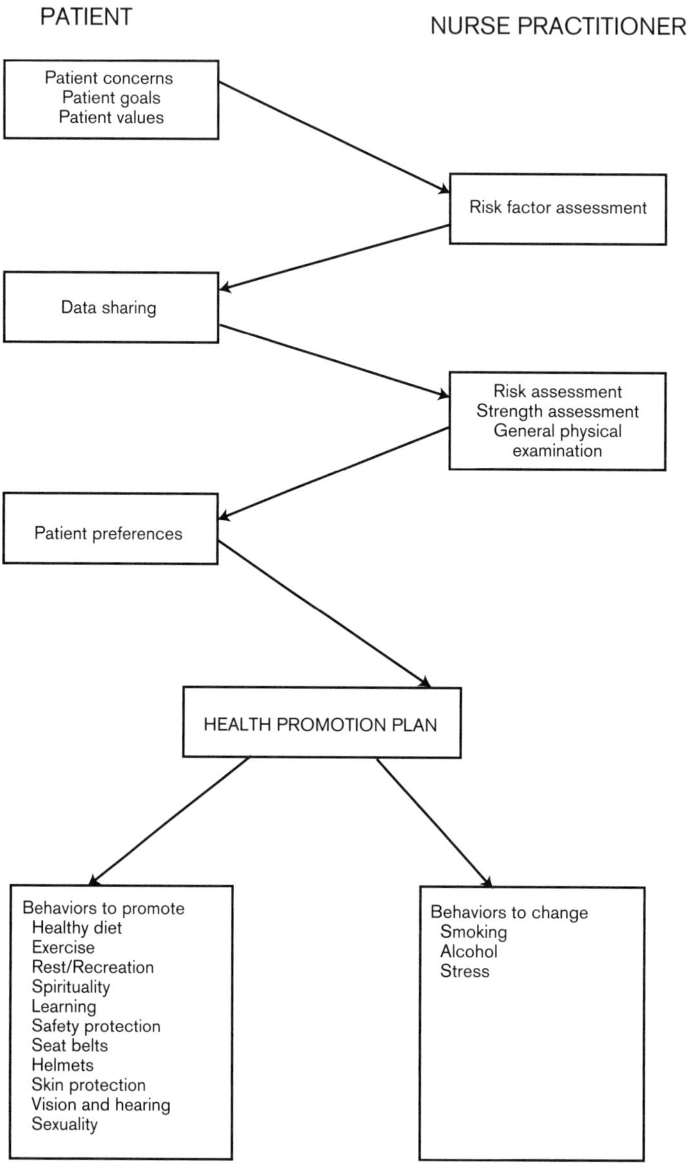

PATIENT   NURSE PRACTITIONER

```
┌─────────────────────┐
│  Patient concerns   │
│   Patient goals     │
│   Patient values    │
└─────────────────────┘
                          ┌──────────────────────┐
                          │ Risk factor assessment│
                          └──────────────────────┘
┌─────────────────────┐
│    Data sharing     │
└─────────────────────┘
                          ┌──────────────────────┐
                          │   Risk assessment    │
                          │ Strength assessment  │
                          │  General physical    │
                          │    examination       │
                          └──────────────────────┘
┌─────────────────────┐
│ Patient preferences │
└─────────────────────┘

            ┌───────────────────────┐
            │ HEALTH PROMOTION PLAN │
            └───────────────────────┘

┌─────────────────────┐      ┌─────────────────────┐
│ Behaviors to promote│      │ Behaviors to change │
│   Healthy diet      │      │   Smoking           │
│   Exercise          │      │   Alcohol           │
│   Rest/Recreation   │      │   Stress            │
│   Spirituality      │      │                     │
│   Learning          │      │                     │
│   Safety protection │      │                     │
│   Seat belts        │      │                     │
│   Helmets           │      │                     │
│   Skin protection   │      │                     │
│   Vision and hearing│      │                     │
│   Sexuality         │      │                     │
└─────────────────────┘      └─────────────────────┘
```

epidemiologic data on what the major health risk for this group might be. The United States Preventive Services Task Force Guide to Clinical Preventive Services (2003) is a useful source of information on heath risks and screening.

The nurse practitioner is interested in knowing the patient's strengths as well as weaknesses. This helps the patient to be known not just as a collection of potential medical problems, but as a vital, unique person. Patient preferences for healthy lifestyles are considered, and the health promotion plan is developed. Health can be thought of as more than the absence of disease. Dunn (1961) defines health as high-level wellness:

> ... an integrated method of functioning, which is oriented toward maximizing the potential of which the individual is capable. It requires that the individual maintain a continuum of balance and purposeful direction within the environment where he is functioning.

Everyone can improve his or her own health. The health promotion plan might include both behaviors to promote and behaviors to change. Health-promoting behaviors include healthy eating, exercise, and a balance between activity and rest. A sense of reverence for one's own life and elements of learning or growth are also important aspects of a person's life and health. Safety is a consideration for every patient. For example, depending on the patient's age and activities, the nurse practitioner should discuss the importance of equipment such as seat belts, car seats, helmets, or other safety gear. Other topics include sunscreen use, vision and hearing protection, and relationships and sexuality, including safe sex practices and violence prevention.

Behaviors that might need to be changed include smoking, excessive alcohol consumption, and sedentary lifestyles. By documenting the health promotion plan, the nurse practitioner or other providers can offer follow-up and continued support. The nurse practitioner is a partner with the patient and family in choosing to maximize health.

⑳ INFLUENCES ON DIAGNOSTIC REASONING

Maxims

Maxims are guiding principles used by experts that have meaning particularly for the situation at hand. Until one gains experience in a particular setting, the maxim may seem trivial or meaningless, but after experiences in the setting, the deeper meaning of maxims becomes apparent (Benner,

1984). New nurse practitioners can gain much from the wisdom of experienced ones by paying attention to the maxims that the experts share.

One maxim of practice is that common things occur commonly. Students are frequently excited to make a diagnosis of a rare or exotic condition. This can be the result of a rich experience in acute or critical care, where the most serious cases are seen. In primary care, however, common problems predominate. For example, the sound of approaching hoofbeats most likely signifies the presence of a horse—not a zebra. In real life, "zebra" diagnoses are rare. They should be considered with the differential list, but their likely probability must be taken into consideration.

An additional maxim revealed in the Brykczynski (1989) study is that real disease declares itself. This means that the evolution of the disease presents varying pictures. The nurse practitioner will not always have enough data present at a particular visit to make the diagnosis. If the disease is serious, however, it will progress and will be easier to recognize. If the nurse practitioner suspects real disease, it is important to instruct the patient how to respond if the symptoms do not resolve, or if they increase. This maxim serves as a response to the uncertainty of clinical practice.

Brykczynski (1989) also described a maxim used by nurse practitioners that follow-up is everything. This means that each lab test that comes back after the visit has a potential meaning and must be evaluated in the context of the patient's situation. Bringing patients back to the clinic to evaluate treatment is important in validating diagnoses and treatment plans and in building relationships with patients. The answers to practice questions come in the follow-up of the situation. This is important to maintain in a busy practice setting where pressure to see more patients and less support for follow-up telephone calls make expert care difficult. The nurse practitioner has an ethical obligation, however, to resist time pressures and remain committed to the patients he or she has seen.

Patterns of Sound Reasoning

New nurse practitioners can focus on increasing the accuracy and efficiency of their clinical judgments by focusing on the processes, uncertainties, and feedback of making and living with decisions. Table 2–2 summarizes habits that promote effective clinical judgment. Quality clinical judgment requires focused attention by both clinician and patient. Attention to surroundings—including lighting level, noise, privacy, and physical comfort—increase the likelihood of open communication. Nurse practitioners increase efficiency and accuracy of diagnostic thinking when they are rested and not rushed or distracted. Time must be planned for

TABLE 2–2 Habits That Support Clinical Judgment	
Phase of Diagnostic Reasoning	**Habits That Support Clinical Judgment**
Data acquisition	Use systematic or hierarchically organized approach (general to specific) Review multiple systems (selective)
Hypothesis formulation	Generate hypotheses early in encounter Develop competing hypotheses Consider life- or function-threatening problems Consider "zebras" but recognize them as such
Hypothesis evaluation	Recognize interrelation of diagnoses Consider probabilities in context Consider likelihood of altering course of problem with treatment Rule out life- or function-threatening problems
Problem naming	Choose most fundamental problem Include multiple perspectives (biopsychosocial, spiritual; medical, nursing) Include illness prevention and health promotion
Goal setting	Include patient in goal setting Make goals explicit and realistic
Therapeutic option consideration	Include modalities from multiple paradigms Consider patient preferences Consider context and cost in economic and human terms
Evaluation	Plan for follow-up visit or phone call Consider symptom or treatment logs or diaries Measure and document the outcome of your practice for the individual Report the effectiveness of your practice in the aggregate

checking literature, collaborating with colleagues, and following up with patients. Reflection on key cases in peer conferences can improve diagnostic efficiency and confidence.

Errors in Diagnostic Reasoning

Errors in diagnostic reasoning result in missed diagnoses and untreated problems as well as costly or risky tests or treatments for problems that do

TABLE 2–3

Errors in Diagnostic Reasoning

Phase of Clinical Judgment	Diagnostic Errors
Data collection	Not obtaining all relevant cues
	Misjudging importance of cues
	Overemphasizing cues that favor top hypotheses
	Ignoring data that disconfirm working hypothesis
	Forgetting that some data are unreliable
	Ignoring pertinent negative findings
Hypothesis generation	Not generating enough competing hypotheses
	Oversimplifying
	Not generating hypotheses early
	Not including correct diagnosis on hypothesis list
	Failing to revise hypothesis list (premature closure)
	Selecting "favorite" hypotheses
	Generating too many hypotheses and getting lost
	Overestimating low-probability situations
	Underestimating high-probability situations

not exist. Table 2–3 describes common errors that are made even by experts in their diagnostic thinking (Hamm & Zubialde, 1995). In the real world of clinical practice, clear diagnoses are not always obvious. The condition might be early in development. For example, early appendicitis does not elicit the classic signs. Patients may be unable to recall essential elements of history. Alternatively, the condition may not be a recognized medical problem. Chronic fatigue syndrome, for example, was not identified as such until the mid-1980s. Not arriving at a diagnosis can be frustrating for clinicians and patients alike. An open communication and a commitment to continue searching for an explanation for the patient's symptoms can help to maintain trust in these difficult situations. Many patients have told stories of not being listened to, or of being treated as fabricators or as malingerers when the problem was with the diagnostic capacities of the caregiver. Patients are usually reassured when conditions that they fear the most are eliminated from consideration.

Specific errors in diagnostic reasoning include superficial data collection, missing essential cues, misreading the importance of cues (often because they are not consistent with the most highly favored hypothesis), and failing to maintain critical thinking about the data that are presented. Not all of it is reliable. The patient might forget sequences or shade the truth because of embarrassment. Laboratory data can be in error.

Problems in hypothesis generation include narrowing the search field too soon in order to minimize the cognitive complexity of diagnostic reasoning. New practitioners frequently engage in a shotgun approach to data collection and fail to generate hypotheses soon enough in the process. As a result, the information collected is disorganized, making it harder for the practitioner to make sense of the whole picture. Generating too many hypotheses, on the other hand, overtaxes the short-term memory capacity of the novice clinician and results in wasted effort. Obviously, not including the correct hypotheses on the first list makes it harder to eventually settle on it. One of the main errors that experienced clinicians are prone to is "premature closure," or settling too soon on the chosen hypothesis. Even in a busy practice, a healthy skepticism about the hypotheses will decrease the likelihood of settling too soon on an obvious answer. Finally, we see what we expect to see. Data are easier to generate to support our most commonly encountered clinical problems.

⟨))⟩ CRITICAL THINKING

Diagnostic reasoning can be seen as a kind of critical thinking. Critical thinking has been defined as reflective thinking in that one questions one's thinking process to determine if all possible avenues have been explored and if the conclusions that are being drawn are based on evidence. This kind of thinking supports clinical judgment in several ways. First, it becomes a habit of mind to have humility about one's thought processes and to know that even the most experienced thinker can be mistaken. Second, it becomes a systematic way of generating creative ways of thinking about problems. Third, critical thinking returns one to an examination of the strength of evidence for a given conclusion. Evidence here means more than "hard" data such as laboratory values. As we will show later, even laboratory values need to be examined critically when they are used to assist diagnostic reasoning. Evidence that is useful to nurse practitioners includes subjective impressions about how patients present themselves (Webber, 2000). For example, the patient's complaint may be fatigue. But if the patient describes it as a bone-chilling inability to generate energy for daily living—as opposed to a fulfilled fatigue that comes after completing a challenge—that subjective description becomes part of the data used by the nurse practitioner to investigate a potentially serious problem.

Critical thinking can be seen to include creative thinking, and in this sense, the nurse practitioner is creative in developing potential problem lists. A patient may complain of abdominal pain. The pattern is unclear or may indicate irritable bowel syndrome. The creative nurse practitioner explores stress management issues as a way of generating diagnostic and therapeutic choices that might include a diet and symptom log, increased fiber in the diet, a walking program, or a quick return visit to check on symptoms. Creativity may also be required in developing goals with patients for their short- or long-term problems. In addition to creative processing, critical thinking includes systematic thinking through which the nurse practitioner evaluates each new piece of data as either supporting or refuting certain diagnostic hypotheses. Critical thinking can be used with individual patients or as the nurse practitioner considers groups of patients. *Does a subset of the patients have increasing difficulty with certain diagnoses? Is there an environmental component to their health problem?* Critical thinking assists us in examining patterns of health across groups of patients. It can lead to the development of new programming or to generating clinical research questions.

⏵⏵ DEVELOPING EXPERTISE

Benner (1984) has done extensive work describing differences in clinical judgment based on experience. Brykzcynski (1989) has extended this work to focus specifically on nurse practitioner performance. Nurse practitioner students, even those who are experts in hospital or specialty care, find it disconcerting to enter a world where they feel like novices again. Even skills that were a part of their old practice feel awkward. Their minds do not generate ideas smoothly, and they focus on their own performance of skills more than on the patient's situation. With the experience of the clinical practicum, however, the nurse practitioner student gains skill, and by graduation is probably functioning at the advanced beginner level. Features of diagnostic reasoning used in the various stages of expertise are summarized in Table 2–4. As a novice, you will find that having a set system to guide your actions in history and physical examination can serve as a structure until the process is firmly stored in production memory. Early on, anxiety about performance frequently makes the practitioner less aware of the context of the patient's life. Experienced nurse practitioners include in their list of questions one for themselves: Do these findings fit together to form a picture that makes sense?

With some experience, the student's sensitivity to more aspects of the situation will increase. Actions are guided more by principles than by rules. Priority setting might still be a problem. By the end of the educa-

TABLE 2–4	
Skill Acquisition in Nurse Practitioner Practice	
Skill Level	Features of Clinical Judgment
Novice	Rule-based actions, unaware of context
Advanced beginner	Sensitive to aspects of the situation, able to formulate principles, needs help setting priorities
Competent	Goal-directed actions, feeling of mastery based on experience, deliberate planning
Proficient	Sees situation as a whole, immediate grasp of meaning, recognizes patterns of normalcy or aberrance, uses maxims to guide action
Expert	Transcends rules, intuitive grasp of the wholeness of situation, creative response to particularities of situation, flexible response to situations

tional program, students may feel a beginning sense of competence, but many graduates have reported that it takes up to 2 years before real proficiency is gained. Proficiency is characterized by seeing the situation as a whole, much like the description of intuition. Finally, experts develop creative responses to patient situations. Preceptors often function at this level. The student's and new graduate's development along this continuum is something to discuss with faculty, preceptor, and peers. Part of developing one's abilities to think critically and grow professionally depends on an open reflection on processes used in clinical situations.

)) LEVELS OF JUDGMENT

"Clinical judgment" is a term that represents a multitude of meanings and decisions that are made as part of the clinical encounter. Clinical judgment is an association of a complaint or finding with a diagnostic label. Computer programs have been developed to simulate this process because, at this associational level, the memory capacity and processing speed of the computer exceed that of the human brain. An example of a low-level association is as follows: A patient complaint of a sore throat for three days with fever combined with physical findings of inflamed pharynx with tonsillar exudates and swollen, tender lymph nodes leads to ordering a test for streptococcus organisms to confirm the hypothesis of streptococcal pharyngitis. Scripted responses are often used for simple, frequently seen problems to maximize efficiency for busy clinicians. For common problems, accuracy is adequate. Appropriate follow-up prevents the occasional error from resulting in harm to the patient.

A middle-range complexity problem requires pattern recognition across several seemingly unrelated domains to develop diagnostic hypotheses that require further investigation. An older person with a recent history of falls and a recent bereavement raises the question of depression, substance abuse, or early dementia. Obtaining supportive data is more sensitive and more involved than the previous case of ordering a simple laboratory test.

At an even higher level, data help the nurse practitioner to develop an understanding of the meaning of a symptom or finding from a patient's point of view. For example, a patient who has elevated blood pressure in the context of a family history of coronary heart disease and early loss of a parent has in increased risk of cardiovascular disease—and is more likely to question the meaning of life and health at midlife. Recognizing the meanings that a clinical condition might have can lead to a deeper, more helpful relationship between the patient and the nurse practitioner and may increase the patient's participation in choosing how to structure his or her life. Even brief office visits present the possibility of complex, high-level clinical judgment if the clinician is open to this possibility (Agruss & Marfell, 2000).

⟫ SUMMARY

In summary, developing expert clinical judgment skills is a rewarding challenge for any clinician. When we focus attention on the processes used in clinical practice, our effectiveness in helping patients meet their health goals can be increased and the process can support care based on a nurse practitioner-patient partnership model.

REFERENCES

Agruss, J. C., & Marfell, J. (2000). Developmental dynamics of clinical decision making. In K. Crabtree (Ed.). *Teaching clinical decision making in advanced practice* (pp. 27–36). Washington, DC: National Organization of Nurse Practitioner Faculties.

Baddeley, A. (1999). *Essentials of human memory*. New York: Taylor and Francis.

Baxt, W. G. (1991). Use of an artificial neural network for the diagnosis of myocardial infarction. *Annals of Internal Medicine, 115*, 843–848.

Benner, P. (1984). *From novice to expert: Excellence and power in clinical nursing practice*. Menlo Park, CA: Addison-Wesley.

Benner, P., & Tanner, C. A. (1987). Clinical judgment: How expert nurses use intuition. *American Journal of Nursing, 87*, 23–31.

Benner, P., Tanner, C. A., & Chesla, C. A. (1996). *Expertise in nursing practice: Caring, clinical judgment, and ethics*. New York: Springer Publishing Company.

Brykczynski, K. A. (1989). An interpretive study describing the clinical judgment of nurse practitioners. *Scholarly Inquiry for Nursing Practice, 3*, 75–104.

Carnevali, D. L., & Thomas, M. D. (1993). *Diagnostic reasoning and treatment decision making in nursing*. Philadelphia: J. B. Lippincott.

Corcoran, S. (1986). Decision analysis: A step by step guide for making clinical decisions. *Nursing and Health Care, 7*, 149–154.

Dunn, H. (1961). *High-level wellness*. Arlington, VA: R.W. Beatty Co.

Dunphy, L. (1999). The wisdom of advanced practice nurses: Approaches to diagnosis and treatment. Unpublished interview data.

Elstein, A. S., Shulman, L. S., & Sprafka, S. A. (1978). *Medical problem-solving: An analysis of clinical reasoning*. Cambridge, MA: Harvard University Press.

Flagler, S. (2000). Recognizing the thinking processes behind clinical decision making. In K. Crabtree (Ed.). *Teaching clinical decision making in advanced practice* (pp. 7–16). Washington, DC: National Organization of Nurse Practitioner Faculties.

Gordon, M. (1994). *Nursing diagnosis: Process and application*. New York: McGraw-Hill.

Hamm, R. H., & Zubialde, J. (1995). Physicians' expert cognition and the problem of cognitive biases. *Primary Care Clinics in Office Practice, 22*(2), 181–211.

Jenny, J., & Logan, J. (1992). Knowing the patient: One aspect of clinical knowledge. *Image: The Journal of Nursing Scholarship, 24*, 254–258.

Lange, S. L., Haak, S. W., Lincoln, M. J., Thompson, C. B., Turner, C. W., Weir, C., Foerster, V., Nilasena, D., & Reeves, R. (1997). Use of Iliad to improve diagnostic performance of nurse practitioner students. *Journal of Nursing Education, 36*(1), 36–45.

Larkin, J., McDermott, J., Simon, D., & Simon, H. (1980). Expert and novice performance in solving physics problems. *Science, 208*, 1135–1342.

Miller, G. (1956). The magical number seven, plus or minus two: Some limits on our capacity for processing information. *Psychological Review, 63*, 81–97.

Newell, A., & Simon, S. A. (1972). *Human problem solving*. Englewood Cliffs, NJ: Prentice-Hall.

Nicoll, C. D., Pignone, M., & Detmer, W. M. (2000). Diagnostic testing and medical decision making. In L. M. Tierney, S. J. McPhee, & M. A. Papadakis, (Eds.). *Current medical diagnosis & treatment* (39th Ed.) (pp. 1598–1608). New York: Lange Medical Books/McGraw-Hill.

Rew, L. (1988), Intuition in decision making. *Image: the Journal of Nursing Scholarship, 20*, 150–155.

Rew, L., & Barrows, E. M. (1987). Intuition: a neglected hallmark of nursing knowledge. *Advances in Nursing Science, 10*, 49–62.

Shaw, J. D., Newell, A., & Simon, H. A. (1958). Elements of a theory of human problem-solving. *Psychological Review, 65*, 151–166.

Tanner, C. A., Benner, P., Chesla, C., & Gordon, D. (1993). The phenomenology of knowing the patient. *Image: the Journal of Nursing Scholarship, 25*, 273–280.

Tanner, C. A., Padrick, K. P., Westfal, U. E., & Putzier, D. J. (1987). Diagnostic reasoning strategies of nurses and nursing students. *Nursing Research, 36*, 358–363.

Tulving, E. (1972). Episodic and semantic memory. In E. Tulving & W. Donaldson (Eds.). *Organization of memory* (pp. 381–403). New York: Academic Press.

United States Preventive Services Task Force Guide to Clinical Preventive Services (2003). *Put prevention into practice.* Rockville, MD: Agency for Healthcare Research and Quality. *http://www.ahrq.gov/clinic/prevnew. htm.* Downloaded June 28, 2003.

Waldorp, M. (1987). The workings of working memory. *Science, 237*, 1564–1567.

Webber, P. B. (2000). Clinical decision making: Components, processes and outcomes. In K. Crabtree (Ed.). *Teaching clinical decision making in advanced practice* (pp. 17–25). Washington, DC: National Organization of Nurse Practitioner Faculties.

White, J. E., Nativio, D. G., Kobert, S. N., & Engberg, S. J. (1992). Content and process in clinical decision-making by nurse practitioners. *Image: Journal of Nursing Scholarship, 24*, 153–158.

CHAPTER 3

Assessment and Diagnosis

CHAPTER OUTLINE

FOCUS ON ELEMENTS OF CLINICAL JUDGMENT

Chapter 2 outlined the processes used in diagnostic reasoning or clinical judgment. Experienced nurse practitioners use a systematic data collection, data clustering, differential diagnosis, and treatment planning approach to clinical judgment. They also sometimes transcend the step-by-step process and come to an immediate grasp of the situation through a process called intuition. Intuition is the result of years of experience and many cases of patterns being developed that are available for matching. This chapter focuses on the beginner's approach to collecting necessary data in order to accurately describe the patient's health condition, strengths, and capacities—all for the purpose of developing an efficient, useful plan for treatment and follow-up. Each source of data for the assessment is considered in detail. This chapter will be useful to students learning health assessment as well as to those beginning their clinical practice as nurse practitioner students. It presumes the condition of conducting a comprehensive history and physical examination. The process is modified if a brief, episodic visit is conducted. For example, the nurse practitioner selects features of this full data collection that seem appropriate to the patient's problem.

Consistent with the focus of Chapter 1 on the relationship between nurse practitioner and patient, this chapter focuses on assessment, a way of understanding the patient situation. The word assessment derives from the Latin verb *assidere*, to sit beside. This view of assessment is quite different from the biomedical term "history taking." "Taking" implies that the power and knowledge reside in the practitioner and that the patient is no more than a passive source of data. The nurse practitioner-patient model chooses the former definition. To assess is to "sit beside" the patient long enough to understand the story of the illness or condition that causes problems and to understand the strengths and capacities of the person's life. Based on a full assessment, the nurse practitioner and patient can develop a full set of diagnostic statements that can direct a management plan to maximize the patient's power over health-related choices.

⟫ HISTORY

Assessment is usually organized into history taking and physical examination, with laboratory testing as an additional consideration. Although many textbooks point to the techniques of physical examination, in actual fact, nurse practitioners rely more heavily on history than on physical findings when making a diagnosis. Some authors suggest that history contributes 60 to 70 percent of the data necessary for accurate diagnosis. The patient's history tells the story of the illness. The narrative of the patient history helps the nurse practitioner to interpret a multitude of data bits and to place them into a coherent picture that leads to accurate diagnosis. The nurse practitioner needs to be careful to remember that the early purpose of the history is to enter the world of the patient to understand his or her unique experience. This requires allowing the patient time to tell the story. Interrupting and asking questions that cut the patient off send the message that the nurse practitioner cares less about the patient than about the medical problem. It also cuts off a chance to see how the patient perceives the problem. When the patient is interrupted with a list of questions, the focus of the interview is shifted from the patient's world to the nurse practitioner's world. When this happens, contextual data are lost and the developing trust between practitioner and patient is threatened.

RULE OF THUMB: Listen for the elements of patients' stories. What factors do they see as important? What is the trajectory of their experience?

When taking a history, nurse practitioners should consider the setting and the body language conveyed. Patients should be allowed to meet their providers and tell their stories with as much dignity as possible. This means that they should be clothed and preferably seated in a comfortable chair rather than placed with their feet dangling off the end of an examination table. Efficiency can be maintained by having patients disrobe and be positioned on the examination table after the initial interview while the nurse practitioner attends to other duties, such as hallway consultations or returning brief telephone calls. Patient dignity must never be violated to serve office efficiency.

RULE OF THUMB: Take the initial history while the patient is clothed. It maintains dignity and helps the nurse practitioner see the wholeness of the patient.

By sitting at the same level as the patient, the nurse practitioner conveys a partnership that works against the power structures inherent in a person consulting a professional about his or her health care. Positioning oneself slightly to one side of the patient—for example, with the clinician seated at a desk and the patient in a chair at the side of the desk—conveys the impression that there is no barrier between patient and clinician. Having the desk as a separation places a visible gulf between the two.

To establish a tone, the nurse practitioner should explain to the patient that notes will be made during the interview so that facts are not lost. This does not mean that the nurse practitioner should focus on paper forms or a computer or dictating machine while collecting patient data because this will make patients feel as if they are a byproduct of a complicated system. It is possible to complete documentation in the room with the patient, but writing and filling out forms should not be allowed to interrupt the flow of the conversation.

The tone that the nurse practitioner tries to achieve varies with the patient and the setting, but in order to establish relationship-centered care, the initial interview is the most important step. Convey genuine interest and concern with the patient situation. Being lighthearted and joking or teasing can work after one knows the patient, but initially, a pleasant business-like manner opens doors. Follow the patient and/or family lead in adapting the tone of the interview. When working with children, a playful, respectful distance can decrease fears. With adolescents, a respectful, no-nonsense, plain-talk attitude often works. Using adolescent language and current catch phrases can show that you understand their world, but because adolescent pop culture changes fast, one can come off looking behind the times easily, and this does not accomplish the purpose of establishing rapport. Keep in mind that older patients frequently have some loss of vision or hearing, which can affect the interview process. Speaking slowly and with a low pitch with good face-to-face contact can help communication with older patients.

Remember that, whatever the age of the patients, their story and their world is of utmost concern to you. Getting to know them and their concerns and strengths is the most important feature of the early nurse practitioner-patient interaction.

> RULE OF THUMB: Initial visits are for more than history taking. They provide a context from which to begin establishing the relationship with the patient.

Demographics

Most clinic settings use patient records that will provide the nurse practitioner with data that might be useful in diagnostic or therapeutic reasoning. The date of the last visit, the thickness of the file, and the data relating to age, sex, marital status, occupation, and insurance coverage are important to consider. Other information such as allergies, current medications, or an active problem list might be available before the patient interview begins.

Chief Complaint

Most nurse practitioner visits, even if for a school, employment, or routine physical, involve some health complaint. Frequently, as the patient makes the appointment or is checked in by the office assistant, a chief complaint is entered on the encounter form or chart. Even if "healthy physical" or "2-month checkup" is listed as the reason for the visit, be open to the possibility that there are health concerns. Sometimes patients are reluctant to share their concerns with office assistants or scheduling secretaries. Nurse practitioners should not assume that they know why patients have come to the office. Always ask, "What brings you here today?" or "Do you have any concerns we can discuss while you are here?" Documenting the patients' chief complaints in their own words is most useful because it records how they perceive their own problem.

RULE OF THUMB: Do not assume that the reason for a visit obtained by the office staff is the patient's only concern. Always ask if there are other concerns.

Be aware that a patient's true concerns might not come to light in the first minutes of the appointment. There may be a ritual of information sharing, caregiving, and response during which patients come to know you as a clinician and during which they decide to reveal deeper concerns. Nurse practitioners learn to pay attention to the "Oh, by the way..." comment that comes out just as you reach for the door handle to end the interview. With experience, nurse practitioners learn to read the silence and the tension in the room, to develop a sense of when there is more going on. For example, an experienced clinician who had a relationship with a female patient visiting the clinic for a routine appointment felt that "something was not right" in the course of the appointment. At the end, after being asked repeatedly if everything was all right, the patient revealed that she had been physically abused. Keeping lines of communication open is important. Learn to develop your "antennae" about whether the whole picture is being revealed.

It is often useful to know why the patient is coming for care today. Sometimes managing a chronic problem becomes difficult when additional stresses in life appear. If the underlying chronic problem cannot be resolved, perhaps the stress associated with the chronic problem can be addressed to restore balance in the person's life. In any case, understanding what prompted the visit reveals how the patient copes with problems and how serious he or she believes they are.

RULE OF THUMB: Develop antennae about whether the whole picture is being revealed.

At times a patient with multiple chronic illnesses may have a laundry list of concerns. However, in most practices, time is a valuable commodity. So if the patient presents new concerns that are not urgent, he or she can be scheduled for a visit to address those concerns specifically. For example, a patient could be complaining of sleep disturbance in addition to being monitored for diabetes. Suggest that the patient keep a sleep log for 2 weeks and return for a visit to focus on that concern. You can also do some quick sleep hygiene teaching during this visit. In 2 weeks, either the problem will be resolved or you will need to evaluate it further, but with the sleep log, you will have more data from which to operate.

Eliciting a history and performing a physical examination are routine for nurse practitioners, but the patient may not understand our routine. Explain how you will proceed and how the patient can participate. For example, "First, I will ask you some questions about this problem and your general health, and then I will do the physical examination. Then we can discuss what we think the problem is and how we can proceed." Establishing the agenda for each visit helps to meet expectations for both the patient and the nurse practitioner. It also supports nurse practitioner decisions about what data to collect that day and how to plan overall follow-up.

> RULE OF THUMB: Together with the patient, establish an agenda for each visit to meet expectations and to focus activities.

History of Present Illness

Once the chief complaint is identified, a deeper exploration of the history of this complaint is conducted. This exploration will form a link between the patient's world of experience and our own understanding of actual or potential problems. This is called the history of present illness, or HPI. The best way to conceive of the HPI is to think of it as a story with a beginning and at least a partial middle. The end will come as the problem is identified and dealt with. In considering the diagnostic possibilities, the chronology of events is very important. For example, cough and fever before nasal congestion point to viral influenza rather than simple viral upper respiratory illness or "cold." Try to help the patient focus the history of events by asking, "When did you start to feel weak?" If the patient responds, "A few days ago," clarify by asking, "Today is Wednesday. Did you feel well on Sunday?" Patients often minimize how long they have been feeling ill. It takes several days before they decide that the condition is troubling enough to warrant calling for an appointment. In your notes, document actual dates as clearly as possible.

Other important elements to consider include starting with open-ended questions and only later moving to closed ended questions. For example, "How did you first know you were becoming ill?" or "Can you tell me more about the pain?" are open-ended questions. "Did you have a cough?" is closed. Closed-ended questions are necessary to bring details to light. But they should be addressed after the patient's story has been told. Consider both quantitative and qualitative questions. Quantitative questions address how long, how much, or how many times an event occurred, whereas qualitative questions ask for a description of severity, type, color, character, and experience. Record particularly descriptive phrases used by

TABLE 3–1	
History of Present Illness: OLDCART System	
O: Onset	When did this problem start? How did it start? Has it changed over time? For an injury, exactly how did the injury occur (the mechanism of injury)?
L: Location	Where exactly are the symptoms experienced? Can a specific location be identified, or is the problem more generalized? Has the symptom moved?
D: Duration	Are the symptoms constant, fluctuating, getting better or worse?
C: Characteristics	How are the symptoms experienced? Dull ache, sharp pain, heat, or electrical?
A: Aggravating	What makes the symptoms worse?
R: Relieving	What makes the symptoms better?
T: Treatment	What have you done so far to try to help the problem?

the patient for future reference. Qualitative questions are useful for distinguishing types of pain such as gnawing, sharp, dull, aching, or prickly. Depending on the differential list, this description can be useful in narrowing the potential problems. If closed-ended questions are overused, the patient can respond only to the agenda set by the nurse practitioner and thus will feel unimportant and disempowered.

There are a number of mnemonics that are useful in completing the HPI. Table 3–1 lists the elements of the OLDCART system. The acronym OLDCART is explained in the table. This is one of many that can be used by new nurse practitioners when directing history taking. The list is also useful for experienced nurse practitioners when they are confronted with a patient picture that is not immediately falling into place. Having a system prevents clinicians from leaving out some essential data because they think they already know what is going on. This prevents the diagnostic reasoning error of premature closure.

As outlined in Chapter 2, clinical judgment is useful not only in forming the final problem list, but in directing every step of the clinical process. For example, what follow-up question to ask is partly determined by the list of diagnostic hypotheses being developed. If the nurse practitioner suspects viral or bacterial upper respiratory illness, questions will focus on symptoms of the eyes, ears, throat, and chest. Less attention will be paid to musculoskeletal or neurological symptom evaluation. On the other hand, a headache will necessitate questions about eyes and visual changes, ears, consciousness, and muscle weakness. Diagnostic reasoning begins before the first word of the interview is spoken. After the patient's story is elicited, specific questions are asked that help to distinguish between competing diagnostic hypotheses. For example, the question, "Do you feel the pain more often on an empty stomach or several hours after eating?" helps to distinguish between ulcer and gallbladder disease. Eliciting the patient's story will help the nurse practitioner to understand the illness experience from the patient's perspective.

The nurse practitioner continues to clarify the patient's story until a clear picture of the illness appears. This can require patience because patients do not know which facts "fit together" to support our diagnostic hypotheses. Patients may get the chronological order confused or not recall the onset of their problems. They also might have more than one problem and not be able to distinguish which symptoms cluster together. At times the picture is not completely clear at this point of history taking and several possible hypotheses exist. Other areas of history can fill in some gaps of knowledge and point to one or two hypotheses more than others.

Periodically, the nurse practitioner can restate the emerging understanding of the story in order to clarify and summarize. This allows the patient to rectify any misunderstandings that the nurse practitioner may still hold. One important issue to include in the HPI is what the patient thinks may be wrong. Patients know their own bodies better than anyone and may have important insights to share. On the other hand, by understanding patients' fears, the nurse practitioner can explain reasons why many of those fears may be unfounded. This is particularly true when dealing with children. Parents know their children, and a parent's perception that "Something is not right with my child" should get the focused attention of the nurse practitioner until the problem is identified and resolved.

Visits for periodic health screening, to establish a new patient-provider relationship, or to follow up on an existing problem do not use the HPI in the same sense unless a new problem is also identified. One can ask, "What do you want to accomplish today?" or "What is the most important issue for us to deal with today?" This is particularly useful for the patient with a long list of problems or complaints. Be sure to make a plan for follow-up on other problems.

Past Medical History

The past medical history (PMH) is the section of the assessment process that develops background data for the health patterns of the person. This information is useful in three ways. First, the PMH may help to refine an active hypothesis list. If the patient had a cholecystectomy in the past, typical gallbladder disease is an unlikely cause of abdominal pain. On the other hand, a history of diabetes mellitus predisposes the patient to vascular, renal, and retinal disease and helps to adjust the risk factor or disease under consideration. Second, other active problems related or unrelated to the chief complaint are encountered and assessed (Coulehan & Block, 1997). Third, in the case of a healthy visit, the PMH is the chief indicator of risk factors for targeted risk reduction strategies for the future. One can truly be involved in primary prevention when one uses past medical history to guide health teaching and reduce risks of health problems.

Significant Events

PMH includes childhood and other illnesses, surgical history, other hospital admissions, history of trauma, pregnancies, medication, allergies, exposures to toxic substances, and psychiatric diagnoses. Travel outside the United States and any possible exposure to infectious or toxic agents can also be explored. Patients frequently forget that they have been diagnosed with specific conditions. Many practices use a questionnaire that the patient completes before the face-to-face visit. Nurse practitioners should review this form carefully to clarify the data and fill in essential information. The patient might record mastectomy as a previous surgery. It would be important to know whether lymph node dissection had occurred, what the findings were, if known, and whether the patient received chemotherapy and/or radiation therapy after the procedure. Patients frequently forget conditions that happened in the distant past or that seem completely resolved. One way to double-check the past medical history is to ask about medications.

Past medical problems can be queried by a direct question: "Do you have other health problems?" In the absence of past medical records, the patient's report of problems has the potential for misinterpretation and error. Another approach is to ask about hospitalizations or important diagnostic workups such as stress tests, x rays, or emergency room visits. Accidents and injuries are as important to consider as medical problems. If the past problem is unclear, it sometimes helps to ask how the condition was treated. This will help to differentiate between asthma and pneumonia if all that the patient recalls is a "lung problem."

RULE OF THUMB: Patients often forget significant health events. Asking about significant diagnostic workups and hospitalizations will remind them of problems in the past.

Medications

Ask patients about all medications that they take, including prescriptions, over-the-counter medications, vitamins, and herbal remedies. Ask if they take any medications that have been prescribed for other members of the family as well. Even for patients who are well known to the practice and whose medications are listed on the chart, ask what medications they are currently taking. This helps to determine if the medications that were ordered are really being taken. Patients can also be asked if they are having trouble obtaining or remembering to take their medications. Economic factors play a role for patients who take expensive medications and who do not have health insurance coverage for medications. This review of medications also gives the nurse practitioner information about patients' understanding of their medication and helps to determine any difficulties that they are having with the prescribed regimen. Information about alcohol, tobacco, and illegal drugs can be elicited here or included in the social history. Do not presume by age or appearance which patient is likely to be using illegal substances. The National Household Survey on Drug Abuse (Wright, 2002) reports that up to 11.4 percent of those surveyed reported illicit drug use in the previous year in the state with the highest rate of use.

Factors other than availability and cost can also affect medication delivery. A clinical example illustrates this point. A non–English-speaking patient was under treatment for hypertension that was not well controlled. The nurse practitioner was considering a dosage increase and asked the patient, through an interpreter, if she was able to take the medication as ordered. The patient reported that she frequently forgot her late-day dose. After asking the patient where she stored her medication on a typical day, the nurse practitioner recommended that the patient store the medication in her bathroom, where she got ready for bed. This increased her ability to obtain all her doses, resulting in improved blood pressure control at the original dose.

Immunizations

Immunization status should be reviewed. It is an important part of the history, reflecting continuity or discontinuity with health-care providers, and it is part of the healthy visit for children and adults. Many parents bring their child's immunization cards with them to office visits. This allows any additional immunization series to be documented. Adults also have several immunizations that are important to follow as well. For example, many adults are unaware that they need a tetanus booster every 10 years. Older adults and those with chronic disease need a pneumococcal immunization (United States Preventive Services Task Force, 2003). This is a good time to inquire about the use of complementary and alternative methods such as chiropractic, naturopathy, Reiki, meditation, or other ways to maintain health.

Allergies

Allergies can be discussed and reviewed at this time. Always ask what kind of reaction the medications or food caused because patients often mistake a side effect with an allergy. One should note the side effect, but not as an allergy, which would be characterized by rash, hives, wheezing, or other hypersensitivity reactions. Most patient records have several places for prominent display of allergies to food or medication. This helps to prevent a provider from ordering medications that might cause an adverse reaction for the patient. Take time to check for allergies on records that have been used for some time and note any new allergies or reactions.

Family History

Family history provides additional information that helps to determine the risk factor pattern for a patient. The most efficient way to represent the family history is to draw a genogram, as shown in Figure 3–1. This method of representation can be used to record family patterns of births, ages at death, and causes of death and can also reflect with whom the patient currently lives. Try to include information at least two generations back and any children and their health status. The genogram can be used to reflect difficulties like alcoholism or the quality of relationships in the family by drawing slashes across the relationship lines that are troubled or heavy lines for the relationships that are strongly supportive. Judgment is required to determine if this level of information is useful. Do include information about conditions that are known to have familial patterns of inheritance. If there is no room for a genogram, reflect the major diseases that have familial patterns, such as diabetes, heart disease, arthritis, psychiatric problems, alcoholism, and cancer, in the list.

The definition of family may affect the data collected. Some conditions, such as heart disease, diabetes, and cancer, have definite familial risk factors. Blood relatives in this case are most significant. Other conditions, such as exposure to tuberculosis, might be shared by anyone living in the household. It may be important to clarify who lives with the patient and how his or her health might affect the patient.

Eliciting the family history can enhance understanding of the patient's life. For example, while being interviewed, an adolescent in a substance abuse recovery program revealed that a sibling had died of cancer. In

Figure 3–1
GENOGRAM OF FAMILY HISTORY

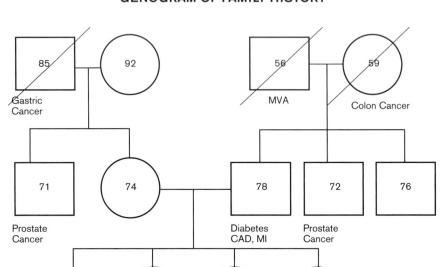

tracking his substance abuse history, it was learned that much of his substance abuse began soon after the death of that sibling. Paying attention to dates can expose recent losses with which the patient may be dealing and can indicate important anniversaries or ages. A man whose father died of a heart attack at age 39 may be anxious about his own health. That anxiety might assist him in making a health promotion appointment, or his anxiety could make it difficult to enter the health-care system. Understanding the meaning that the patient makes of the event is key to establishing a helping relationship.

Social History

Social history is the section of the assessment phase in which the nursing approach differs the most from the medical approach. Even if the nurse practitioner uses the medical category headings as the standard medical record—which this author argues against—the nursing perspective brings out a clearer picture of the patient's everyday living situation, builds an understanding of the person at a deeper level, and can be reflected in the social history section. The purpose of the social history is more than simply to identify risk factors for disease. The social history serves as a way of imagining how to support the person in developing patterns of life that support health. The social history taking by nurses therefore differs in both content and intention from the standard medical database.

Traditional elements of the social history include ethnic background, religion, marital status, education, work history, and lifestyle issues such as nutrition; activities; and tobacco, alcohol, and illegal substance assessment. Simply indicating marital status by category (married, divorced, etc.) does not reflect the quality of support or demand that is involved in the family situation. Specifically ask where the patient obtains support and what burdens, such as the care of an older relative, that he or she might be experiencing. Information about religion may be important in determining preferences for treatment, but do not assume that a religious category is important in determining the patient's values. Other elements include key relationships and supports from sources that might not be considered family, such as a faith community.

Ethnic background is important for understanding the patient's values and cultural heritage. Being careful to avoid stereotyping, one can consider what is known about ethnic groups in planning care. For example, Hispanic families are very close, and important health issues are usually addressed with that in mind. Hispanic women may have preferences for certain methods of family planning. Asian families also tend to make decisions together using an adult male as the spokesperson for the family. Just as Anglo families operate in unique ways, families from other cultures do also. Immigrants might hold very tightly to the values and traditions of their home country, or they might be transitioning to adopt the values of what they see in the culture of the United States. Be sensitive to the range of possibilities when getting to know the patient and family. The clinician is sensitive to possible differences and treats each situation with respect.

Educational background can be important in considering potential resources as well as ways in which people learn new material. Nurse practitioners must be careful not to "talk down" to patients who may be as educated as they are, albeit in other academic areas. Even very well-educated patients cannot be assumed to have mastered health-related information. On the other hand, nurse practitioners must not assume that any patient can read written instructions on medication and other health-related material. When dealing with health issues, even educated patients are anxious, and high anxiety levels can impede learning.

Work patterns are an important facet of the social history. If the patient is retired, include the type of work that he or she performed.

Worksite exposures can be risk factors for many potential problems. Work background also gives the nurse practitioner a sense of how patients might handle new information and what kind of resources they might have at their disposal. Nursing histories are more expanded in this area and include such information as leisure-time activities, again for risk factors and exposures as well as a reflection of resources and activity level.

Nutrition and diet patterns are best assessed by asking for a 24-hour recall. If asked a simple question such as "How is your diet?" patients are likely to say "Okay." Asking about yesterday's eating pattern or a typical day's eating pattern, especially if illness has altered the intake pattern, can shed light on whether the person always eats alone, is hurried, has access to healthy food, or has a knowledge or preference pattern that must be accommodated.

Activity assessment includes typical energy expenditures such as housework or yard work, and also sports and recreational activities. Activities related to work or sports can inform diagnostic decisions regarding repetitive stress and other potential injury situations. It is important to ask people what they believe their exercise capacity to be and how they respond to increased levels of activity, for example, "How far can you walk before getting short of breath?" or "Can you climb two flights of stairs without stopping?"

Substance use, which may have been addressed with medications, can be a sensitive topic when interviewing patients. Many patients fear that clinicians will respond judgmentally about their use of substances that they know are harmful or illegal. The best approach is to maintain an open communication style, to explain why you are asking (because tobacco, alcohol, and illegal drugs might affect prescribing decisions), and to emphasize that you are concerned about the person's whole health, not just disease problems. A useful and easy tool to use in primary care when asking about alcohol is the CAGE questionnaire:

1. Have you ever felt the need to Cut down on your drinking?
2. Have you ever felt Annoyed by criticism of drinking?
3. Have you ever had Guilty feelings about drinking?
4. Have you ever had a morning Eye opener? (Mayfield, McLead, & Hall, 1974).

Similar questions can be asked about use of marijuana, cocaine, or heroine. If patients report using illegal drugs, inquire about the drug delivery modes used. Risk factor patterns differ if the patient uses intravenous access (shoots), skin injection (pops), or nasal delivery (snorts).

Substance use patterns can be described by first use, amount of use, and last use.

Asking about the patient's family constellation is important and can be addressed with family history, but the purpose for asking here is different from looking at disease risk patterns. The nurse practitioner needs to develop a picture of the patient's demands and supports. Asking, "Who lives with you?" can be the start of exploring this circumstance. Beyond the actual domicile, ask whether patients are responsible for the care of anyone who may live separately from them. Many adults are responsible for aging parents who may live independently and who make up a large part of the social demands placed on patients' lives. Also, many grandparents are sole caretakers for their grandchildren. Developing a picture of the human environment for patients helps to individualize treatment plans.

Domestic abuse is a topic often avoided by health-care workers. One cannot make the assumption that, because the person is well dressed or lives in an affluent community, there is no risk of domestic abuse. One way to find out about this sensitive area is to be direct and ask, "Has anyone ever pushed or hit you?" Sexual abuse is closely related and can be asked in a similar way, such as, "Has anyone ever forced you to do anything sexual that you did not want to do?" More general questions about safety in the home and the neighborhood can get the patient talking about difficult areas. If threat or abuse is revealed, ask if the person has a safe place where he or she can go or if he or she knows the number of abuse hotlines. Patients who are truly afraid will not be willing to carry these numbers on their person for fear that they may be discovered. Patients frequently deny their fears, but by asking, the nurse practitioner opens doors, and on subsequent visits the patient might be more willing to discuss the problem. Many clinics and private offices post the numbers for local shelters and hotlines in the women's bathroom so that patients can receive information anonymously.

Sexual histories often cause anxiety both for new nurse practitioners and for patients. It often helps to explain why you want the information that you are seeking. Explain that sexuality reflects health for the whole person and introduces an element of risk with certain sexual practices. Certain diseases and medications can also affect sexual patterns, and patients may be afraid to bring up their questions if the nurse practitioner does not open the discussion. One question to ask is whether there has been a change in sexual patterns lately. Do not assume that all patients are heterosexual. Asking, "Are you sexually active? With men, women, or both?" opens the question. Explain that you ask everyone the same question. Also ask about safer sex practices and family-planning techniques used.

The social history reveals much about how the patient lives his or her life and what problems other than physical ones the person may be dealing with. Patients report that nurse practitioners are open and thorough when caring for them (Benkert et al., 2002). This approach depends on practicing from a database that is broader and more personal than that of the traditional medical model. The next section portrays a way of combining the nursing and medical models in building an understanding of the patient.

Nursing/Functional Health Pattern Assessment

Functional health patterns were developed by Gordon (1994) to serve as a database for determining nursing diagnoses. Nurse practitioners engage in some activities that require making medical diagnoses, but their practice base is always nursing. The value that nurse practitioners bring to a practice relates to an improved ability to assist patients with lifestyle changes and an ability to support them as they cope with illness. The openness and thoroughness that patients report when cared for by a nurse practitioner is dependent on practicing from a database that is broader and more personal than that of the traditional medical model. Even in practice settings that function from a medically dominated model and record only medical terminology, the nurse practitioner has an obligation to include the type of data reflected in the functional health pattern in the medical record. If a full functional health pattern will be collected, much of this information can be included there. If the documentation system used in a particular setting does not accommodate functional health patterns, expand the social history section to reflect nursing issues.

When a patient is in the clinic for an episodic visit, it is important to prioritize the information needed for the purpose of the visit. As a clinical example, a man presents to the employee health clinic with a complaint of sore throat. Important data would relate to:

1. Nutrition—Is the patient able to eat and drink sufficiently?
2. Sleep/rest—Is sleep interrupted?
3. Activity/exercise—Does the patient feel fatigued?
4. Role/relationship—Is the patient able to work? Are there children in the home?

The purpose of the functional health pattern is to determine the extent to which illness is affecting the person's life. What accommodations must be made even for a self-limiting condition? This is nursing's central question. What is the human response to the health problem? Table 3–2 reflects

TABLE 3–2

Functional Health Patterns and Questions to Elicit Data

Pattern Area	Sample Questions
Health Perception/	Do you have a regular health-care provider? How often do you go?
Health Management	What do you do to stay healthy?
Nutrition/ Metabolic	What did you eat yesterday or on a typical day? What do you drink? How is your appetite? Any skin problems?
Elimination	How often do you move your bowels? How many times do you empty your bladder at night? Is there unexpected loss of control?
Activity/Exercise	How far can you walk before feeling tired? Do you have energy to do the things you want? Do you need any assistance with feeding, bathing, toileting, dressing, or getting around (activities of daily living)? Do you need any help with cooking, shopping, cleaning (instrumental activities of daily living)?
Sleep/Rest	How many hours do you sleep? Any trouble falling asleep or with early wakening? Do you feel rested?
Cognitive/ Perceptual	Any hearing or vision problems? Any memory changes? How do you like to learn new things? Any pain or discomfort?
Self-Perception/Self Concept	How would you describe yourself? Do you feel good about yourself? Any changes in how you feel about your body? Do you get angry or down at times?
Role Relationship	Who lives with you? Do you have friends? What kind of work do you do? Do you have other responsibilities?
Sexuality/ Reproductive	Any problems with your sexuality? Any changes? If sexually active, do you practice safe sex? Do you use birth control? What mode of birth control do you use?
Coping/Stress Tolerance	How do you cope with stress? Any use of alcohol, drugs? Do you have someone to talk things over with?
Value/ Belief	What is most important to you in your life? Are you religious? Any values about life that health-care providers should know about? Have you a health-care proxy or living will?

Source: Modified from Gordon, M. (1994). *Nursing diagnosis: Process and application* (3rd ed.). St. Louis: Mosby.

TABLE 3–3

Comparison of Nursing and Standard Medical Database

Medical Database Elements	Nursing Database (Functional Health Pattern Elements *Italicized*)
Demographic Data	Demographic Data
Chief Complaint	Chief Complaint–Patient's Agenda
History of Present Illness	History of Present Illness–Patient's Story
Past Medical History	Past Health History
Childhood diseases	Elements of medical history (as on left)
Hospitalizations/surgeries	*Health Perception/Health Management*
Obstetric history	*Nutrition/Metabolic*
Accidents/Injuries	*Elimination*
Serious illnesses	*Activity/Exercise*
Medications	*Sleep/Rest*
Immunizations	*Sexuality/Reproductive*
Allergies	
Family History	Family Medical History
Medical illnesses	Household/Work Exposures
Exposures	*Role/Relationships*
Social History	Social History
Work	Work
Health beliefs	Health and Cultural Beliefs and Practices
Travel	Typical Day
Lifestyle	*Cognitive/Perceptual*
Nutrition, activities,	*Self Perception/Self Concept*
tobacco, alcohol, drugs	
Relationships	*Coping/Stress Tolerance*
Family composition	*Value/Belief*
Sexual history	
Review of Systems	Review of Systems

the 11 functional health patterns with sample questions that can be used to elicit data for each pattern area. Table 3–3 shows how the functional health pattern data parallel and expand the traditional medical database.

Review of Systems

This section of the history is often completed immediately before the physical exam, and is organized by body systems Reviewing health data in a head-to-toe systematic way makes a transition from "whole person" information to a focus on bodily concerns. In some settings, patients complete questionnaires that reflect these data before they enter the examination room. Table 3–4 displays sample questions that can be used to elicit the review of systems. Whenever a questionnaire is completed, it should include symptoms that are current or related to past medical history and prompt the patient to report any past difficulties. The review of systems also helps to remind patients of conditions that they may have forgotten. Knowing about these conditions can help the nurse practitioner to further refine the hypothesis list or screen out potential new problems. For each body system, start questions in general terms and then proceed to include more specific items. When documenting this section, students frequently forget that this information is reported from the patient's point of view and should not include observational data.

At this phase of history taking, the hypothesis list is taking shape. The initial diagnostic possibilities that are generated are weighed as each new

TABLE 3–4

Sample Questions for Review of Systems

System	Suggested Questions
General	How is your general health? Are you sleeping restfully? Is your appetite good? Have you had any recent weight changes? Any fever, chills, or night sweats?
Skin	Any rashes, moles, itching, changes in color, easy bruising, changes in hair?
Head	Any headache, dizziness, fainting, history of head trauma?
Neurological system	Any weakness or paralysis? Any feeling of needles and pins, or other loss of sensation? Any trouble walking? Any seizures? Any trouble with memory or speech? Any nervousness or depression?
Eyes, ears, nose, and throat	Any eye problems, blurring, loss of vision? Any trouble hearing, ringing in ears, pain, discharge, or itching? Any problem with runny nose, change in ability to smell, nosebleeds, or sinus trouble? Frequent sore throats, trouble swallowing, hoarseness?

(Continued)

TABLE 3–4

Sample Questions for Review of Systems *(Continued)*

System	Suggested Questions
Mouth	Any mouth sores, dental problems?
Neck	Any pain, swelling, or stiffness in the neck?
Lymph nodes	Any swelling or painful lymph nodes in armpits, groin, neck?
Breasts	Any lumps, pain, or discharge? Do you check your breasts regularly?
Chest	Any chest pain, cough, difficulty breathing, shortness of breath? How far can you walk before becoming breathless?
Cardiovascular	Any chest pain, palpitations?
Gastrointestinal tract	Any stomach pains, indigestion, nausea, or vomiting? Any blood in your stool? Have your bowel movements changed? Any diarrhea or constipation? Any rectal itching, pain?
Endocrine	Any intolerance of heat or cold? Frequently thirsty?
Urinary tract	Any trouble passing urine, burning, itching, odor, frequency, loss of control, or pain?
Genitalia	Female: Any vaginal discharge, itching, or odor? When was your last menstrual period? What is the length of your cycle, the length and amount of flow? Do you engage in sexual relations, with men, women, or both? What method of contraception is used? Is your sex life satisfying? Male: Any urethral problems such as discharge, burning? Do you do testicular self exam? Do you engage in sexual relations, with men, women, or both? What method of contraception is used? Is your sex life satisfying?
Extremities	Any leg pain or cramping, joint pain or stiffness? Do your feet get cold easily? Do you have vein problems? Any back pain?

piece of data is elicited. Some data serve to support one hypothesis in favor over another; some data are noncontributory. Some data serve to rule out specific hypotheses. The problem list might contain clear physical disorders that are visible, other physical disorders that are presumed based on the story, emotional distress related to specific disorders, general emotional disorders, family or social disorders, or even spiritual distress. The patient's problem list may contain more than one diagnosis from any of the biological, psychosocial, or spiritual realms. The nurse practitioner can obtain further data to help refine the hypothesis list by performing the physical examination and ordering diagnostic tests.

> RULE OF THUMB: Write the current diagnostic hypotheses on a list and think critically about whether all the data so far collected are potentially explained by the list. If not, consider other hypotheses.

)) PHYSICAL EXAMINATION

When making the transition from history to physical examination, explain clearly to the patient how to prepare for the examination. Be specific about what clothing to remove and provide privacy and appropriate draping for physical warmth and comfort. The physical examination serves to clarify diagnostic hypotheses and detect unanticipated problems of which the patient is unaware.

In primary care, there are many ways of performing the examination. Textbooks of physical assessment outline a general head-to-toe model that is useful for an initial visit or a periodic reassessment. In most practices, an initial patient visit is scheduled for longer time blocks. This type of visit may be reimbursed at a higher level because of its comprehensiveness. Students in nursing or medical school learn to perform the head-to-toe exam in an organized way. In actual practice, however, nurse practitioners must learn to focus their physical assessment skills and make the examination appropriate to the patient's complaint and history. If the patient complains of headache, a review of head, eye, ear, nose, and throat and a neurological examination are indicated. For joint pain, a review of musculoskeletal tenderness, range of motion, and strength might be indicated. The body systems that are examined depend on the working hypothesis list that the nurse practitioner has generated. Examination skills need to be organized at a surface, general screening level, with subroutines of examination techniques that can be adapted to specific findings and complaints. Positive or negative findings that serve to refine the hypothesis list must be noted and recorded using the clinical documentation system. Even though a diagnosis is not clear, the rich data reporting from that visit can enhance later diagnostic accuracy when the condition has evolved further. Full documentation serves to protect both patient and provider. (See Chapter 5, entitled Documentation, for more information.) The physical examination can also be a time to provide feedback and teaching about findings and about self-care.

The differential list is further refined based on data from the physical examination. In many cases, the nurse practitioner is sufficiently confident of the problem that empiric treatment can be considered without further testing. In other cases, even though the problem is identified, it is a good opportunity to perform routine screening testing as recommended by the Preventive Services Task Force. Understanding the nature of diagnostic testing and how to appropriately use data from testing will be considered next.

> RULE OF THUMB: Include appropriate prevention and screening activities on the differential list based on the patient's risk factor assessment.

)) LABORATORY TESTING

Diagnostic tests can be used to confirm or rule out diagnostic hypotheses or as screening devices for conditions with subtle presentations that need to be picked up early, such as lead poisoning in children or diabetes in adults. Diagnostic tests vary in their usefulness based on their sensitivity, specificity, and predictive value. Furthermore, the predictive value varies by the prevalence of the condition. When considering or evaluating a test, remember that there are patient, test, and disease factors that affect the interpretation of individual diagnostic tests.

No test is perfect. In a given population, a positive reading is found with some people who have the condition and with some that do not. On the other hand, a negative test is found with people who do not have the condition and with some that do. Table 3–5 indicates the characteristics of all tests.

A test's sensitivity is defined by the following formula:

TABLE 3–5
Tests: Characteristics and Diseases

Test Reading	Disease Present	Disease Absent	Total
Positive	True positive (TP) A	False positive (FP) B	All positives A+B
Negative	False negative (FN) C	True negative (TN) D	All negatives C+D
Totals	All diseased A+C	All healthy B+D	Grand Total

$$\text{Sensitivity} = \frac{\text{The number of true positives}}{\text{The number of people with the disease who are tested}}$$

or   A/A+C where A= true positives and C=false negatives

A highly sensitive test has few false negatives (FN). With a sensitive test, negative test results mean a low likelihood that the patient has the disease. It is useful in screening a condition that might not otherwise be detected.

A test's specificity is defined by the following formula:

$$\text{Specificity} = \frac{\text{The number of true negatives}}{\text{The number of all tested individuals who do not have the disease}}$$

or   D/D+B where D= true negatives and B= false positives

A highly specific test has few false positives (FP). It is useful for ruling in a specific diagnostic hypothesis. If the test is positive, the patient very likely has the disease.

Of course, if a given test is positive for an individual patient, the nurse practitioner does not know if the test is true (A) or a false positive (B). The nurse practitioner must consider the probability of the condition under consideration for a person in similar demographic and risk groups to the patient being evaluated. The positive predictive value (PPV) is calculated using the following formula, which includes true positives (TP) and false positives (FP):

$$\text{PPV} = \text{TP/TP+FP}$$

Similarly, the negative predictive value (NPV) is reflected in the following formula, which includes true negatives (TN) and false negatives (FN):

$$\text{NPV=TN/TN + FN}$$

Predictive values are proportional to the prevalence of the disease in a given population. If the disease is highly probable for a person, the positive test carries more weight. On the other hand, if the condition was unlikely in the first place, a positive test does not guarantee that the disease is present. Another consideration is that if the condition is highly likely but the test result is negative, the nurse practitioner is less confident of the diagnosis, but considering that false negatives are possible, the diagnosis might still be made.

When deciding whether to order a test, the nurse practitioner considers cost, convenience, sensitivity and specificity, and risk of missing a condition. One should ask whether the test result would affect the treatment plan being considered. If not, the test might not be necessary. Tests should not be ordered to increase one's own confidence and comfort. Appropriate screening for life-threatening or life-altering conditions must be considered. Nurse practitioners can use the Clinical Preventive Services Guidelines or other research-based guidelines for deciding on screening tests for specific patients. Always consider the individual patient's situation. For example, at the time of this writing, mammography every 1 to 2 years is recommended for women aged 40 and over by the U.S. Preventive Services Task Force (2003). However, if the patient has a strong family history of breast cancer, the nurse practitioner would be justified in ordering annual mammograms earlier for that patient.

> RULE OF THUMB: When ordering a test, ask yourself if management will potentially change based on the information gained. If not, refrain from ordering tests for your own comfort.

A sample clinical problem that combines our discussion of decision analysis in the last chapter with our understanding of test characteristics in this chapter is one where there is a real choice between management strategies and one where the outcome is uncertain. The sensitivity of the prostate specific antigen (PSA) in detecting prostate cancer with a PSA > 4 ng/ml is 0.67. The specificity is 0.97. The chance of a false positive test (3 for every 100 patients tested) is greater than the chance of a true positive test (Presti, Stoller, & Carroll, 2000). One such example is the decision whether to test a specific 50-year-old man with the PSA test. The patient is resistant to invasive testing, which would be required if a positive test result were to be obtained. Therefore the decision analysis indicates that the benefit of testing this man is less than the risk of testing. You would perform a digital rectal screening examination of the prostate and wait until he reaches age 65 or shows symptoms suggestive of prostate cancer before offering the PSA blood test. Decision analysis allows patient preferences and values to be entered into testing and treatment questions and therefore, in spite of its seeming objective mathematical approach, it can actually involve the patient in decision making in a very active way.

))) DIFFERENTIAL DIAGNOSIS

An evolving problem list can become quite long, even on an initial visit. The process used to assemble the data into a picture occurs simultaneously with ongoing data collection. The first piece of data opens certain diagnostic possibilities. New data can be used to support or refute the hypothesis

---

Box 3–1 Words of Wisdom

I think I assess the situation from a practical standpoint. I sometimes have to say to myself, "O.K. this is a normal child with reactive airway disease who now has chicken pox," or you know, whatever disease they have, and I have to sometimes separate these pieces out before I can bring them all together if that makes any sense. I have to look at what's good for each individual piece of this and then say, "How do these all marry together so that this parent can leave here and take care of this child?" You know, in a holistic, safe way, that this child is going to get well. I do that to a much lesser degree in pediatrics than I did with adults when you have multiplicity of complexities going on. With the adult, when you have hypertension and diabetes and a peptic ulcer and chronic obstructive pulmonary disease and all these things, and [you think] of all these pieces, and then bring these pieces together. I guess I think about this a lot because I am a preceptor and I am trying to make my student aware of each of these individual pieces and how they fit together and how, it's overwhelming to the students. Students ask me how I learned and I don't honestly know.

Source: Dunphy, L. (1999). The wisdom of advanced practice nurses: Approaches to diagnosis and treatment. Unpublished interview data. Used with permission.

---

or begin a parallel line of reasoning considering a separate problem. As the evolving picture develops, the relative weight of competing hypotheses shifts. As a precaution against premature closure, using a systematic approach will uncover data that lead in new directions.

As nurse practitioners learn to make diagnostic statements, they frequently begin by seeing discrete problems (Box 3–1). With experience, the wholeness and interrelationship among problems merge into a more complete picture. For example, a patient with type 2 diabetes may be experiencing high blood sugar as reflected in HgbA1c readings. In questioning the patient about lifestyle factors, the nurse practitioner learns that the patient has been under much recent job stress, causing him to work longer hours than usual and change his eating patterns. His sleep has been disturbed, which has resulted in difficulty concentrating at work. One way to view this man's problems is from the purely physiologic model, and the resulting decision might be to increase antidiabetic medication. By seeing the wholeness of the patient's life, the nurse practitioner can help the man make a connection between his stress, his dietary lapses, his lack of exercise, and his poor sleep quality (Fig. 3–2). By addressing the lifestyle

Figure 3-2

PATIENT-NURSE PRACTITIONER LINKAGES: CASE EXAMPLE

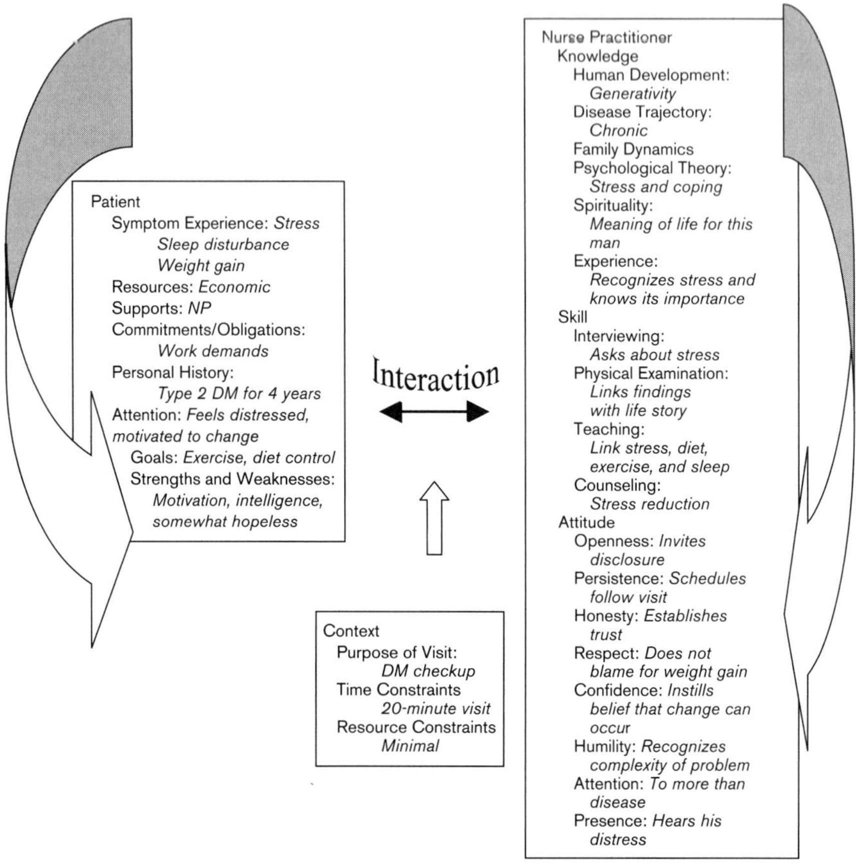

Patient
Symptom Experience: *Stress*
   Sleep disturbance
   Weight gain
Resources: *Economic*
Supports: *NP*
Commitments/Obligations:
   Work demands
Personal History:
   Type 2 DM for 4 years
Attention: *Feels distressed,*
motivated to change
   Goals: *Exercise, diet control*
Strengths and Weaknesses:
   Motivation, intelligence,
   somewhat hopeless

Interaction

Context
Purpose of Visit:
   DM checkup
Time Constraints
   20-minute visit
Resource Constraints
   Minimal

Nurse Practitioner
Knowledge
   Human Development:
      Generativity
   Disease Trajectory:
      Chronic
   Family Dynamics
   Psychological Theory:
      Stress and coping
   Spirituality:
      Meaning of life for this
      man
   Experience:
      Recognizes stress and
      knows its importance
Skill
   Interviewing:
      Asks about stress
   Physical Examination:
      Links findings
      with life story
   Teaching:
      Link stress, diet,
      exercise, and sleep
   Counseling:
      Stress reduction
Attitude
   Openness: *Invites*
      disclosure
   Persistence: *Schedules*
      follow visit
   Honesty: *Establishes*
      trust
   Respect: *Does not*
      blame for weight gain
   Confidence: *Instills*
      belief that change can
      occur
   Humility: *Recognizes*
      complexity of problem
   Attention: *To more than*
      disease
   Presence: *Hears his*
      distress

factors and scheduling a visit in 2 weeks, the nurse practitioner can assess the effectiveness of lifestyle modification in controlling the patient's blood sugar. If necessary, medication adjustment can be made at that time. Medical and nursing diagnoses can reflect the patient situation (Table 3–6).

The nurse practitioner may not record all the possible diagnoses, but establishing a plan that reflects the full range of the patient's situation will be more supportive of him as a human being and will be more effective in controlling his blood sugar. The most elegant diagnosis is the one that incorporates the issues raised in several others. In this case, the diagnosis Ineffective Therapeutic Regimen Management and Coping: Readiness for Enhanced (NANDA, 2003) can incorporate diet, exercise, and stress management activities.

TABLE 3–6

Case Example of Medical and Nursing Diagnoses

Data	Medical Diagnoses	Nursing Diagnoses
HgbA1c 9.6	Uncontrolled Type 2 diabetes mellitus	Ineffective Therapeutic Regimen Management
Body weight 196, up 8 pounds Frequent fast food choices		Imbalanced Nutrition: More than Body Requirements
Poor sleep quality		Disturbed Sleep Pattern
Stress at work		Coping, Readiness for Enhanced
Reduced exercise		Deficient Diversional Activity

⟩⟩ MANAGING A NEW PATIENT

Here is how it looks and sounds in real clinical practice. The following excerpts come from a set of interviews with nurse practitioners (Dunphy, 1999). A family nurse practitioner describes her approach to a new patient:

> My initial diagnosis at that time just by speaking with him, without any labs and examining him physically was this. His diabetes was in poor control. His hypertension was in poor control. He had some rhinitis, probably allergic, but he wasn't having a problem. He had known unequal pupils since he had surgery and had damage to the pupillary musculature, but it does not affect his vision, but if you didn't happen to know that, you know.... It's real important to put that in the problem list. He'd had a TURP for BPH. He had a real bad pars planis with secondary hip pain, and he kept going to people with back pain and nobody ever stood him up and looked at his feet. Seborrheic dermatitis. The guy is an Irishman with pale skin and washed out blue eyes, never used sunscreen. Had had lots of skin cancers. The doctor kept calling him back to cut out the skin cancers but never told him to use sunscreen.

> (From Dunphy, L. [1999]: Unpublished interview text. Used with permission.)

For the patient described above, the nurse practitioner outlines her approach to diagnostic test ordering. Note that the hypotheses precede the test consideration. She goes on to describe her initial treatment plan (Dunphy, 1999).

OK, first thing you need is your laboratory parameters to check the problems that you just defined, so I would do blood counts, chemistries, thyroid function, glycohemoglobin, urines, PSA. The first time I see a patient I always do the whole gamut. The guy also had bilateral total hip replacement, so I reviewed the SBE prophylaxis because he had never been told about it. I started him on Prinivil, an ACE inhibitor, because he is a diabetic and had previously been on Hytrin, and it wasn't doing the trick, as well as it wasn't protecting his kidneys...Started him on Glucotrol, he'd not been on anything other than Micronase which he quit because he really didn't know how to use the stuff. Talked to him about his seborrhea and sunscreen.

(From Dunphy, L. [1999]: Unpublished interview text. Used with permission.)

The nurse practitioner sees the wholeness of the patient's situation. This is a different approach than treating discrete problems as they come up (Dunphy, 1999).

He had had previous healthcare and he thought he was doing fine. He just had never had it all put together. As far as he was concerned, he happened to have some elevated blood pressure and some elevated blood glucose, but nobody had ever put it all together as a whole body. He went to someone for his glucose and he went to somebody for his blood pressure. The guy wasn't a train wreck; at least until he saw me and somebody (me) made a list. He had not had a recent eye exam and being a diabetic, I make sure they get it every single year. And that's how I started. His wife is also a patient of mine, a great cook, which is a tragedy for a diabetic, and he, like most husbands, will eat what he is given. So she needed some education as to what's the proper thing to eat and when to cheat.

(From Dunphy, L. [1999]: Unpublished interview text. Used with permission.)

The nurse practitioner is able to pull all of the patient's concerns and problems together n a way that honors his wholeness and his family dynamics. Her concern is for preventing future problems that are likely with his pattern of risk factors. Her method of collecting data and clustering it together to form a comprehensive picture of his life results in an effective, personal plan.

The differential diagnosis list should always include any conditions that are life, organ, or function threatening. The nurse practitioner interviewed previously, describing a different patient situation, stated (Dunphy, 1999):

> I always think in terms of the most dangerous, the most serious thing first, not necessarily the most catastrophic, the most serious. Say I know somebody who has a AAA and he comes in with abdominal pain and it's sensitive. Well, he probably has diverticulitis, but if I blow it and if I go that way and he is dissecting, then he's dead. So I will treat his diverticulitis and get the ultrasound right now. I consider the most urgently deadly thing. Cancer is not an emergency. It will kill you, but it's not going to kill you tomorrow. But an AAA, it can blow at any time. I had someone blow in here once. Had the surgeon waiting. The OR team was waiting in the ER for him because we knew we had one. I put my hand on his belly and it was throbbing and he was hypotensive and he was sweating and he was ready to go on vacation and just wanted to check this out before he left. I said, "Well, you are going on vacation but you're going in a different direction." So, you think of the most life-threatening situation.
>
> (From Dunphy, L. [1999]: Unpublished interview text. Used with permission.)

The nurse maintains a level of suspicion about what could be happening with the patient. By considering the worst possible situation and proving it not to be true before the patient leaves the appointment, the nurse controls his or her own anxiety about the situation and does everything possible to intervene if the condition is life threatening.

Beyond life-threatening medical diagnoses, Brykczynski reported that nurse practitioners conceived of problems that they saw in two ways: first, the disease and second, the illness. "What can I do to help facilitate the diagnosis and treatment of the real disease and what can I do to help the patient psychologically deal with it in the brief time that the patient is with me?" (1989, p. 93). Life experience questions from the history related to "What is going on in your life right now?" help to focus on the response aspect of care. Brykczynski relates a vignette shared by a participant in her study of a 38-year-old man who complained of chest pain. The history did not indicate that coronary artery disease was a high likelihood, and no other pattern emerged. She noted that he had mentioned his wife repeatedly, and when she asked "How is your wife?" he revealed that because of her diabetes she had just had the last of several stillbirths. The man reported that he had had another child die during a previous marriage. The nurse practitioner recognized that the man did not have coronary disease. "He has HEART disease." (1989, p. 94). Once the problem is seen, an approach that is appropriate can be developed.

⟩⟩ PROBLEM LIST IDENTIFICATION

Thinking in terms of both disease and illness is consistent with the observation of Engel (1977) that the biomedical model has limits. Much of human suffering dealt with in primary-care practice relates to the illness aspect of the patients' lives. Both illness and disease deserve attention as potential diagnoses groups in nurse practitioner practice. Nurse practitioners are free to select from the standard list of medical problems and from standardized lists of nursing problems as they consider planning care for their patients. Even if encounter forms or computerized documentation systems make it difficult to record nursing concerns in nursing language, nurse practitioners can enter their concerns under health promotion, adjustment, patient education, or other codes. The optimal practice is one that allows recording and following both medical and nursing concerns for patients over time. Nurse practitioners who are unfamiliar with nursing diagnoses because they have never been exposed to them or because they disliked the old "nursing process" way of thinking should familiarize themselves with the diagnostic labeling systems currently in use to identify labels for issues they are dealing with in primary care.

Medical problems are recorded as symptoms when no clear diagnosis is established, or as medical diagnoses if data support making a specific diagnosis. These can be acute, self-limited conditions or chronic ongoing problems. There can be social situations listed as problems, such as alcoholism in the family or unemployment. Emotional factors, such as bereavement or depression, and adjustment issues related to life changes, such as risk for injury because of visual deficits or potential hypoglycemia, should also be noted. Nursing labels such as Social Isolation, Altered Family Processes, Activity intolerance, Sleep Pattern Disturbance, Body Image Disturbance, Hopelessness, Impaired Memory, Pain, and Post-trauma Syndrome can individualize the problem list for patients in primary care and assist the team in addressing problems other than medical ones (NANDA, 2003).

A recent study reported student nurse practitioner practice patterns for more than 8000 patient encounters at practice sites across the United States (Crabtree, Hameister, Warren, & Allan, 1999). The most frequently reported medical problems were hypertension, normal pregnancy, diabetes, sinusitis, and upper respiratory infection. The most frequently reported nursing diagnoses were Health Maintenance, Altered Health Maintenance, Health Seeking, Health Management Deficit, Knowledge Deficit, Pain, Impaired Tissue integrity, and Potential for Infection.

ONGOING MONITORING

The collection of data after the initial treatment plan is established is typically used for evaluation, but in the clinical setting, a follow-up visit can serve simultaneously as evaluation and adjustment of the current plan as well as identifying new problems. Similar processes of keeping a questioning attitude about "What is really going on here?" can be used for initial and follow-up visits. Often the way in which a patient responds to a particular treatment plan offers data about whether the initial diagnosis was correct.

SUMMARY

Nurse practitioner practice adds elements of medical care to the nursing base on which all nurses practice. Conceiving of patient problems in the broadest possible terms is the most cost-effective and useful approach to the person's life. The purpose of the assessment process used in nurse practitioner practice is to arrive at a full understanding of the patient situation. The problem lists are generated from the basis for developing the treatment plan.

REFERENCES

Benkert, R., Barkauskas, V., Pohl, J., Corser, W., Tanner, C., Wells, M., & Nagelkirk, J. (2002). Patient satisfaction outcomes in nurse-managed centers. *Outcomes Management. 6,* 174–81.

Billings, J. A., & Stoeckle, J. D. (1999). *The clinical encounter: A guide to the medical interview and case presentation.* St. Louis: Mosby.

Brykczynski, K. (1989). An interpretive study describing the clinical judgment of nurse practitioners. *Scholarly Inquiry for Nursing Practice, 3*(2), 75–104.

Coulehan, J. L., & Block, M. R. (1997). *The medical interview: Mastering skills for clinical practice.* Philadelphia: F. A. Davis.

Crabtree, K., Hameister, D., Pohl, J., Warren, B., & Allan, J. (1999). Analysis of student nurse practitioner primary care practice patterns in the northwest, midwest and south. *The American Journal for Nurse Practitioners, 3*(5), 9–11, 13–14, 17–18, 23–24.

Dunphy, L. M. (1999). The wisdom of advanced practice nurses: Approaches to diagnosis and treatment. Unpublished raw data.

Engel, G. L. (1977). The need for a new medical model: A challenge for biomedicine. *Science, 196,* 139–136.

Gordon, M. (1994). *Nursing diagnosis: Process and application* (3rd ed.). St. Louis: Mosby.

Mayfield, D., McLead, G., & Hall, P. (1974). *American Journal of Psychiatry, 131,* 1121.

North American Nursing Diagnosis Association (NANDA). (2003). *Nursing diagnoses: Definitions & classification* 2003-2004. Philadelphia: Author.

Presti, J. C., Stoller, M. L., & Carroll, P. R. (2000). Urology. In L. M. Tierney, S.J. McPhee, & M.A. Papadakis (Eds.). *Current medical diagnosis & treatment 2000* (pp. 917–958). New York: Lange Medical Books/ McGraw-Hill.

Rakel, R. E. (1995). *Textbook of family practice* (5th ed.). Philadelphia: W.B. Saunders.

U.S. Preventive Services Task Force (2003). *Put prevention into practice.* Rockville, MD: Agency for Healthcare Research and Quality. *http://www.ahrq.gov/clinic/ppipix.htm.* Downloaded September 25, 2003.

Wright, D. (2002). State estimates of substance use from the 2000 National Household Survey on Drug Abuse. DHHS Publication #SMA 02-3731, NHSDA Series H-15. Rockville, MD: Substance Abuse and Mental Health Services Administration.

CHAPTER 4

Planning and Interventions

CHAPTER OUTLINE

◯ CLINICAL JUDGMENT IN INTERVENTION SELECTION

Previous chapters have shown that clinical judgment is part of every phase of nurse practitioner practice. This chapter focuses on the judgments that nurse practitioners make about treatments and interventions designed to improve the patient's health status. The range of interventions available for selection by nurse practitioners includes all of the interventions that registered nurses are licensed to perform as well as those that only licensed advanced-practice nurses are authorized to carry out, such as medication selection and prescription writing. Because the scope of interventions varies according to each state's nurse practice act and regulations, it is the responsibility of advanced-practice nurses to maintain knowledge of their local regulations. Many nurse practitioners are active in local, state, and national professional organizations in order to promote authorization for them to fully exercise their expanded role. Each year in its January issue, *The Nurse Practitioner: The American Journal of Primary Care* publishes an updated list of privileges granted by each state. At this time, some states provide full independent prescriptive authority, whereas others require physician supervision of prescription writing. Some states also limit the types of medication that can be prescribed independently.

Prescription writing is an important aspect of expanded practice, but it is not the focus of all clinical encounters. Early in the course of a student's education, these expanded-role activities absorb much focused attention, but experience indicates that nurse practitioners' effectiveness is often attributable to such interventions as teaching and support, which all nurses are authorized to perform. This chapter focuses on helping nurse practitioners develop a method for including all these different kinds of interventions in their range of options. Student nurse practitioners are sometimes surprised that there are no "right answers" when it comes to intervention selection. Just as making a diagnosis is a probability statement, choosing a specific intervention does not necessarily guarantee a specific outcome. Students who are gaining experience in more than one practice setting are frequently surprised to see that, in different settings, the same condition may be managed in different ways. This contributes to students' uncertainty as they learn new modes of practice. Flexibility is key in learning new skills. Very often, environmental, social, and economic factors affect management selections. Judgment in intervention selection requires more than just making the diagnosis and applying a simple solution.

> RULE OF THUMB: If you see different management practices used by different preceptors, ask your preceptors how they decide to manage conditions. They often have good reasons based on their experience in particular settings or with particular patients.

⦾)) LINKAGES BETWEEN INTERVENTIONS AND OUTCOMES

All interventions are selected strategically. That is, they are selected to accomplish a certain goal. At times that goal is implied. For example, a decision to treat a skin rash with a topical steroid cream has the goal of eliminating the rash without damaging the underlying skin structure. At other times, the goal of treatment might be more complex, requiring specific conversation to clarify both the nurse's and the patient's thinking. For example, the decision to treat mild hypertension with diet, exercise, and smoking cessation must be balanced against the benefits of medication management.

Practice guidelines assist this decision-making process, but the patient's preferences and capacities must be included in both ends and means considerations. The importance of establishing a trusting relationship with the patient is evident here when treatment options are considered. The Patient-Nurse Practitioner Linkage Model reflects the elements of the encounter that support efficient and appropriate intervention selections (Fig. 4–1). Be sure that you clarify the patient's goals and the types of interventions that individuals and families find acceptable (Box 4–1).

RULE OF THUMB: Explore patient preferences for treatment before establishing a plan.

Figure 4–1
PATIENT-NURSE PRACTITIONER LINKAGES
IN INTERVENTION SELECTION

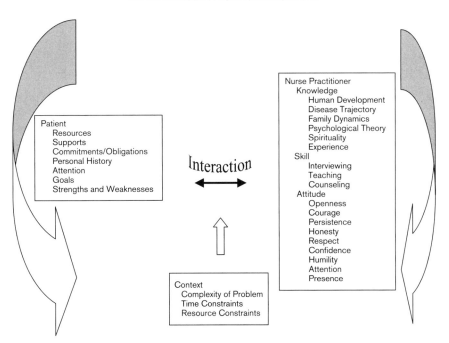

Box 4–1 Sample Communication

NP: How has the medication that we started for you last month for your hypertension been working for you?

PT: Pretty good.

NP: I notice your pressure is pretty close to where it was when we started. Have you been taking the medication every day?

PT: Well, most of the time. Sometimes I don't.

NP: Is there a particular reason why you don't? Do you forget or is it something else?

PT: Well, you see, when I have to take the bus, like to come here, or when I go to church, I don't take it, because, you know, it makes me have to go to the bathroom.

NP: OK, I understand. Well, on days that you can't take it in the morning like today, you can take it in the afternoon when you get back home. It might interrupt a nap, but at least you will get it.

PT: Oh, I didn't know I could do that.

NP: Sure, but if you take it just before bed it might keep you awake. You can always call and ask me or the nurse for advice on how to change your medications. We really like hearing from you! And we really want to help you control that blood pressure.

PT: OK. I'll try taking them when I can.

Nurse practitioners need to be aware that goals and preferences can change over time. For long-term patients, it is important to review annually (at least) the goals of therapy and such things as advance directives. When goals of treatment are specified ahead of time, attainment of these goals can be discussed by both patient and nurse practitioner during follow-up visits. This kind of conversation can support the partnership mode of working together that often characterizes nurse practitioner practice.

))) PLANNING PROCESS

The planning process proceeds seamlessly as part of the patient encounter. Just as patient problems vary in their complexity, the resulting set of plans will vary in complexity. A classic article reflects the scope of problems and how solutions relate to them (Getzels, 1982). Table 4–1 displays different types of problems encountered in clinical practice and the types of solutions that are used in addressing them. It shows that, as the nurse practitioner grows in skill, different approaches to intervention selection can be developed.

TABLE 4–1

Typology of Problems

Type of Problem	Type of Solution	Example
Problem presented by patient	Solution clearly evident	Strep throat, no penicillin allergies
Problem presented by patient	Solution unknown to caregiver, but may be evident to others	Stress incontinence, in practice where this is rare occurrence
Problem presented by patient	No known solution	Terminal cancer
Problem present but not discovered	No solution considered	Undiagnosed prostate cancer
Problem discovered by NP	Solutions exist if diagnosed	Breast cancer
Problem discovered by NP	Standard solution exists but may not be known by NP	Depression
Problem discovered by NP	No standard solution exists	Sedentary lifestyle
Concept of problem created by NP	Solution must be created	Chronic sorrow Developmental delay Dysfunctional grieving

Source: Modified from Getzels (1982).

Planning for different types of problems will vary. For the clear-cut problem, the planning process involves a matching of acceptable solutions, which have been learned with experience or at formal and informal educational settings or with the use of guidelines for practice available from the National Institutes of Health. For problems that are beyond the scope of practice for a particular nurse practitioner, consultation with other healthcare providers, individual study, and referral would be appropriate processes.

Some problems remain unclearly defined even after a full assessment. In this case, nurse practitioners set up a treatment plan using interventions that will improve the most likely cause of the problem and not cause or mask other problems by their use. This situation requires closer monitoring to determine if the treatment plan was successful. At times, only after

noting the effectiveness of a particular treatment plan is the diagnosis con-
firmed.

Other problems are more existential in nature. For example, a patient
may have sleep disturbance, reduced social engagement, and difficulty concentrating at work. The patient may present to the primary-care setting
with vague complaints that do not coalesce in a clear clinical picture, but
by including consideration of daily life patterns and a holistic assessment,
the nurse practitioner may uncover dysfunctional grieving and conceptual-
ize the patient's problems in this way. Many of the North American Nursing Diagnosis Association (NANDA) diagnoses would fall into this
category. The planning that this type of problem requires involves considering a wide range of interventions that will be discussed later in this chapter.

For all patients, as problems are identified, the nurse practitioner envi-
sions an optimal outcome. This could be as simple as resolved infectious
disease or as complex as lifestyle change to reduce body weight and manage type 2 diabetes mellitus. There might also be intermediate outcomes
such as acceptance of the disease state and increased knowledge about
medication. For all outcomes, the nurse practitioner considers choices of
interventions that the patient can manage cognitively, financially, and emo-
tionally. The person's life should not be disrupted unnecessarily. In addition to addressing overt problems, the nurse practitioner addresses risk
reduction using such devices as smoking cessation counseling. Throughout
the relationship, as it is developed, the nurse practitioner works to support
the person as a human being and to honor the person's concerns and capacities. Additional decisions are made as to when to return to clinic and
what type of monitoring is required and useful. For chronic conditions,
monitoring can be supported through the use of flow charts, for example,
to remind the provider when to order ophthalmic screening examinations.
The nurse practitioner's planning abilities will evolve with experience. At
first, simple problem solution matching and application will occupy much
of the student's attention. Later, more complex views of the patient situation will emerge and allow a different level of creative planning.

◎)) TYPES OF INTERVENTIONS

Several authors have contributed to a discussion of nursing interventions.
The Iowa Intervention Project group has published an extensive list of
nursing interventions based on literature and survey work with a wide
range of nursing specialties, including advanced practice (McCloskey &
Bulechek, 2000). They have clustered nursing interventions into six large
domains in the Nursing Intervention Classification (NIC). Table 4–2 pro-

	TABLE 4–2	
	Nursing Intervention Classification (NIC) Domains	
Domain Name	**Sample Interventions**	**Nurse Practitioner Focus**
Physiologic–Basic	Activity and exercise management	Exercise prescription
	Elimination management	Incontinence evaluation
	Immobility management	Referrals for physical therapy
	Nutrition support	Diet prescription
	Physiologic comfort promotion	Comfort measure teaching
	Self-care facilitation	Evaluation of activities of daily living
Physiologic Complex	Electrolyte and acid base management	Laboratory test orders
	Drug management	Prescription writing
	Neurological management	Specialized physical examination
	Perioperative care	Preadmission evaluation
	Respiratory management	Asthma management
	Skin and wound management	Suturing/wound management
	Tissue perfusion management	Managing vascular disease
Behavioral	Behavior therapy	Short-term health counseling
	Cognitive therapy	Cognitive function testing
	Coping assistance	Referrals in community
	Patient education	Health education
	Psychological comfort promotion	Support
Safety	Crisis management	Crisis management and referral
	Risk management	Reduction of medical error
Family	Childbearing care	Prenatal care/Nurse midwifery
	Life span care	Family care: Birth to death
Health System	Health system mediation	Third-party payor negotiations
	Health system management	Systems design in care setting
	Information management	Documentation, communication

Source: Adapted from McCloskey, J.C. & Bulechek, G.M. (Eds.). (2000). *Nursing intervention classification (NIC)* (3rd ed.). St. Louis: Mosby-Year Book. Used with permission.

vides a description of these domains with an explanation of nurse practitioner focus.

Hospital-based practice has adopted the NIC more extensively than ambulatory centers, but advanced nursing practice still incorporates general nursing practice. A review of the NIC can remind all nurse practitioners of interventions that are part of the domain of nursing. An examination of the practice patterns of nurse practitioner students reviewed the assessment database and the intervention selections for 3733 patient visits. Students reported nursing interventions from each of the domains and classes described by the NIC. Most frequently used were patient education (57%), drug management (51%), information management (32%), risk management (25%), nutritional support (23%), activity and exercise (23%), communication enhancement (19%), coping assistance (19%), physical comfort promotion (15%), and health system management (14%) (O'Connor, Hameister, & Kershaw, 2000). The NIC provides practical interventions that nurse practitioners can use in caring for patients.

Reporting the nursing basis for practice and coding the interventions using Current Procedural Terminology (CPT) codes enable study of the unique contribution that nursing makes to patient care. Ambulatory care sites tend to choose the CPT system (American Medical Association, 2002) for documentation, but that system was developed by the American Medical Association and may omit many of the nursing activities captured in other taxonomies. Chapter 5 on documentation will discuss ways to document nurse practitioner activities for full reimbursement.

Levels of Interventions

Another way of conceiving interventions was proposed by Eisenhauer (1994). She points out that any given intervention might be used for more than one diagnosis and that a specific diagnosis might have more than one intervention selected as appropriate. She also points out that, just as human problems can present at several levels, from the simplest symptomatic complaint to deeper life pattern issues and finally to the deepest life processes, so interventions can be selected to deal with these multiple levels of problems. A nurse practitioner can use this typology in working with patients over a long term. Box 4–2 offers a case example. Interventions that alter home and work environments are deeper and require sustained involvement. Table 4–3 illustrates Eisenhauer's Typology of Interventions used by nurses. The complexity of the levels increases as one reads down the table.

Engebretson has presented another conceptualization of nursing interventions (1997). She studied the way that nurse healers conceived of their work and developed a model of nursing interventions that includes more than one paradigm or model for practice. She pointed out that the biomedical model of therapeutics is a powerful force in health care, but that it is

---

Box 4–2 Case Example: Intervention Selection

A patient's nasal allergy symptoms were not alleviated by a simple antihistamine prescription. On follow-up visit, the nurse practitioner performed a deeper assessment of environmental factors and life patterns. He asked, "Is anything unusual going on in your life right now?" The patient replied that it has been stressful because her father had recently been discharged from the hospital after a heart attack and she was spending every evening at her family home, returning late to her apartment and having trouble sleeping. Her nasal congestion was making sleeping difficult.

The nurse practitioner recognized that the nasal allergy is only part of what is causing distress. He asked for more information and learned that the patient's father was near death for part of his hospitalization, but after successful bypass surgery, he was recovering at home. The nurse practitioner asked, "Would you feel comfortable taking an evening off from visiting at home?" The patient replied that she thought she could but had not even considered it. The nurse practitioner suggested that she spend at least one evening at her apartment with an early bedtime using diphenhydramine for allergy-symptom control. If she felt the need, she should make a telephone call to say hello to her father. She was instructed that if the family had real concerns about the father's progress, it was the professionals' responsibility to manage it and not the daughter's. The nurse practitioner called the next day to see how the patient was doing. The patient reported a good night's sleep and better energy. Follow-up visits determined that the patient would benefit from short-term counseling, for which she was referred. By addressing deeper life patterns, the patient was able to learn new ways of relating with her family and was able to achieve symptom control also.

---

often held in opposition to other less materialistic views of the world. For example, spiritual and energy work are often seen as being at odds with the medical model. Her way of bringing multiple modes of interventions together in one large view holds much promise for nurse practitioners. Research has shown that patients are interested in nontraditional forms of treatment. The number of visits to complementary and alternative medicine (CAM) practitioners was greater than the number of visits to primary-care physicians in 1997 (Eisenberg et al., 1998). In response to this increasing interest in alternative or complementary therapies, the National Institutes of Health have developed a National Center for Complementary and Alternative Medicine (NCCAM) to support research in this area. A recent survey of family nurse practitioner programs reflected that 98.5

TABLE 4–3

Eisenhauer Typology of Nursing Interventions

Intervention Level	Intervention Examples
Level A Alter symptoms	Pain medication Topical agents
Level B Alter response to potential problems	Diet teaching Exercise promotion
Level C Alter health patterns	Coaching for exercise habits Constipation management
Level D Alter life patterns	Cognitive therapy Therapeutic Touch
Level E Alter life processes	Spiritual support Psychotherapy

Source: Adapted from Eisenhauer, L. A. (1994). A typology of nursing therapeutics. *Image: The Journal of Nursing Scholarship, 26*, 261–264. Used with permission.

percent included some content in CAM. There was a wide variety in how this content is delivered and in the range and depth of CAM competencies. The study's author recommends incorporation of a holistic philosophy in implementing CAM activities (Burman, 2003).

Engebretson's (1997) model shows the broad range of interventions that nurse practitioners can choose in working with their patients. Table 4–4 expands Engebretson's model to include social and environmental factors that nurse practitioners might consider in selecting interventions. Be aware that many of the modalities noted in Table 4–4 require specialized training. Engebretson's model shows that, in addition to the list of physical, psychological, spiritual, and energy interventions, one can consider the goals or methods of therapy as mechanical, purification, balance, and supranormal.

> RULE OF THUMB: As a nurse practitioner, you may want to develop a list of alternative modalities practitioners to whom you can refer patients.

Strong advantages of this model are that it includes patients' cultural health practices in the broader framework of health care. The model also shows that there are many more options available than medication pre-

TABLE 4—4

Nurse Practitioner Interventions Based on Engebretson's Multiparadigm Model

Modalities	Mechanical	Purification	Balance	Supranormal
Physical manipulation	Suturing Splinting Therapeutic exercise	Soaks	Range of motion Yoga	Intuitive body work
Applied or ingested substances	Prescription medications Topical agents	Irrigations Wound management	Therapeutic diets	Homeopathy Aromatherapy
Energy	Laser treatments Hot packs Icing	Phototherapy	Acupressure Acupuncture	Therapeutic Touch Reiki
Psychological	Cognitive repatterning, teaching	Psychotherapy	Counseling	Guided imagery
Spiritual	Ritual and worship participation	Repentance, purification rituals	Meditation	Prayer
Social	Group participation	Forgiveness	Group therapy	Art therapy Music therapy
Environmental	Safety Environmental modification as for children of Alzheimer's patients Allergen reduction	Environmental toxin control Sanitation	Feng Shui	Nature rituals (Native American)

Source: Adapted from Engebretson (1997). A multiparadigm approach to nursing. *Advances in Nursing Science, 20*(1), 21–33. Used with permission.

scription and patient teaching. It is interesting to note that, as one moves down and to the right in the framework, the provider becomes less important in directing the practice and the patient or group becomes more important. This model provides options for nurse practitioners to empower patients to assume control of their own health. It is necessary for the nurse practitioner to be knowledgeable about these modalities, but not necessarily to be skilled in each area of the model. Just as with traditional medical care, consultations and referrals are used to expand the therapeutic judgment and options in planning care. For example, a patient could be referred for acupuncture or psychotherapy. The nurse practitioner continues to follow the patient, keeps informed about the results of therapies carried out by others, and monitors the overall results of a range of therapies.

))) SOURCES OF INTERVENTION IDEAS

Evidence-Based Practice

Nurse practitioners deliver care consistent with national standards and select interventions that are research based. A recent move in health-care planning has been that of evidence-based practice. The evidence-based practice model is driven by the belief that all patients deserve optimal care and that interventions that have been supported by research should be available to all patients, whether they are in an academic medical center or a free-standing rural health clinic. The federal government has supported this effort through its Agency for Healthcare Research and Quality (AHRQ, formerly Agency for Health Care Policy and Research), whose interdisciplinary teams have developed clinical practice guidelines. These teams rate research support for interventions based on the strength of research evidence. Randomized clinical trials are the strongest evidence. If interventions were not tested at this level, other forms of research, such as observational studies and case reports, are also considered. As the guidelines are published, the study team rates the strength of the evidence supporting specific interventions.

There has been some controversy regarding the implementation of evidence-based practice guidelines. Some fear that it will lead to a "cookbook" approach to practice that ignores the individual needs of patients. Others fear that interventions typically chosen by nurse practitioners, such as health education or counseling, might lack empirical evidence of success and therefore will not be reimbursed under strict evidence-based guidelines. The wise clinician will find a balance between "shoot-from-the-hip" individual solutions, which lead to unnecessary variation in care delivered, and rigid "cookbook" approaches. It is often overlooked that one of the principles of evidence-based practice is to bring a range of evidence to the clinical judgment situation and to promote conversation between provider and patient about treatment preferences with a consideration of risks and benefits of various options. If this conversation is preserved and the patient's part of implementing evidence-based practice is preserved, then evidence-based practice has the potential for increasing the quality of care.

In a busy practice, two situations come to mind in which the use of guidelines is beneficial. First, examine your patient base. Are there medical or social problems seen frequently in your setting? Standardizing care for these problems can lead to efficiency and the highest quality of practice. For example, if your practice in an occupational setting has many middle-aged patients at high risk for hypertension and hypercholesterolemia, practice guidelines can help to establish routine screening schedules and flowsheets for following individual patients. In a different setting, such as one with a large group of Central American immigrants, diabetes care may be important, and cultural influences are an important part of diabetes management. Central American families eat together and have a diet with rice and beans as a staple. Pictures of sample menus that emphasize fruits and vegetables and fresh drinking water rather than sweetened drinks are important. Standard meal plans can be developed for the specific populations of the practice. Specific resources can be found at such websites as *http://www.hispanichealth.org*. Using guidelines for diet teaching and scheduling follow-up care can support high-quality practice.

On the other hand, you may have a patient with a condition rarely seen in your practice. Researching guidelines for patient management from web-based resources can keep your practice up to date and offer intervention suggestions. Most major diseases have websites and advocacy groups that can provide resources for individuals or for the practice. Along with appropriate consultation, your practice can offer high-quality care for rare conditions through the use of such guidelines.

Guidelines Clearing Houses

The federal government also supports such Web-based resources as the National Guideline Clearinghouse (*http://www.guidelines.gov*). This website allows searching for guidelines for specific conditions and supports comparison of guidelines when more than one is available. The Cochrane Library (*http://www.update-software.com/cochrane/*) is another source of guidelines. The proliferation of guidelines has made it time consuming to sort through all the possible sets. The individual nurse practitioner will need to decide how frequently to check guideline updates. The best way to use these guidelines is to consult them for assistance with individual patient situations as well as for expertise on conditions with which the practice has limited experience. Intervention selection is based on a clinical judgment that includes an understanding of the patient's situation as well as an understanding of physiology, pharmacology, human responses to illness, and research evidence. Putting all these factors together in developing a treatment plan requires more than knowledge. It requires art. A nurse practitioner can spend a career developing this art.

⟲ NURSE PRACTITIONER INTERVENTIONS

This major section describing nurse practitioner interventions is organized according to the Engebretson (1997) Typology of Interventions (see Table 4–4). It covers the major interventions used in nurse practitioner practice from a holistic perspective.

Physical Manipulation

Nurse practitioners in many settings perform physical interventions that many registered nurses do not perform. These include suturing, cast application, endometrial biopsy procedures, and others. It is important to remember that nurse practitioners must limit these modalities to those for which they have been specifically trained. Specific settings may require the nurse practitioner to present credentials showing evidence that he or she has been appropriately trained. In all these areas, nurse practitioners should clearly identify the limits of their use of these modalities. For example, suturing the face of an adult might be in the area of training, whereas suturing the face of a child might not.

Therapeutic massage can relieve musculoskeletal complaints, and recommendations for therapeutic or aerobic exercise are important for many patients. Exercise programs are useful for reducing blood pressure, cholesterol, and blood sugar, and are important to weight management programs. For sedentary patients, a stress test can screen for coronary artery disease. Many patients benefit from organized exercise programs such as those associated with rehabilitation programs. Knowing individual patients and how they will respond to such suggestions is important. Some will appreciate a specific exercise prescription. Others will prefer a self-guided approach. The Worldwide Web offers exercise suggestions, some for a fee (*www.ediets.com*). In any case, monitoring the patient's response to exercise is just as important as suggesting it (Kennedy, 2001). Remind patients that not everything available on the Worldwide Web has quality information. Have patients bring information they have received from the Web into appointments so that you can review its content.

Exercise Prescriptions

The lack of exercise in the average American's lifestyle contributes to many long-term health problems, including obesity, cardiovascular disease, deconditioning, and muscle weakness, which in turn can contribute to falls and perhaps also depression. The benefits of exercise for all age groups have been reported widely (United States Department of Health and Human Services, 1996). All this being true, one must ask why more Americans do not participate in regular physical exercise. Several possibilities, including fear, ignorance, and avoidance of pain, are probably the major causes. Patients may have a reason to fear exercise. They may fear that they will have a heart attack or stroke if they begin an exercise program. They may live in neighborhoods where they do not feel safe walking alone and may not have considered safe places where they can exercise in all kinds of weather, such as shopping malls. Nurse practitioners should explore resistance to exercise to help uncover likely solutions. Older people may believe that they are too old to benefit from exercise, but even a mild strength-training program can improve stamina, decrease falls, and improve quality of life.

> RULE OF THUMB: Keep in mind that many patients begin an ambitious exercise plan only to experience aches and pains, leading them to drop their programs. To avoid this problem, encourage patients to strive for gradual increases in endurance and strength.

Different kinds of exercise need to be considered in establishing the treatment plan. First, aerobic exercise contributes to cardiovascular fitness. It includes walking, swimming, or any exercise that raises the heart rate for time periods longer than 20 minutes. Exercise after meals can help decrease insulin resistance. Starting a program with 3 sessions of 20 minutes in length per week is recommended for sedentary patients. The second type of exercise is strength training. This important form of exercise is not limited to young body builders, but can be protective of injury for every age group. Even older patients who are able to increase their strength experience a sense of well-being and are less likely to fall. Finally, stretching exercises can minimize stiffness and enhance flexibility, which can prevent pain or injury from falls.

Cardiovascular Clearance

For patients with cardiac risk factors, a stress electrocardiogram can provide clearance for exercise. Unfortunately, many patients who would benefit from cardiopulmonary rehabilitation are not referred to such programs. These programs provide supervised progressive exercise and include patient education. Determine where such programs exist in your area and determine also what third-party payors require by way of referral before such programs can be ordered. Programs in community agencies such as senior citizens centers, town recreation programs, and YMCA programs need not be prohibitively expensive.

Even patients with orthopedic problems can participate in some form of exercise. For example, those with hip or knee pain can do upper-body workouts. For patients with cost concerns, food cans or plastic bags filled with water can be used in place of expensive free weights. Help patients strategize about how they can include exercise in daily activities such as gardening, shopping, or house and yard work.

Medications

Prescription Writing

Perhaps the most notable difference in nurse practitioner practice as compared with the staff nurse role is prescriptive authority. Nurse practitioners are responsible for complying with their own state laws and regulations. Most boards of nursing make regulations easily accessible from a website. This book assumes that the nurse practitioner has full prescriptive authority. In individual states, if a physician co-signature is required, the principles of prescription writing remain the same.

Nurse practitioners prescribe for a range of health problems. A recent study of nurse practitioner prescribing practices in Colorado examined 53 clinicians who kept prescription logs for 2 weeks. A total of 4024 patients were seen, averaging 15 patients per day. A total of 4998 prescriptions were written for an average of 94 per nurse practitioner, or about 7 prescriptions per day. Seventy percent were new drugs for the particular patient. The most frequent diagnoses for which prescriptions were written were respiratory (991), women's health (744), mental health (703), eye or ear problems (422), and musculoskeletal problems (356). Also considered were dermatological (345), cardiovascular (341), gastrointestinal (281), endocrine (241), and genitourinary (168) problems. Infections accounted for many of the conditions in different body systems. Other problems were allergic rhinitis, contraception, hormone replacement therapy, anxiety and

TABLE 4–5

Drug Classification by 1970 Comprehensive Drug Abuse Prevention and Control Act

Class	Definition	Example
Schedule I	Highest possibility for abuse and with no acceptable medical use	heroin marijuana hallucinogens
Schedule II	Acceptable medical uses but have high potential for abuse and dependence	morphine codeine methadone
Schedule III	Less potential for abuse but may lead to low physical but high psychological dependence	some barbiturates, benzphetamine glutethide
Schedule IV	Low potential for abuse and limited chance of dependence	phenobarbital, benzodi- azipines chloral hydrate propoxyphen
Schedule V	Less potential for abuse	dextromethorphan Lomotil

Source: Modified from Rakel (1998), *Essentials of family practice* (2nd ed.). Philadelphia: W. B. Saunders Company.

depression, pain, hyperlipidemia, and hypertension. In addition, gastroesophageal reflux, diabetes mellitus, and thyroid disorders required prescriptions (Gutierrez & Sciacca, 2000).

Drugs are classified according to the 1970 Comprehensive Drug Abuse Prevention and Control Act into five different schedules, reflecting different potentials for abuse. Table 4–5 reflects the classification and gives some sample medications. In addition to being sensitive to the potential for dependence on drugs, the nurse practitioner must also consider the risk of some drugs to the fetus if a pregnant woman takes the medication. A classification that rates the risk of specific drugs based on the adequacy of evidence is reflected in Table 4–6.

Medication errors are a growing concern and can be decreased through clear and accurate prescribing practices. At the simplest level, legibility is essential for safe prescribing. Take the time to make your handwriting legible, even in the midst of a busy practice day. According to the National Coordinating Council for Medication Error and Reporting, illegible handwriting contributes to some 15 percent of errors (Stepanian, 2000).

TABLE 4–6

United States Food and Drug Administration Classification of Drugs in Pregnancy

Category	Pregnancy risk	Examples
A	Studies with pregnant women have not shown risk to fetus in first trimester and no evidence of risk in later trimesters.	
B	Animal studies have not shown risk to fetus, but no adequate studies in pregnant women have been reported. OR animal studies have shown an adverse effect but human studies have not shown risk to fetus in first trimester and no evidence of risk in later trimesters.	Hydrochlorothiazide Dramamine Amoxicillin Erythromycin Flagyl
C	Animal studies have shown an adverse effect on fetus but no adequate human studies, but benefits may outweigh risk; OR no animal studies and no adequate-human studies.	ACE inhibitors SSRIs Bactrim Cipro
D	Positive evidence of human fetal risk but benefits may outweigh risk.	Depakote
X	Animal or human studies have shown fetal abnormalities or toxicity, and the risk outweighs the benefits.	Accutane Statins

Prescription Pads Prescription pads should be treated as carefully as a personal checkbook. If blank prescriptions get into the hands of unauthorized people, the chance of abuse is high. Prescriptions can be forged, placing the provider or practice group at legal risk. The prescription should be printed with the names, addresses, and telephone numbers of key members of the practice. Even in states where supervision is not required, listing the name of the head of the practice can minimize delays when prescriptions are filled in pharmacies where the nurse practitioner may not be known. Some nurse practitioners may feel that listing their name alone is a means of professional recognition and that it moves the practitioner beyond a suggestion of medical dominance. On the other hand, a pragmatist might argue that whatever form increases the efficiency of filling patients' prescriptions is acceptable. These issues will need to be addressed individually in each practice setting, consistent with states' practice regulations.

Elements of the Prescription A prescription is a communication between provider and pharmacist that is intended to convey information clearly and precisely. When writing the prescription, think of making the communication easy for the pharmacist to decipher. Under unusual circumstances, telephoning the pharmacy can minimize delays in filling prescriptions and increase patient satisfaction with the entire process. Written documentation to the pharmacist must follow the telephone call. Table 4–7 summarizes the elements of a prescription (Rakel, 1998).

Patient Information Include the patient's full name, address, and date of birth on the prescription. Many names are common and can lead to confusion if the name is the only data provided. Having complete information will help the pharmacist to establish clear records for your patient and to screen for the individual's allergies and drug interactions for medications that may have been prescribed by others. Filling out the address portion of the prescription not only helps avoid confusion among patients with the same name, it also minimizes the chance of diversion. In some instances,

TABLE 4–7	
Elements of a Prescription	
Patient Information	Name
	Address
	Date of birth
	Body weight for pediatrics
Provider Information	Names of providers
	Address of practice
	Supervising physician (If required)
	Space or license of DEA number
Drug Name	Generic or trade name
	Designate if substitution allowed
Dose	Metric system
	No trailing zero
Formulation and Route	Concentration or mix
	Ointment versus cream
	Oral, transdermal, suppository, rectal, or vaginal
Directions to Patient	Clear directions
	Avoid "as directed"
Amount Dispensed	Write out number (e.g., "thirty") to avoid tampering
Number of Refills	How often the prescription can be refilled without contacting provider

when several families share an address or there is no permanent address, this requirement may be difficult to meet. For example, homeless people will not have an address, but they may be linked to a shelter system that can serve as their "medical address." For pediatric patients, include the body weight on the prescription to safeguard against your own miscalculation or the accidental misreading of your prescription by the pharmacist.

Provider Information Prescription pads are frequently printed with the names and addresses of the key players in the practice. A nurse practitioner's prescription pad can include the nurse practitioner's name as well as the name of a supervising physician, which may be required in certain states. The address and telephone number of the practice are printed on the prescription pad. The license or Drug Enforcement Agency (DEA) number is printed or written in, and the signature is required.

Drug Name All prescriptions contain the symbol Rx. This is Latin for *recipe*, which means "take." The name of the drug can be written in either its proprietary or generic form. Many prescription pads have a box designating whether substitution with generic form is allowed. In these days of managed care, third-party payors may contact providers to authorize substitute prescriptions from the same group of drugs. These substitutions are made based on pricing and effectiveness. The individual provider must decide whether there is justification to override the third-party payor's recommendation. Some drugs have variable bioavailability, and a specific proprietary form over time will help to maintain even blood levels of the drug. Thyroid replacement hormones are examples of drugs with variable bioavailability.

> RULE OF THUMB: When writing a prescription, avoid using the form of drug name that is easily confused with another drug name.

Dose Dosage errors are as potentially harmful as drug substitutions. The metric system is standard. Be clear in differentiating milligrams from micrograms. Avoid the use of abbreviations such as U for units, which can be confused with a 0 (zero). When using decimals, precede the decimal with a zero, but do not trail with a zero. For example, write "0.25 milligrams," not ".250 mg." The abbreviations for milligrams and micrograms are confusing; spell the words out.

Formulation and Route The formulation and concentration of a drug are important, particularly with pediatric suspensions or syrups. For example, amoxicillin comes in dosages of 125 mg/5 mL, 200 mg/5 mL, or

400 mg/5 mL. For topical preparations, the strength of the medication, as well as the base preparation, can affect drug delivery. Specify cream or ointment formulations. In both label and patient instructions, be clear about the route of administration. Have the patient (or the parent for pediatric patients) repeat the instructions to ensure understanding, particularly for medications that are not simple oral tablets or capsules.

Directions to the Patient The term "SIG." refers to directions to the patient. For example, the amount, the timing, and whether the dose should be taken with meals or on an empty stomach are specified. For safety, also include the reasons for taking the drug so that the patient can remember what the specific drug is for. Avoid the use of "take as directed." Many patients are anxious about their health and will have a hard time remembering specific instructions. In special circumstances, the clinician can specify to not use a childproof container, such as when prescribing medication for a person with arthritis.

Amount Dispensed The pharmacist needs to know how much of the drug to dispense. This number is preceded by a "#" sign to indicate number. Writing out the number will prevent tampering. For example, "30" can be changed to "300" simply by adding a zero. However, writing "thirty" prevents this tampering. One month's supply is usually a good amount to consider. In the case of a drug that is needed for a shorter time, such as a course of antibiotics, the full amount needed to control the infection should be dispensed. In some cases, when a new drug is being tried, particularly if it is expensive, less than a full month's supply can be dispensed on a trial basis. If the drug works well and does not produce side effects, then a telephone reorder can be made.

Number of Refills The provider's judgment determines how many refills to allow. For ongoing regular maintenance medications, a full year's supply can be ordered. The pharmacy enters the dates into the computer and the patient can refill the prescription monthly without having to contact the provider's office. For drugs that might need to be adjusted, however, writing a prescription for a full year could cause confusion. For example, the person could continue to receive the old drug from one pharmacy and obtain the new drug from a different pharmacy, resulting in drug interactions or overdosing.

Prescription writing is an important responsibility for the nurse practitioner. Learning the laws and regulations as well as the conventions of prescription writing encourages good communication among patients, providers, and pharmacists.

Nutrition and Diet Therapy

Many health conditions require the modification of a patient's diet for optimal recovery. This can be one of the most difficult recommendations we can make to a person. Food habits are overlaid with meaning. For example, food can signify love, embody the flavors of the old world, provide comfort, or supply social support. Placing a person on a restricted diet and focusing on the restrictions more than the allowances can deprive someone of much daily pleasure. On the other hand, small adjustments that do not interfere with the person's values and enjoyment might be all that is necessary to improve health.

Frequent diet recommendations include restrictions in fat, carbohydrates, and sodium. Many patients will benefit from referral to nutrition counseling. If that is not possible in your setting, some general principles of diet therapy include starting with patient preferences. The patient's reported dietary intake can be reviewed, and then the nurse practitioner can suggest small adjustments that move the patient toward a healthier pattern. Patients themselves might be able to make suggestions that will be easy for them to accomplish. For example, patients who are employed outside the home can pack their own lunches to decrease reliance on machine or lunch-wagon foods, which are frequently high in fat. When reviewing diet history, include a consideration of alcohol intake, which can be a hidden source of calories for many.

> RULE OF THUMB: Have the patient keep a 72-hour food intake diary to determine the pattern of eating. Often this self-awareness exercise can help patients see for themselves their patterns of eating.

Nursing theories can help in setting up lifestyle change approaches. Pender (1987) described a health promotion model that examined patients' perceived risks of not changing, perceived barriers to following advice, and perceived benefits of following advice. Depending on other resources, stresses, and strains in a person's life, timing for lifestyle change might be something to consider. Choosing which lifestyle factor to adjust might be important too. Any patient who smokes needs support to stop smoking, and many need to increase exercise and improve their diet. All these changes can overwhelm a person and his or her family. By establishing a team approach, you can help patients prioritize their efforts.

For some patients, having a preprinted diet to follow can get them on the right track for change. This decreases the number of decisions they must make regarding food in a week and can train their tastes and expectations to a new way of eating. After a few weeks, patients can ease up and adapt the diet to their preferences while maintaining the parameters of the diet. Recent research on behavior change with middle-aged women with diabetes showed that this technique was successful in supporting long-term behavior change (Whittemore, Chase, Mandle, & Roy, 2002).

When dealing with dietary changes or other lifestyle adjustments, be careful to avoid a tone of scolding or blaming. Patients frequently feel that they have been "bad" or have let you down because they have not strictly followed recommendations. Work to establish a team or coaching relationship in which you and the patient work together toward small improvements that last a long time. Use terms such as choices, negotiations, or adjustments. Avoid terms such as cheating, being bad, or slipping. One way to do this, ironically, is to avoid praising good behavior. If they are "being good" for you, they are not making choices for themselves. Focus on the feeling of increased energy, improved symptoms, and small pleasures.

Psychological and Cognitive Support

Many patients come for relief of pain that is not all physical. Most nurses function from a model that assumes that body, mind, and spirit are connected. It is not unusual for emotional strain to be expressed in physical muscle strain or gastrointestinal disturbance. Spiritual crises often also bring on other problems, such as depression. Patients with problems in any realm will need support as they either take steps to recover, accept a diagnosis that is long term and progressive, or face ultimate losses. Nurse practitioners should have access to a list of referrals for patients who need ongoing counseling or therapy, but some principles of counseling can be incorporated into office visits of any type.

Health Counseling

Health counseling, as described by the Current Procedural Terminology guidelines (American Medical Association, 2002), is health-related teaching and guidance. Psychotherapy is the term used for the emotions-based work that requires specialized training. Much work in assisting patients to make long-term health choices does relate to exploration of meanings and fears. A basic principle of counseling is to help patients express thoughts and feelings of which they may not be aware in response to specific situations. Box 4–3 offers a case example. Table 4–8 lists communication techniques that enhance the patient's expression of thoughts and feelings.

Box 4–3 Case Example: Health Counseling

A 21-year-old college student was diagnosed with genital herpes. Her women's health nurse practitioner met with her when the diagnosis was made in order to do health counseling. The goals for the counseling were to: (1) teach the patient about self-management; and (2) help the patient to explore feelings about now having a lifelong condition. The patient quickly understood the treatment guidelines and reported that she understood the benefit of reporting any new flare-ups early. Her feelings about having a lifelong condition centered on feeling embarrassed to discuss the condition with potential sex partners in the future. The nurse practitioner noted that for this patient, sex would be very intentional, which was not a completely negative experience. The nurse practitioner and patient role-modeled the conversation of sharing the patient's condition with a potential intimate partner, and the patient reported feeling more comfortable after she had said the words aloud. Follow-up visits with her women's health nurse practitioner included monitoring both herpes symptoms and personal feelings and relationships.

A study of nurse practitioner and physician documentation of health risk and health promotion counseling conducted in an emergency and urgent care area reflected that neither discipline documented opportunities for health promotion. Despite the fact that 59 percent of the 305 patients screened had at least one health risk, such as smoking, high blood pressure, or overweight, only 22 percent received documented health counseling. Nurse practitioners were slightly more likely than physicians to counsel on smoking cessation, but otherwise did no better than physicians in health promotion counseling. There is much more that health-care providers can do to assist the public in considering healthy choices (Sheahan, 2000).

Safety

Nurse practitioners need to be aware of a patient's risk for harming himself or herself or another person. Contrary to common fears, direct questions about suicide will not give a patient an idea that he or she does not already have. If a patient appears suicidal, the nurse practitioner should ask and document the following three questions:

1. Have you considered hurting or killing yourself?
2. Do you have a plan for how you would do it?
3. Do you have the means to carry out that plan?

TABLE 4-8	
Communication Techniques	
Technique	Rationale
Self-awareness	Be aware of your own emotions and thoughts and personal communication style.
Awareness of others	Be aware of the effect that you have on others. Be sensitive to the comfort level of the patient.
Be flexible	Tailor your communication style to suit the person with whom you are working. Use appropriate terminology that he or she can understand.
Be aware of timing	Be sure the patient is comfortable, can pay attention, and is not distracted.
Use simple, clear messages	Do not give more detail than is needed to explain your message. Leave time for questions and answer them.
Use appropriate self-disclosure	Share something of yourself without overburdening the patient in order to establish a relationship.
Ask for validation	Repeat your understanding of what the patient is saying to be sure you are on track.
Be aware of nonverbal communication	Sit at the same level as the patient and delay answering pages and phone calls during your communication.

Individual state laws vary in how long patients can be hospitalized for threat of suicide. If a patient is suicidal in your presence, get help immediately from coworkers and call appropriate emergency teams to transport the patient to safety. Do not leave the patient alone. You do not break confidentiality if you act to protect the patient or a person to whom the patient might inflict harm.

Some patients may have considered suicide but have neither a plan nor the means to carry it out. Some of these patients would benefit from agreeing to a safety contract after evaluation by a mental health professional (Box 4–4). This contract states that if the patient begins to develop a plan, he or she will call an appropriate support person. The patient can sign the contract, and both you and the patient can keep a copy. Again, appropriate referral and documentation is important. Patients who act impulsively or have chronic suicidal thoughts should be referred to a specialist (Oakley, 2001).

Other safety considerations include the safety of older patients living at home alone. If the nurse practitioner has concerns about the patient's ability to perform activities of daily living and to maintain a safe home

Box 4–4 Safety Contract

I, _____, agree to the following conditions:

(1) I will bring all prescription medications to my clinic this afternoon for review.

(2) I will not stay in a home that has a gun or firearm.

(3) I will attend all therapist sessions.

(4) I will take public transportation and refrain from driving.

(5) If I am unable to complete any of these obligations, I will notify my clinic at (phone number).

(6) If I feel overwhelmed, I will call my clinic (phone number) or go to the emergency room.

(7) If I begin to develop a plan to hurt myself, I will call my clinic or go to the emergency room.

Signed _____

Date _____

Witness _____

environment, a referral for home evaluation by a home health agency can be made.

Education

Education is an important part of every primary care visit. Patients can be encouraged to maintain health practices and might benefit from instruction in new health practices. Patients with chronic health problems involving long-term management require special programs, such as diabetic teaching, whereas those with other concerns (cardiovascular risk factor management, pulmonary disease, arthritis) can benefit from a variety of educational approaches. To follow the principles of adult education, the nurse practitioner should:

◎ Start with what the patient already knows.
◎ Offer material at appropriate reading levels.
◎ Provide time for practice and questions.

Research has shown that low levels of health literacy are related to poor glycemic control for patients with type 2 diabetes (Schillinger et al., 2002). High-school graduates read at an eighth-grade reading level, on avcrage. Reading-level scales are available; use them to determine the reading level of pamphlets and other written material that you use frequently. One recent study showed that literacy testing for patients can lead to discussion of the best ways to learn, but that it must be done with respect for patient privacy and dignity (Brez & Taylor, 1997).

Providing material in appropriate languages for your patient population is another consideration. If you have a large Asian population, obtain Asian-language pamphlets. If they do not exist, partner with a local cultural agency to secure translators. A principle of translating material is to back translate so that misunderstandings can be picked up. For example, have one person translate from English to Mandarin. Then have another person translate from the Mandarin to English. Check to see if facts and the sense of the message are correct.

Asking patients to undertake lifestyle modification can be one of the most difficult aspects of nurse practitioner practice. Brykczynski's (1989) study related an example of an approach to addressing smoking cessation. The nurse practitioner had noted that the patient, an otherwise healthy 70-year-old, continued to smoke and was resistant to hearing more about approaches to stopping. She responded by sharing honestly that her impression of the patient was that he had a lot to live for and that smoking was contradictory to his otherwise active and healthy lifestyle. She had not "preached" at the patient; she had shared her honest observation based on knowing him. He responded that he had never thought about the problem in that way and was able to rethink his smoking decision.

Spiritual Support

Many nurses feel inadequate discussing spiritual issues. They feel that a person's spiritual life is too personal to be violated or that one must have similar religious views in order to discuss these issues. If spiritual issues come up, they want to refer immediately to clergy for support, which is not in itself a bad thing to consider. Many patients, however, are estranged from their religious background. Spirituality is a concept that is broader than religion. It involves issues such as the meaning of life or suffering. It includes a connection to a higher purpose or involves transcending the here and now and connecting to the timeless or ultimate. Many people who do not believe in God still operate with spiritual principles and experience spiritual crises. These most typically occur at life's major transitions, such as the death of a loved one or the birth of a child, but can also occur at such times as retirement or loss of health. By being willing to explore what the event means to the person, the nurse is engaging in spiritual care. Many patients are seeking a person who will listen to their concerns.

Nurses can enhance their comfort in dealing with patients' spiritual issues by developing their own sense of spirituality. Being a nurse exposes one to the highs and lows of human existence. Each nurse needs to develop a way of making sense of what he or she sees and how he or she contributes. Being grounded in one's own sense of meaning can help one stay open to discussion of such matters with others. Particular religious beliefs rarely intrude on such conversation.

Religious beliefs, however, might affect the nurse practitioner's judgment about interventions. During the assessment process, asking if particular religious beliefs affect health practices can lay the groundwork for discussing intervention selections. Particular beliefs might affect decisions about contraception, end-of-life treatment, the use of blood products, dietary restrictions, or animal-sourced medications. Again, a network of providers to whom one can refer patients for interventions that are beyond the scope of one's practice will be invaluable. For example, there might be a particular priest who works well with "lapsed" churchgoers. A rabbi or clinical nurse specialist in your area might be particularly good with interfaith marriage problems. Knowing your community's resources will help you offer the most appropriate interventions for your patients.

A research study designed to examine the relationship of spirituality and symptom distress for women in shelters showed that spirituality as measured by the Spiritual Perspectives Scale was valued highly. The women reported that using spiritual resources such as prayer provided them with a sense of peace. The quantitative measures showed that a negative correlation was found between use of spiritual resources and scales such as hostility, obsessive-compulsive behavior, and interpersonal sensitivity (Humphreys, 2000). Patients are using spiritual resources but may not understand that nurses care about and support these resources unless the nurse practitioner opens the conversation.

Social Interventions

Stress and Relaxation

A major contributor to illness and suffering is the experience of stress. It is not only the harried business executive who experiences stress. The parent of small children, the caregiver of an aging spouse or parent, the recent immigrant—all of these individuals can be expected to be experiencing stress. One modality that can assist patients in learning to respond to the stresses of life is relaxation. Many people are not aware of how much tension they carry in their muscles, particularly in the shoulders and neck. Patients can be referred to meditation groups or body-mind centers where relaxation can be taught. Yoga or spiritual meditation can be useful in learning how to slow down the mind and body. One patient once re-marked to me that meditation helped the mind slow down to become in rhythm with the body. As a result, he experienced more control over his symptoms. Patients often benefit from group support by learning relax-ation or other health techniques.

A brief guided imagery experience can introduce a person to a relax-ation experience. This can even be done in an office visit. The environment must be conducive to quiet. Slow, rhythmic breathing can begin the experi-ence. The patient can be instructed to systematically focus on relaxing one part of the body. One technique is to begin with the feet and work up to the scalp and face. Sometimes, imagining a walk through a favorite place or a place of beauty can help the person transcend the moment and achieve relaxation. As with all techniques, relaxation requires practice. The nurse practitioner must be adept at finding a quiet center in himself or herself and from that place of peace inviting the patient to an experience of quiet (Keegan, 2001).

RULE OF THUMB: Consider learning meditation for yourself; incorpo-rating relaxation techniques into your practice can then flow naturally.

Energy Work

Research has shown that one in four Americans uses complementary and alternative medicine (CAM), with expenditures for these modalities close to those for traditional medical care (Eisenberg et al., 1998). Many pa-tients do not tell their physicians that they use these modalities, fearing ridicule or dismissal. Nurse practitioners are ideally suited to blend the tra-ditional and alternative approaches to health care because of the body-mind-spirit model that they use.

The most common modalities used are acupuncture, chiropractic care, and massage. Not surprisingly, the conditions most often treated with al-ternative methods are back and neck problems, anxiety, and depression (Caulfield, 2000). The National Center for Complementary and Alterna-tive Medicine, a branch of the National Institutes of Health, serves as a clearing house for research on the effectiveness of CAM. It also funds re-search and assists the dissemination of findings.

One area of holistic care that many nurses are including in their prac-tice includes interventions related to energy flow. The most accepted form in the nursing world is Therapeutic Touch, researched and taught by nurse Delores Krieger (1979). The nurse theorist Martha Rogers was known for saying that human beings do not *have* energy patterns; they *are* energy patterns. The theory of illness using energy modalities is that health requires a constant flow of energy, commonly considered as through acupuncture meridians. The idea behind most energy modalities is that the universe is made up of energy in varying waves and patterns. In order to learn to perform Therapeutic Touch, the nurse centers and then passes his or her hands close to but not touching the patient's body. Sensing for energy patterns, which may feel like heat or cold or like a kind of magnetism, one detects imbalances in energy flow. Focusing energy and clearing blockages restore a balance in energy flow. The patient usually describes a pleasant feeling of relaxation when experiencing Therapeutic Touch. Other energy work may involve Reiki therapy, a similar technique designed to restore balance and flow (Dossey, Keegan, Guzzetta, & Kolkmeier, 1995). Specialized workshops can provide essential skills for performing energy therapies. Most holistic modalities have training programs in which one can learn the technique and become certified. As a new nurse practitioner, you may want to develop a referral list. Later, as you find time, become prepared to offer these modalities yourself.

Nurse practitioners can augment the practice by gaining skill in providing interventions such as relaxation techniques, Therapeutic Touch, biofeedback, counseling, or continence training. Workshops and training opportunities exist to increase specific skills. Investigate billing requirements for the major payors for your practice as well as certification requirements for certain therapies. Nurse-managed clinics might be more open to providing alternative therapies than the standard private practice or health maintenance organization setting, but in any setting, the therapy must have demonstrated benefit and be cost effective to the practice setting. Practices might offer some therapies on a private-pay basis if patients desire them, but generally, they are not reimbursable by third-party payors. Many patients are willing to pay out of pocket for complementary methods that provide them with comfort. Nursing functions from a framework that is built on the assumption that body, mind, and spirit work together to produce health. Alternative therapies might offer new ways of supporting health for patients.

Environment

Many people have reported the experience of entering a place of worship or art museum and noting the "energy" of the environment. Certainly the energy of a sports arena is palpable. All spaces collect energy from the people and objects in them and form the pace and activities that occur there. When you have control over the environment where you practice, consider how the use of color, art work, or plants can help to construct a healing environment. Even Florence Nightingale wrote about the importance of the order and the art work present in the "sick room." Our practice environments create a space for communicating and for healing. Consider the message that your environment sends to the patient. One women's health practice has each room decorated in a different theme from a popular designer. The environment cares for patient and provider both. A popular Eastern movement called Feng Shui considers designing spaces for optimal energy flow. Your patients may already be designing their home spaces with energy in mind. What is the quality of energy they encounter in your practice? The waiting room is particularly important because most patients spend more time in this area than the rest of the office.

)) PUTTING IT ALL TOGETHER

Isolating the various types of interventions that nurse practitioners can use sets up a false set of categories. Nurse practitioners deal with the wholeness of people's lives. Being flexible in intervention selection is key to individualizing care. Brykczynski (1989) noted that the nurse practitioners participating in her study reported using low-technology, nonpharmacologic interventions in addition to prescribing medication. One nurse practitioner reported that a colleague remarked on the frequency with which she had recommended vitamins and normal saline nose drops. Sometimes a supportive visit, although not supported by cost-effectiveness research (yet), can keep a patient on track and mobilized to take action for health.

By considering the real-life world of patients, the nurse practitioner can devise low-tech solutions to improve care. One of Brykczynski's participants related a story of a patient who repeatedly complained of back pain. The nurse practitioner noted that the patient was very short and that she worked at a desk job. The nurse practitioner demonstrated some ergonomic principles; the patient made a change in her desk chair height; and her back pain was relieved, all without expending the cost of diagnostic testing.

)) PLANNING FOR FOLLOW-UP

Whether the interventions selected for an individual patient include prescriptions for medication, adjusted diet or lifestyle, the use of relaxation or other techniques, or simply comfort measures to assist in healing and re-covery, all patients need to understand clearly how to monitor their own progress. The nurse practitioner must clearly explain when the patient is to return for follow-up, what signs of progress to expect, and what to do if progress does not occur or health worsens. Encouraging patients to call with questions is important. Many patients are reluctant to "bother" their providers with their questions, and suffer in silence until their next sched-uled appointment. This can be dangerous. All clinical judgments have an element of uncertainty. We, as clinicians, can be wrong about our diagno-sis or treatment selections. Furthermore, the selected treatment might cause allergies previously not identified, or new conditions could emerge that need attention. Several items will need evaluation, including the re-sults of laboratory tests that are not yet available, the effectiveness of the treatment plan, and any side effects caused by the plan. In these days of time pressure for all levels of providers, it is important to have a system that allows patients to reach providers with questions or feedback.

The specifics of follow-up vary by the issues being addressed, but they should include self-care and comfort measures that can be used, such as encouraging fluids and increasing humidity for upper respiratory condi-tions, gentle stretching exercises for back strain, or dietary adjustments for gastroenteritis or constipation. They should also include specific instruc-tions for medication administration. Discuss the names of the drugs being ordered. This can help to reduce medical error. If the patient expects to re-ceive a diuretic, he or she should know how it can be expected to work. If the pharmacist dispenses a medication designed for something else, the pa-tient can catch the error before harm is done.

Furthermore, the plans for follow-up should include reasons why the patient should call the office or engage in emergency care that is specific to the condition. For example, if a fever persists after 2 days on antibiotics, the patient should call the office to be seen again or to have medication ad-justed. The plan should also include the timing of the next office visit. De-pending on the severity of the condition, the visit could be in days, weeks, or months. Even for self-limiting conditions, the timing of the next well-patient visit should be discussed.

If management plans are complicated, written instruction should be given. Many offices have patient instruction sheets for comfort measures for common problems. This saves time during the visit and ensures that complete instructions are given. The sheets must be in a language that the patient can understand. Plans for follow-up should also be documented in the patient record for several reasons. First, your office system can remind you about patients whom you want to call because of concern for their recovery. Secondly, continuity of care is improved when patients return, particularly if they see a different provider.

Patient Self-Management

Patient self-management is a concept describing the need for patients to make management decisions for themselves based on responses to the management of long-term conditions. Two examples of conditions that are appropriate for patient self-management include diabetes mellitus and asthma, which provide for monitoring of response to treatment plans. Diabetic patients can adjust medication, diet, and exercise by following frequent blood glucose checks at home. Allison Page (2000) describes a self-management program for asthmatic patients that includes patient education to support the day-to-day management decision that patients and families make. The plan involves care by a team of providers and includes assessment using a standard history form, pulmonary function testing, and tracking of education so that reinforcement and follow-through are possible. Specific skills for parent and child are listed for a set of five visits so that the educational program is standardized. The key to self-management for asthmatics is the use of a peak flow meter and proper recording and interpretation of the findings.

◯⟩ EVALUATING OUTCOMES

After establishing the treatment plan, evaluation is the next judgment that the nurse practitioner makes. Because most diagnoses are at least somewhat uncertain and because treatment options vary in their effectiveness in dealing with a particular problem, the nurse practitioner has many reasons to be curious about how well the treatment plan is proceeding. Evaluation can be considered from several perspectives. First, is the plan effective? Are desired outcomes being met? Is the blood pressure decreasing? Is the glucose under better control? Is the pain relieved? Secondly, the "costs" for treatment must be considered. Does the medication cause side effects? Is the treatment regimen too expensive to continue because of drug costs? Is the treatment plan inconvenient in the context of this particular person's life? Now is the time to consider adjusting the treatment plan to better meet the patient's needs. For some patients, making changes is in itself stressful. For these patients, a wider margin of acceptable response might be considered. Other patients are active in shaping their own treatment plan, and several adjustments to a treatment plan are considered before a stable plan is put into effect. The ongoing assessment of chronic conditions was discussed briefly in Chapter 2.

As an example of a way that treatment plans can be evaluated, a student once reported the case of a man whose blood pressure was not under good control despite the prescription of an ACE inhibitor. He mentioned in passing that, since his retirement, his wife "kicked him out of the house all day" and did not allow him to return until dinnertime. When asked about how he managed his three-times-a-day medication schedule, he admitted that he was taking all the pills at the same time just before bed. An adjustment in the medication schedule improved his blood pressure control. Understanding the day-to-day aspects of patients' lives makes treatment plans more effective.

Another way to consider evaluation of treatment plans is to look across patients. For example, if your practice has many hypertensive patients, how are they faring as a group? Would group support or teaching serve the needs of these patients and increase efficiency of practice? This examination can be done as an audit for quality improvement. Another consideration of patient groups might include noting the major cultural or ethnic groups in the area and providing culturally appropriate supports, such as family appointments or traditional consultants. Thinking of patients in groups will help you to demonstrate the value your interventions have for the practice and for the entire community. This kind of data is useful when negotiating a salary raise or when writing grants to agencies for community-based care.

One benefit that nurse practitioners have in community-based care is the long tradition of community health from which they can draw. Start small by choosing one important group from your practice and make a plan for developing resources and approaches for this group. Measure your effect, and in the following year, add an additional focus. Over time, you can build a rich network of community-based connections that support clinical effectiveness.

Documentation of patient instructions and telephone follow-up is important from a legal perspective. It also forms the basis for billing and supporting continuity of care. Clinical judgment about intervention selection is not complete until outcomes have been achieved. In some cases, the patient may not return for additional care, implying the resolution of an acute self-limiting condition. In many cases, however, such as chronic conditions, outcomes are intermediate and can be reflected in such measures as body weight for congestive heart failure patients, blood glucose levels for diabetics, or peak flow measurements for asthmatics. Outcome determination and documentation require teamwork between nurse practitioners and patients. Satisfaction with care is enhanced for both parties as outcomes are followed and documented. Chapter 5 discusses at length documentation systems for all aspects of the clinical-judgment process.

⏺ SUMMARY

This chapter has demonstrated the wide range of interventions available to nurse practitioners and has shown several systems for organizing intervention choices. The process of forming clinical judgments about intervention selection is based in a good assessment of the patient situation and a holistic view of the person. The model for Nurse Practitioner-Patient Linkages forms the basis of continuing the relationships to support open discussions about treatment and outcome preferences. Nurse practitioners often use prescription writing as a way of supporting patient health, but interventions are not limited to this form of care. Evaluation of intervention effectiveness can form the basis for practice evaluation and for research. Nurse practitioners continue to grow in their judgment processes and in their range of options as they gain experience.

REFERENCES

American Medical Association (2002). *Current procedural terminology: CPT 2003*. Chicago: American Medical Association.

Brez, S., & Taylor, M. (1997). Assessing literacy for patient teaching: Perspectives of adults with low literacy skills. *Journal of Advanced Nursing, 25*, 1040–1047.

Brykczynski, K. A. (1989). An interpretive study describing the clinical judgment of nurse practitioners. *Scholarly Inquiry for Nursing Practice, 3*, 75–104.

Burman, M. E. (2003). Complementary and alternative medicine: Core competencies for family nurse practitioners. *Journal of Nursing Education, 42*(1), 28–34.

Caulfield, J. S. (2000). The psychosocial aspects of complementary and alternative medicine. *Pharmacotherapy, 20*, 1289–1294.

Dossey, B. M., Keegan, L., Guzzetta, C. E., & Kolkmeier, L. G. (1995). *Holistic nursing: A handbook for practice* (2nd ed.). Gaithersburg, MD: Aspen.

Eisenberg, D. M., Davis, R. B., Ettner, S. L., Appel, S., Wilkey, S., Van Rompay, M., & Kessler, R. (1998). Trends in alternative medicine use in the United States, 1990–1997: Results of a follow-up national survey. *Journal of the American Medical Association, 280*, 1569–1575.

Eisenhauer, L. A. (1994). A typology of nursing therapeutics. *Image: The Journal of Nursing Scholarship, 26*, 261–264.

Engebretson, J. (1997). A multiparadigm approach to nursing. *Advances in Nursing Science, 20*(1), 21–33.

Getzels, J. W. (1982). The problem of the problem. In R. Hogarth (Ed.). *New directions for methodology of social and behavioral science: Question framing and response consistency*, no. 11. (pp. 37–49). San Francisco: Jossey-Bass.

Gutierrez, K., & Sciacca, S. (2000). Prescribing behaviors of Colorado advanced practice nurses. *The Nurse Practitioner: The American Journal of Primary Health Care, 25*(11), 14–15.

Humphreys, J. (2000). Spirituality and distress in sheltered battered women. *Journal of Nursing Scholarship, 32*, 273–278.

Keegan, L. (2001). *Healing with complementary and alternative therapies.* Albany, NY: Delmar.

Kennedy, J. M. (2001). Health promotion. In L. M. Dunphy, & J. E. Winland-Brown (Eds.). *Primary care: The art and science of advanced practice nursing* (pp. 57–83). Philadelphia: F. A. Davis.

Krieger, D. (1979). *The therapeutic touch.* Englewood Cliffs, NJ: Prentice Hall.

McCloskey, J. C., & Bulechek, G. M. (Eds.). (2000). *Nursing intervention classification (NIC)* (3rd ed.). St. Louis: Mosby-Year Book.

Oakley, L. D. (2001). Psychosocial problems. In L. M. Dunphy & J. E. Winland-Brown (Eds.). *Primary care: The art and science of advanced practice nursing* (pp. 1025–1092). Philadelphia: F. A. Davis.

O'Connor, N. A., Hameister, A. D., & Kershaw, T. (2000). Developing a database to describe the practice patterns of adult nurse practitioner students. *The Journal of Nursing Scholarship, 32*(1), 57–63.

Page, A. (2000). Improving pediatric asthma outcomes using self-management skills. *The Nurse Practitioner: The American Journal of Primary Health Care, 25*(11), 16, 18, 27–30, 32–33, 37.

Pender, N. (1987). *Health promotion in nursing practice* (2nd ed.). Norwalk, CT: Appleton & Lange.

Rakel, R. F. (1998). *Essentials of family practice* (2nd ed.). Philadelphia: W. B. Saunders Company.

Schillinger, D., Grumbach, K., Piette, J., Wang, F., Osmond, D., Daher, C., Palacios, J., Sullivan, G. D. & Bindman, A. B. (2002). Association of health literacy with diabetes outcomes. *Journal of the American Medical Association, 288*, 475–482.

Sheahan, S. L. (2000). Documentation of health risks and health promotion counseling by emergency department nurse practitioners and physicians. *Journal of Nursing Scholarship, 32*, 245-250.

Stepanian, C. (2000). Waving goodbye to confusing medication orders: Prescription for change. *Massachusetts Nurse, 70*(6), 17.

United States Department of Health and Human Services. (1996). Physical activity and health: A report of the Surgeon General. Atlanta, GA: Centers for Disease Control and Prevention, National Center for Chronic Disease Prevention and Health Promotion.

Whittemore, R., Chase, S. K., Mandle, C. L., & Roy, C. (2002). Lifestyle change in type 2 diabetes: A process model. *Nursing Research, 51*(1) 18–25.

Documentation

CHAPTER OUTLINE

Documenting Nurse Practitioner Services
  Documentation Pointers
Problem-Oriented Record
  Subjective Data
  Objective Data
  Assessment
  Plan
Standardized Language and Classification Systems
  International Classification of Disease
  Current Procedural Terminology
Medicare Billing and Documentation
  Ensuring Compliance and Avoiding Fraud
  Special Situations
Privacy of Health Care Records
Computerized Records
Summary

DOCUMENTING NURSE PRACTITIONER SERVICES

Documentation of the nurse practitioner-patient encounter serves several useful purposes. This chapter reviews those purposes and examines commonly used documentation systems, including computerized record keeping. It also shows how documentation is useful to various audiences, such as other health-care practitioners, accrediting agencies, and third-party payors such as insurance companies or Medicare. Because documentation is a complex process that will be mastered over time, student nurse practitioners should initially focus on recording the data collected and ensuring that the plan and interventions carried out in the encounter are accurately reflected in the patient's chart.

Documentation provides a record of the patient's symptoms, physical signs, and laboratory findings; the nurse practitioner's decision-making process; and the selected treatment plan and its results. Within a group practice, documentation serves important communication functions. For example, it records the nurse practitioner-patient encounter to remind the practitioner what happened during the visit. Many times, practitioners must refer to the patient record to refresh their memory of data collected or of treatment recommended. Documentation also ensures good communication among members of the health-care team. For instance, if the patient receives follow-up care from another practitioner, the patient record provides information that is essential to maintain continuity of care.

Accurate patient documentation also aids quality improvement efforts or clinical research. For example, a nurse practitioner might ask whether drug-resistant infections have increased within certain patient groups. To answer this question, the nurse practitioner could review the records of all patients who received specific antibiotics to assess their recovery rates or the need for additional antibiotic coverage. For example, one study reported by Sheahan (2000) investigated how physicians and nurse practitioners in an emergency room setting documented health risk factors and health promotion counseling. After reviewing 305 records, the study determined that 59 percent had at least one health-risk factor such as smoking. Only 22 percent of these had health counseling documented in the record, with nurse practitioners being slightly (odds ratio 0.16, $p=.02$) more likely to provide smoke-cessation counseling. This can serve as a baseline for improving practice.

In addition, patient records can indicate the effectiveness of interventions that have been used by nurse practitioners but have not been subjected to rigid clinical trials. For instance, a nurse practitioner might try a new teaching method for patients who were recently diagnosed with diabetes, then evaluate the patient records for beneficial outcomes related to the new intervention, such as improved glucose control or better return to clinic for appointments. One study of 100 records from a nurse-managed clinic reflects the absence of outcome data regarding health perceptions or quality of life in patient records that would allow improvement of health services (Davis, Holman, & Sousa, 2000). As these examples show, good outcome documentation can help improve the care given to future patients. Research that uses patient records is now more tightly controlled because of HIPAA regulations, which will be discussed later in this chapter.

Another important reason for accurate documentation is to communicate with audiences beyond the practice itself. Third-party payors are increasingly vigilant in deciding what kind of care to reimburse. Many Health Maintenance Organizations (HMOs) require documentation to justify length of visit, frequency of follow-up, and even the particular drug that is allowed for prescribing. Accurate documentation ensures that the practice and the nurse practitioner are reimbursed for care that was provided. Medicare has strict documentation guidelines that determine levels of reimbursement (see Medicare Billing and Documentation, further on in this chapter, for more information). Accrediting agencies such as the Joint Commission on the Accreditation of Health Care Organizations or rating organizations such as the National Committee for Quality Assurance examine documentation to verify that care standards are met.

Finally, one more reason for good documentation is to provide legal protection in the event of a lawsuit. The patient's medical record is a legal document that can be used as evidence in malpractice cases. Good documentation not only shows the quality of care provided, but also offers a defense in court.

> **RULE OF THUMB: Assume that the patient and his or her lawyers might some day read the notes that the nurse practitioner is writing.**

All of the purposes of recording the nurse practitioner-patient encounter described above—communication, research, reimbursement, and legal protection—are served by clear, accurate, and complete documentation. Documentation is an opportunity for nurse practitioners to review the level of their thoughts.

> **RULE OF THUMB: Not documented = not done.**

As nurse practitioner practice evolves, a debate continues about what to record and whether medical diagnoses and treatments should be the only elements included. Documenting nursing's unique contribution to care and the nurse practitioner's mastery of advanced nursing practice requires the use of the language that includes concepts specific to nursing. A survey of 197 nurse practitioners found that 47 percent reported that they documented assessments differently from physicians. Those nurse practitioners also reported that they recorded different patient outcomes, such as patient satisfaction and increased patient involvement in decision making. One participant commented, "We look at the situation differently, more holistically (Chase & Leuner, 2000, p. 301). Comments from participants in this data set indicate the difference that their practice provides to individual patients and to the practice setting through such skills as consultation and coordination. The majority (64%) of the nurse practitioners in a related data set (Leuner & Chase, 1997) noted that they did not record all their interventions. One respondent reported, "There is so much that goes on in a visit that it's virtually impossible to record it all. I am especially thinking of a physical exam visit because with adolescents, even younger kids, behavioral issues, psychosocial problems" do not get recorded (Chase & Leuner, 2000, p. 302). Another nurse practitioner reports, "I consider much of what I do a nursing intervention, for example, teaching health promotion activities, anticipatory guidance" (Chase & Leuner, 2000, p. 302). Nursing's language is not foreign to the primary-care setting. Nurse practitioners who limit their language to medical terminology only limit their ability to measure nursing's unique contribution to patient care.

Documentation Pointers

1. Write in a clear, direct, nonjudgmental way, but include the richness of detail of the visit and how the patient is managing health problems.
2. Ensure that patients' records are available to them to review. This supports accurate clinical judgment that is sensitive to the individual needs of patients. Sharing records with patients can increase their participation in their own care and can increase a sense of trust for some. The Health Insurance Portability and Accountability Act (HIPAA) has provisions that limit sharing electronic information about patients, but it does not prohibit sharing information with the patient (Buppert, 2002b).
3. Ask patients how much information they want or need.
4. Ask patients which members of their family or perhaps friends they are comfortable sharing information with.
5. Develop a system for maintaining current, accurate records. Saving up hastily scratched notes and documenting at the end of a busy day is not ideal. Dictation, voice recognition, and computer systems allow complete record keeping with minimal time spent on the task.
6. Develop an outline form for your documentation that includes all essential data elements in a way that is retrievable; avoid writing in full sentences and paragraphs, which does not allow other providers to easily retrieve data (Fig. 5–1). An outline template can also serve as a memory tool.

⟩⟩ PROBLEM-ORIENTED RECORD

The organization of medical records has undergone many changes. By understanding the background for the systems in use, the nurse practitioner

Figure 5–1

SAMPLE OUTLINE FOR TAKING NOTES DURING HISTORY AND FOR DOCUMENTATION

Subjective Data

Demographics: Sex _____ Age _____ Living situation _____ Key contacts _____
Insurance status _____ Other providers of health care _____

Chief Complaint:

History of Present Illness:

Past Medical History:
Significant Events: Surgeries, diagnostic workups such as cardiac catheterizations, etc.

Menstrual, pregnancy history:

Medications (List all reported medications and ask about natural or herbal remedies used):

Immunizations (age-appropriate):

Allergies to drugs or food:

Family History: M		F	Siblings	Grandparents

Social History: Work history and exposures
Substances: How long, how much

Tobacco use		ETOH	Illegal substances	

Nursing/Functional Health Pattern
Assistance required:

Review of Systems
General: Weight change, fevers, lymph node swelling or tenderness
HEENT: Migraines, sinusitis, hearing loss, visual problems, frequent sore throats, head trauma, dizziness, syncope, dental problems
CV: MI, chest pain, palpitations, dyspnea, varicose veins
Respiratory: Asthma, COPD, TB, pneumonia, exercise capacity, orthopnea, cough
GI: Heartburn, ulcers, constipation, gallbladder
Endo: Thyroid, DM, heat or cold intolerance
GU: UTIs, breast exam, breast problems, incontinence, sexual problems
Neurological: Muscle weakness, CVA, numbness, tingling, balance, seizures, memory
Musculoskeletal: Joint pain or stiffness, muscle weakness
Skin: Rashes, wounds, pigment change, hair and nail change

Objective Data

Physical Examination
HEENT:
Neurological:
Cardiovascular:
Pulmonary:
Abdominal:
Genitourinary:
Skin:
Laboratory testing (Record here data that are useful in making diagnosis):

Assessment

Differential Diagnosis (Record here your thinking about possible diagnoses. You can then organize the data collected above into problem-oriented sections):

Plan

Diagnostic tests:
Teaching (content, follow through):
Medication (record med, dosage, amount to dispense):
Other treatments or recommendations (Record here initial plan developed. This can be modified after conversation with patient) (Diet, activity):
Return for follow-up:
Referrals:

can be a contributor in shaping systems for the future. A revolution in medical charting came as a result of the Problem-Oriented Record, introduced by Dr. Lawrence Weed at the University of Vermont (1971). This system introduced the concept of the "SOAP" note, which is described in the following paragraph. The system was designed to assist students in learning to make and record health-related decisions. Before this, health information was recorded based on its source. In that way, history and physical examination data were grouped together, as were all laboratory data, and different providers documented in their own sections. All this separation made it difficult to synthesize data, which are necessary for good clinical judgment. Consequently, many problems remained unidentified or poorly tracked. For example, in a hospital chart, the nurse's notes might clearly document signs of a developing infection, whereas the surgical resident's notes might only record lab findings. It would take full-blown infection to occur before the pieces were put together and treatment was begun. In primary care, data come from many sources as well. Grouping data and judgments around identifying and tracking problems improves the accuracy of nurse practitioners' decision making.

This section applies documentation principles to the charting format known as SOAP (**S**ubjective data, **O**bjective data, **A**ssessment data, and **P**lan). If other formats are used, the principles learned by "SOAPing" a problem still apply.

Subjective Data

The Subjective (S) portion of the record includes all data from the patient's report, such as history of present illness, past medical history, family history, social history, functional health patterns data, and review of systems. These data include reported medications, immunization status, allergies to foods or medications, and past hospitalizations, if appropriate. For women, include last menstrual period and menstrual cycle information. Using an outline format with data organized by the headings listed above can make data more retrievable. Even for simple problems, a woman's pregnancy status must be known when prescribing certain medications. The patient's responses to the Review of Systems are organized by body systems, but as it reflects patient report of history, it belongs in the Subjective section. If the patient's particular way of describing a problem seems important, include direct quotes. This is not necessary, however, if the description is simple and without nuance. Table 5–1 reflects the hypotheses that are generated by the particular way in which the patient describes the condition.

TABLE 5–1

Sample Documentation of Subjective Data

Patient Statement	Nurse Practitioner Inference
"I have this burning that comes back every evening. It's here in the middle of my chest."	Characteristics of pain, pattern, and location that the patient reports indicate that she may fear cardiac disease. NP can address this concern as part of the workup.
"My wife says I need to come and see you about my cough."	The patient is not coming of his own accord. He may not be motivated to participate in his own care. NP can assess for this as interview proceeds.
"My back hurts so much I have not been able to work."	Back pain can have many causes, including stress and ergonomic factors. The NP can assess for what the patient does at work and whether there is stress either at work or at home. Many patients are more comfortable expressing physical than emotional pain.

Objective Data

The Objective (O) section of the record includes all data obtainable through objective means, but is not limited to numeric data. Begin the objective portion of the record with a brief description of the overall impression of the patient. Such phrases as "tired looking," "energetic," or "worried" can convey information that is useful in forming clinical judgments. Include vital signs and pertinent physical examination findings as well as available laboratory data. Do not reflect clinical judgments that you are considering in this section.

> RULE OF THUMB: The Objective section is "just the facts, ma'am."

The S and O sections are performed with reasonable skill, even for advanced beginner students. At first, students are unable to focus on which pieces of data are significant to a problem, and tend to include every piece of data available. This can make it difficult to track the clinical judgment of the nurse practitioner or to efficiently retrieve information at a later time.

Making this even more complicated, it is important in both the Subjective and Objective sections to record two kinds of data: positive and negative. Positive data are indicators of a problem that are present or reported. Negative data are indicators that one would expect for a given condition, but that are not reported or present. In order to know what data are expected, the differential diagnosis list that is being developed must be considered. Chapter 2, on clinical judgment showed that data are used to predict the likelihood of a list of possible diagnoses. The elements of history and physical that get recorded are not the same as a direct recording of the process used in considering diagnostic hypotheses. This can be confusing to the nurse practitioner student.

> RULE OF THUMB: After making your diagnosis, you must decide what to document. In choosing what to document, "work backwards." Start by deciding which conditions you want to show that you considered. Decide what data are most important to reflect for each condition. One good way is to show first the data that support your diagnosis. Then show data that refute the competing diagnoses.

Another documentation consideration is that, for any presenting problem, there is a possibility that a serious or potentially life-threatening process could be at work. It is always a good policy to record data that show you have evaluated the patient for the serious condition and that data do not confirm that possibility.

Flow sheets are another way of recording subjective and objective data in the patient record along with the SOAP note described above. When following patients over time, flow sheets can be useful for tracking data. For example, a flow sheet can show the effect of a change in medication management of hyperlipidemia, obesity, or hypertension over months or years. Other flow sheets can be developed for specific practices, such as health screening for pediatric practices by age group (Powers, Gillett, & Goldblum, 2000).

Assessment

Although the Assessment (A) portion of documentation varies greatly from patient to patient, it must always include active problems that are being managed in the particular visit as well as chronic problems that might affect the treatment plan. For the problem list to serve both patient and practitioner well, the simple problem label may not be enough. For example, if the patient has hypertension and has been managed by lifestyle modifications and medication for some time, the nurse practitioner should reflect on the effectiveness of control in the Assessment section. Rather than simply repeat "Hypertension" in the A section, it is more useful to write, "Hypertension well controlled with medication." Many practices include a health promotion line on the problem list to reflect the preventative focus of that practice. Reassessment is ongoing in the management of health problems. For example, a problem list might read: (1) Hypertension stage 2, well controlled; (2) Type 2 diabetes mellitus, poorly controlled; (3) obesity, unchanged. This kind of information directs evaluation and helps the nurse practitioner adjust interventions more effectively than a simple list of "HTN, DM, obesity."

In some cases, a clear problem name cannot be identified. For example, abdominal pain that does not fit a clear diagnostic pattern can be reflected in the problem list by simply naming the complaint. The nurse practitioner can reflect the uncertainty of the diagnosis by writing "abdominal pain, R/O irritable bowel syndrome." Or "Cough, viral bronchitis vs. allergy." Nurse practitioner students are often reluctant to disclose that they cannot name the problem. The uncertainty of clinical judgment is a feature of primary care that differs from many acute-care situations. It is a mistake to name a problem in error, simply to have a problem on the list, as well as to fail to reveal competing diagnostic hypotheses. In primary care, uncertainty is reasonable and expected. If the patient's problem does not resolve, consultation or referral may be necessary.

One way to organize a clinical record is to maintain an active problem list near the front of the patient record. This is particularly useful when

TABLE 5–2

Sample Problem List

Patient: Sam White   **DOB 3/15/1948**

Date	Problem	Disposition	Outcome
2/15/97	New patient		
	Obesity	Ongoing, diet counseling	
	Smoker	Ongoing, smoke cessation recommended	Stopped smoking 4/98
4/30/97	Acute bronchitis	E-mycin	Resolved
10/24/97	Acute bronchitis	E-mycin	Resolved
4/25/98	Hypertension	HCTZ, recommend walking	Controlled on meds 8/98
5/24/98	Acute bronchitis	E-mycin	Resolved
8/98	Chronic bronchitis	Pulmonary rehab Proventil prn	

dealing with chronic conditions. The nurse practitioner can initiate such a tool in any practice, even if a blank progress note sheet is filed at the beginning of the Progress Notes section. Table 5–2 shows a sample problem list. The running problem list in this example allowed the recognition of the pattern of frequent episodes of bronchitis. This provided the impetus for evaluating the patient for chronic bronchitis.

> RULE OF THUMB: When reviewing the Assessment part of the record, ask yourself: Are all data that were used to justify the naming of a problem included in the S and O sections of the note? Are all data accounted for in the Assessment section?

Plan

The problem list should drive intervention selection in the Plan (P). The Plan, which includes detailed and specific descriptions of the interventions, contains four general sections:

1. *Diagnostic testing.* This section includes a list of all tests to be conducted. The results of these tests will help to clarify the assessment but are not yet available to the provider.
2. *Therapeutic plans.* This section includes prescriptions, therapies, consultations, counseling, activity promotion or restriction, dietary changes, or any of the therapeutics discussed earlier. When recording prescriptions, be sure to include all the data that were written on the prescription itself, including number or volume to dispense and number of refills allowed. This information clearly shows how the patient was managed and is vital to other providers who may sometimes handle patients' calls for prescription refills. In addition, this information is particularly important when prescribing drugs that are prone to abuse. Patients might call and ask for a refill on a prescription sooner than is allowed. By being clear about how much has been prescribed, you can avoid premature refills. Even though it is time consuming, record teaching that is done so that its effectiveness can be evaluated on subsequent visits and so that other providers can reinforce what you have done.
3. *Education.* This section specifies educational approaches to be used. Every visit is a teaching opportunity. Education might include information related to the problems being managed, such as symptom control for upper respiratory infections, medication teaching, diet and activity recommendations, and risk reduction strategies, such as information on smoking cessation or seat belt usage.

4. *Plan for follow-up.* When should the patient be seen again? Under what circumstances should the patient call back? For example, when treating a viral infection, remind the patient to call back if he or she is not better in 2 days or if fever develops. Documenting follow-up instructions also allows other providers to effectively manage patients if they call in when you are not available.

Plans can include a sense of the goal for treatment. For simple, self-limiting conditions, this may be obvious and may not need to be stated. For chronic or complex problems, however, the short- and long-term goals of therapy should be considered. By engaging the patient in this discussion, the nurse practitioner can clearly see the choices that the patient makes in altering lifestyle and in following a treatment plan. For example, the patient with hypertension, diabetes, and obesity described previously might set a goal to lose 4 pounds in a month. The intervention might be walking 3 times a week for 20 minutes and eating at least 5 fruits or vegetables every day. The feedback on the short-term goal can help to keep the patient motivated to sustain lifelong change.

Now that the elements of a SOAP note have been presented, Box 5–1

Box 5–1 Sample Documentation

S: CC:"I think I have pinkeye."

HPI: Woke with itchy, red left eye yesterday morning. Just returned from trip on a bus. Eye exudate sticky. No reported change in vision. Denies eye pain or photophobia. Denies fever or malaise.

ROS: No history of hay fever. Does not wear contact lenses.

FSH: No exposure to family member or roommate with eye complaints or recent sexual contact.

O: T: 98.4. Inflamed conjunctiva left eye with crusting. Pupils equal and reactive to light and accommodation. Clear cornea, no scratches evident on fluorescein staining. Fundoscopic exam reveals optic disc with clear margins. No periorbital edema or erythema; no preauricular lymph node adenopathy. Visual acuity 20/20 both eyes.

A: Conjunctivitis, probably bacterial.

P: Flushed eye during office visit. Ciloxan 0.3% 1–2 drops every 2 hours while awake day one. 1–2 drops every 4 hours days 2–5. Warm compresses with sterile saline. Discontinue all eye makeup. Frequent hand washing.

Call if not improved by day 2.

---

shows the documentation for an 18-year-old female college student who has been seen in the clinic in the past. This example shows that signs of viral conjunctivitis (fever, preauricular lymphadenopathy, and bilateral involvement) were not present. Glaucoma is unlikely at this age, and there is no visual loss. Signs of uveitis (iritis, eye pain, blurred vision) were also not present. Foreign body is unlikely because of the clear cornea and generalized injection.

In general, a good principle is to write the note in such a way that the patient could agree with what was stated. For example, reflect any disagreements in nonjudgmental terms. If you and the patient disagree on a treatment plan involving the use of certain medications, you might write: "Patient requested prescription for muscle relaxants, which was discussed as being unlikely to benefit the shoulder pain described." This kind of note can assist in determining patterns of behaviors or difficulties.

Some documentation systems include Intervention (I) and Evaluation (E) data, expanding SOAP to SOAPIE. This allows for re-examining a treatment plan, particularly for a chronic problem. For example, medication side effects and patient success in changing diet or adding exercise can be included in the Subjective data for the next visit, but it reflects Evaluation of the previous Plan.

Other considerations in establishing documentation systems are for legal purposes, to be sure to reflect missed appointments and patient refusal of treatment plans, and to have a system for tracking laboratory data (James, 2000). Table 5–3 reflects some principles of laboratory data management that will improve the quality of care and decrease exposure to liability.

When a urine culture result comes in, how will office staff members know who needs to review the results? These principles not only support quality care, but also protect the provider if a lawsuit ever develops (Starr, 1999).

In summary, the elements of the documentation system should support excellence in clinical judgment and patient care (Box 5–2). The system should be a support to the nurse practitioner's practice and should provide the basis for appropriate reimbursement and legal defense.

RULE OF THUMB: When reviewing your documentation, ask yourself whether the note you wrote conveys the scope and tone of the visit. Was this an enthusiastic health promotion support visit, or was the visit characterized by sharing bad news or risks of serious problems? Does it reflect the way in which the patient is responding to his or her health problem? Does it truly represent the type of visit that occurred?

TABLE 5–3

Key Elements in Laboratory Tracking Systems

Suggestion	Rationale
Keep a running list of pending lab data either by provider or on general practice list.	If the lab data are lost and no report is returned, someone will need to follow up.
File data as it arrives in patient chart.	This allows incorporating the data into the full patient picture.
Have a system for recording who evaluated the data.	This will minimize the risk of data being returned but not evaluated.
Share data with patient and document.	This supports active involvement by the patient in his or her own care.

))) STANDARDIZED LANGUAGE AND CLASSIFICATION SYSTEMS

Standardized language is essential for clinicians to communicate effectively with one another, and for payment and research to continue. For example, if clinicians used different terms when managing patients with similar conditions, it would be impossible to determine whether appropriate care had been given, ensure adequate payment, or compare cases for population research. The feature of labeling and coding that receives the most attention on a day-to-day basis is the billing aspect. It is important to remember, however, that the activities of nurse practitioners are not governed by reimbursement systems. They are controlled by state nurse practice acts. Getting reimbursed for patient-care activities, however, depends on meeting guidelines of third-party payors.

Box 5–2 Words of Wisdom

All documentation systems are designed by the practice, the setting, or the system. If you, as a nurse practitioner, find that elements of your care are invisible in the record because of restrictive coding or limited space, plan a meeting with the head of the practice or clinic to discuss what you feel is missing. Most systems in which nurse practitioners work are dominated by the medical model. Be certain that your contributions that come from a nursing model are not invisible. Claim credit and billing for the care you actually provide.

International Classification of Disease

The World Health Organization developed the International Classification of Diseases (ICD) to classify morbidity and mortality information in a way that communicates consistently. The ICD was originally designed to classify reasons for hospitalizations, but has been extended to also classify reasons for outpatient office visits. The most recently published version is the ninth edition with Clinical Modifications (ICD-9-CM). Since 1988, providers have been required to use the ICD-9 when submitting claims to Medicare under provision of the Medicare Catastrophic Coverage Act. The Centers for Medicare and Medicaid Services (CMS) (formerly Health Care Financing Administration) have designated ICD-9 as their accepted coding system. The Clinical Modifications applied to ICD-9 were designed for including information necessary for classifying morbidity data or indexing medical records, and for the review of medical care in ambulatory settings. It is also useful for basic health statistics. Clinical systems must have sufficient detail to be truly useful.

The ICD-9 has both an alphabetical index and a numeric (tabular) classification system. The basic classification system consists of a 3-digit code. Additional detail is required for most reimbursement mechanisms. A fourth digit reflects etiology, site, and causes or complications. A fifth digit reflects further detail, such as whether the condition is controlled or uncontrolled. For example, diabetes mellitus is coded 250.0, but this is not sufficiently specific. Uncontrolled type 2 diabetes with nephropathy would be 250.42. Controlled type 1 diabetes would be 250.x1 (Castillo, Hopkins, & Aaron, 1998).

When coding a visit, first identify the reason for the visit. This is usually done in an office practice on an encounter form. Clinics such as pre-admission clearance visits attached to a hospital might include services covered by acute-care payment systems and therefore are not coded or billed separately. In ambulatory care, be aware that encounter forms list only the high-frequency reasons for visits and the full list needs to be consulted for accuracy of coding. For example, in an OB/GYN practice, the encounter form lists common reasons for OB/GYN visits. The provider is not limited to the codes on any particular encounter form. The reason for the visit can include specific diagnoses; if an accurate diagnosis is not possible, then symptoms or signs or findings are listed. Without a clear diagnosis, the sign or symptoms are coded. For example, generalized abdominal pain is coded 789.x7. Table 5–4 reflects the disease coding of a visit for a leg ulcer.

TABLE 5–4

Case Example of Coding for Disease

A 64-year-old woman is seen in your office for an initial visit for an "open sore on her leg." In your assessment you note a 3 cm by 4 cm open ulcer on the medial malleolus of the right lower extremity.	454.0 Varicose veins of lower extremity with ulcer
The skin surrounding the ulcer is discolored brown with hemosiderin deposits, which also exist on the left, and sensation of the foot is intact.	Data support selection of varicose veins of lower extremity.
Leg has a hard, nonpitting edema. The ulcer has persisted for 2 months. Edema is greater on the right than the left.	Data support selection of varicose veins of lower extremity.
There is no redness of the skin surrounding the ulcer and the exudate of the open area is straw colored.	454.1 with inflammation or 454.2 with ulcer and inflammation is not appropriate because there is no sign of inflammation.
Pedal pulses are palpable and there is no loss of hair.	Data support selection of varicose veins of lower extremity, not arterial disease.

RULE OF THUMB: To specify the coding, consult the alphabetical index of the ICD-9. This minimizes coding errors and helps to specify a code before going to the classification list. Pay attention to any notes listed with index entries, such as those describing how to classify multiple fractures (distal ulna alone: 813.43; distal radius alone: 813.42; lower radius with ulna: 813.44). Check cross-references to determine the most appropriate code. Determine the highest level of specificity possible, consider age or sex exclusions, then assign the code.

Nurse practitioner practice is not always disease focused. Additional codes are useful for visits in which screening or focused assessment occurs. For example, such visits may involve screening or assessment of patients who have been exposed to a disease such as tuberculosis, but who are found not to have the disease. It would be an error to classify the reason for the visit as tuberculosis because the patient in question does not have this diagnosis. Nevertheless, the visit is justified. Reasons for visits other than diseases use V Codes, "Supplementary Classification of Factors Influencing Health Status and Contact with Health Services." These codes allow classification of visits for many nurse practitioner activities such as counseling, teaching, and support. See Box 5–3 for a suggested list of V codes used by any health-care provider. Nurse practitioners spend much of their practice handling nondisease situations. They need to be fully aware of V codes so that the care they provide is recognized and so that the practice is appropriately reimbursed. V codes may not be reimbursed at the same level as disease-related visits.

In many practices, office staff members are assigned the duty of coding medical conditions. It is the responsibility of professionals, including nurse practitioners, to determine accuracy of coding and to provide sufficient information to the office staff so that their coding can be as accurate as possible. This is important to avoid fraudulent billing. Many practices hire specialized service providers who are expert in billing and coding. Clear,

---

Box 5–3 V-Codes Commonly Used by Nurse Practitioners

V01.1 Contact with or exposure to communicable diseases: Tuberculosis

V03 Prophylactic vaccination

V23.0 Pregnancy with a history of infertility

V25.0 Procreative management

V40 Mental or behavioral problems

V50.1 Plastic surgery visits if not needed for remedying a health state

V59.3 Bone marrow donor

V60 Homeless care

V61.4 Family problems

V62.0 Unemployment

V62.89 Stress

V65.1 Personal consultation on behalf of another person

V65.41 Exercise counseling

V68.0 Issuing medical and work permits

V76 Screening for malignancy because of personal or family history

Source: Modified from Castillo, S. A., Hopkins, C. A., & Aaron, W. S. (Eds.). (1998). *St. Anthony's ICD-9-CM Codebook for physician compliance,* Vols. 1 & 2. Reston, VA: St. Anthony Publishing.

complete documentation of the assessment data, diagnoses, and treatments rendered is the basis for good coding. Periodic discussions with the billing and coding personnel can improve billing revenue and accuracy.

Current Procedural Terminology

Standardized language is essential for naming the disease or condition requiring health care. In addition to this, the American Medical Association realized the need for standardizing medical treatment for the purposes of billing and to allow for research that measures the effectiveness of interventions. Without a consistent language to describe treatments and interventions, payment cannot be standardized and research is made difficult. The publication that lists the procedures performed by physicians and others, including nurse practitioners, is the Current Procedural Terminology (CPT) Classification (AMA, 2002). Codes for all medical and surgical procedures are included in the CPT list and consist of five-digit numbers. Third-party payors review the linkage between identified diagnoses from the ICD-9 and appropriate interventions from the CPT classification.

Reimbursement levels are determined by a classification known as the *level* of the encounter, ranging from level 1 through level 5. Clear documentation supports the selection of appropriate codes and maximizes reimbursement. There are seven components used in determining the level of service provided. They are: history, examination, medical decision making, counseling, coordination of care, nature of presenting problem, and time spent with the patient. History, examination, and medical decision making are key elements in determining the level of the service provided (AMA, 2002). These elements are displayed in Table 5–5. The most common office visits are covered under Evaluation and Management (E/M) codes. Codes are developed to differentiate between new and established patients because more effort is required in assessing new patients. The definition of established patient is one who has been treated by the provider or other members of the group in the past 3 years (Rapsilber & Anderson, 2000).

The evaluation of the patient's history is an essential element of the E/M code. If the chief complaint is not recorded, the visit may not be reimbursed. A problem-focused history includes chief complaint and brief history of present illness. No review of systems is required. An expanded, problem-focused history includes the elements of the problem-focused history with the addition of a pertinent system review. A detailed history must contain the chief complaint; an extended history of present illness; problem-pertinent review of systems beyond the major one being evaluated; and pertinent past, family, and/or social history related to the patient's problem. A comprehensive history includes all the previous elements with the addition of an extended history of present illness; a review of all additional body systems; and a complete past, family, and social history. If the history is taken as part of a preventive medicine visit, it is not problem oriented and therefore does not include a chief complaint or history of present illness. Prevention visits have unique codes (AMA, 2002). The history of present illness must include eight elements: location, quality, severity, duration, timing, context, modifying factors, and associated signs and symptoms. As an example, when documenting care for a patient with a chief complaint of sore throat, the extended history must include

TABLE 5–5

Levels of Evaluation and Management Visits

History	Data Elements
Problem focused	Chief complaint: 7 elements
	Brief HPI: 1–3 elements
Expanded problem focused	Chief complaint: 7 elements
	Brief HPI: 1–3 elements
	Problem-Pertinent ROS: 1 element
Detailed	Chief complaint: 7 elements
	Extended HPI: 4 or more elements
	Extended ROS: 2 elements
	Pertinent past family and/or social history
	(PFHS): 1 element
Comprehensive	Chief complaint: 7 elements
	Extended HPI: 4 or more elements
	Complete ROS: 10 or more elements
	Complete PFSH: 2 elements for established, 3 for new
Physical Examination	
Problem focused	Limited examination of affected body part or organ system: 1–5 elements
Expanded problem focused	Limited examination of affected and other related body areas: 6 or more elements
Detailed	Extended examination of affected body part and any other symptomatic or related areas or systems: 12 elements
Comprehensive	General multisystem examination: 18 elements from 9 systems

(Continued)

TABLE 5–5

Levels of Evaluation and Management Visits *(Continued)*

Complexity of Decision Making

Straightforward	*Minimal number of diagnoses*: 1 minor or established *Minimal or no additional data*: 1 lab study *Minimal risk of morbidity or mortality*: 1 minor problem, home management
Low complexity	*Limited number of diagnoses*: 2 minor or established or 1 new; 2 or more self limiting, or 1 acute uncomplicated *Limited amount of data*: 2 labs, summarize old records *Low risk*: 2 minor problems or 1 chronic stable, OTC drug recommendation
Moderate complexity	*Multiple diagnoses*: 1 new or 1 worse and 1 minor; 1or more chronic condition with mild exacerbation *Moderate data*: 3 labs or 1 lab and summarize old records *Moderate risk*: 1chronic problem or 1 acute systemic problem, prescription required or new problem with uncertain prognosis
High complexity	*Extensive diagnoses*: 1 new problem requiring workup or 1 new stable and one minor problem *Extensive data*: 4 lab studies or 2 labs and extensive chart review *High risk*: 1 severe, chronic problem or 1 life-threatening acute or chronic problem or acute mental status change; or decision not to resuscitate

such elements as severity, onset, duration, aggravating and alleviating factors, and any history of fever, appetite change, ear symptoms, or cough. Past history might make note of other similar symptoms, and social history might include smoking history or history of bulimia. A Comprehensive history would include review of all body systems and a complete past family and social history. This would be justified only if factors such as immune compromise or other, more serious threat were suspected. The clinician determines the appropriate level of history necessary to evaluate the presenting problem.

Similarly, the extent of the physical examination is considered in determining the level of the visit. A problem-focused examination is a limited examination of the affected body system or area. An expanded problem-focused examination includes some other related organ systems.

A detailed examination includes an extended examination of the affected part and other symptomatic parts or systems. Finally, a comprehensive examination is a full physical examination. The following body areas are counted to determine comprehensiveness of the examination: (1) head and face, (2) neck, (3) chest, including breasts and axillae, (4) abdomen, (5) genitalia, groin, and buttocks, (6) back, and (7) each extremity. Organ systems are identified as eyes, ears, nose, throat, mouth, cardiovascular, respiratory, gastrointestinal, genitourinary, musculoskeletal, skin, neurologic, psychiatric, hematologic, and lymphatic/immunologic (AMA, 2002). Table 5–5 lists the elements by level of examination. So, for our example of the patient with the sore throat, an expanded problem-focused examination would include examination of the throat and cervical lymph nodes and chest auscultation.

Finally, the complexity of the medical decision making is considered in coding the level of a visit. The number of possible diagnostic hypotheses and management options; the complexity of the medical records that need to be reviewed; and the risk of complications, morbidity, and mortality associated with the diagnosis or treatment all affect complexity levels. Four levels of complexity are recognized: straightforward, low, moderate, and high. Table 5–5 lists the elements of complexity of medical decision making.

To determine the level of the visit, the comprehensiveness and complexity are combined. For a new patient, the lowest complexity of any element determines the level of the visit. For example, if the history and physical examination qualify as expanded problem focused based on the number of elements documented, but the medical decision making complexity is straightforward, then the visit qualifies as a level 2. All elements must demonstrate level 3 complexity of the visit to be classified as a level 3. For an established patient, two of the three elements can qualify the visit at a given level. So our previous example for an established patient, in which history and physical are level 3 but medical decision making is straightforward, would qualify as a level 3 visit. The CPT code uses the fifth digit to reflect the level of the visit. Table 5–6 summarizes the elements of the visit necessary at each level.

The most common E&M code for an office visit is 99213, or an expanded problem-focused history, an expanded problem-focused examination with medical decision making complexity rated as low, with 15 minutes of face time with an established patient (AMA/HCFA, 1997; Buppert, 1999a, 2000d). Reporting all aspects of a visit maximizes the likelihood of reimbursement for the patient visit. Table 5–7 reflects commonly used codes with some clinical examples.

TABLE 5-6

Evaluation and Management Code Levels

Level	History	Physical Examination	Medical Decision Making
1	None	None	None
2	Problem focused	Problem focused	Straightforward
3	Expanded problem focused	Expanded problem focused	Low complexity
4	Detailed	Detailed	Moderate complexity
5	Comprehensive	Comprehensive	High complexity

TABLE 5-7

Common CPT Codes Used by Nurse Practitioners with Clinical Examples

Setting	Code	Examples
New patient, office or outpatient	99201	Office visit for out-of-town patient needing refill of topical steroid Initial office visit for 15-year-old boy with rash and itching after contact with poison ivy
	99202	Initial office visit for 14-year-old girl with severe acne
	99203	Initial office visit for 32-year-old man with painless hematuria
	99204	Initial office visit for 8-year-old girl, new to area, recently diagnosed with diabetes mellitus
	99205	Initial office visit for 25-year-old homosexual man with fever, cough, and shortness of breath
Established patient, office or outpatient	99211	Office visit for 78-year-old woman with pernicious anemia for monthly B_{12} injection
	99212	Office visit for established patient who was recently swimming in a lake and now presents with ear pain and purulent drainage
	99213	Established patient, 45-year-old man, presents with acute prostatitis

(Continued)

TABLE 5-7

Common CPT Codes Used by Nurse Practitioners with Clinical Examples *(Continued)*

Setting	Code	Examples
	99214	Office visit for established 32-year-old woman with new RLQ pain
	99215	Office visit for established 72-year-old man with diabetes and hypertension whose wife reports recent confusion, agitation, and short-term memory loss
Comprehensive nursing facility assessment	99301	Annual examination with MDS/RAI for 84-year-old woman who has been resident for 2 years, with multiple stable health problems
	99302	Assessment with MDS/RAI of nursing home resident for whom you will assume responsibility; previously stable on oral hypoglycemics, now requiring insulin
	99303	Nursing facility readmission for 82-year-old man who is discharged from acute facility after GI bleeding and transient delirium, now with protein depletion, debilitation, and Stage III coccygeal decubitus ulcer
Subsequent nursing facility care	99311	Scheduled monthly visit for stable 84-year-old woman with Alzheimer's disease, ambulates with walker
	99312	Monthly visit for 86-year-old man with CHF and CRF on digoxin for medication management
	99313	Nursing facility visit for patient with congestive heart failure who is developing new confusional state requiring medical management
Prolonged office visit	99354	Asthmatic patient requiring multiple nebulizer treatments with frequent observation over 2 hours' time
Prolonged service without patient face-to-face contact	99358	After office visit for older patient with multiple medical problems, extended conversation with family members and referrals to community agencies with coordination of care

Source: American Medical Association. (2002). *Current Procedural Terminology.* All rights Reserved.

Returning to the previous example of the college student who is diagnosed with conjunctivitis (see Box 5–1), coding that visit is described in
Table 5–8. She is an established patient for the practice, and therefore,
even though her level of complexity is low, the visit can be coded level 3.
A new patient would need to meet all three levels at level 3.

Nurse practitioners do more than evaluate and manage patient conditions. Interventions such as patient teaching are included in the E/M system and are billable using CPT codes. The CPT uses the term health
counseling for activities that include patient teaching. Health counseling
includes sharing and explaining diagnostic test results, discussing risks and
benefits of treatment, giving self-care or medication management instructions, and teaching families the appropriate care. If more than 50 percent
of a visit is spent on such concerns, the level of the code is determined by

TABLE 5–8

Coding for Case Example

Data	Coding Element	Level
18-year-old female college student who has been seen in the clinic in the past:	New or established	Established patient
History		
S: CC:"I think I have pinkeye."	Chief complaint present	Any level
HPI: Woke (1) with itchy, red (2) left eye (3) yesterday morning (4). Just returned from trip on a bus (5). Eye feels sticky (6). No reported change in vision (7). Denies eye pain (8) or photophobia (9). Denies fever or malaise (10).	HPI: 7 elements	Detailed
ROS: Does not wear contact lenses (11). No history of hay fever (12).		Detailed but not comprehensive
FSH: No exposure to family member or roommate with eye complaints (1) or recent sexual contact (2).	ROS: 2 elements	Detailed (not comprehensive because 2 elements present but not complete)
	FSH: 2 elements	
		(Continued)

TABLE 5-8

Coding for Case Example *(Continued)*

Data	Coding Element	Level
Physical Examination *O: T: 98.4(1). Inflamed conjunctiva left eye (2) with crusting (3). Pupils equal(4) and reactive to light and accommodation (5). Clear cornea (6), no scratches evident on fluorescein staining (7). Fundoscopic exam reveals optic disc with clear margins (8). No periorbital edema (9) or erythema (10); no preauricular lymph node adenopathy (11). Visual acuity 20/20 both eyes (12).*	12 elements	Detailed
Medical Decision Making *A: Conjunctivitis, probably bacterial*	One new diagnosis; considered foreign body, gonococcal and viral conjunctivitis	ICD-9 Code 372.00 Conjunctivitis, unspecified
P: Flushed eye during office visit. Ciloxan 0.3% 1–2 drops every 2 hours while awake day 1. 1–2 drops every 4 hours days 2–5. Warm compresses with sterile saline. Discontinue all eye makeup. Frequent hand washing. Call if not improved by day 2.	Prescription: Home management	One diagnosis with one diagnostic evaluation, low risk, but requiring prescription
		Overall code for established patient: 99213

the amount of time spent. Documentation of the counseling visit needs to include length of time of the encounter, so that if you are audited, you can demonstrate that you and the patient were there at that time (Buppert, 2000c). Document also the reason for the counseling and include a brief note on the topics discussed. This will help with continuity of care for return visits in addition to meeting documentation requirements. For example, if more than half of the visit is spent in health counseling, a note could read, "health counseling visit 10:20–11:00 AM, to discuss diagnosis of diabetes, carbohydrate counting, blood sugar testing, and medication administration." The extra time in this visit would be coded as 99354. For counseling groups of patients with established illness, such as a diabetes group, the code 99078 can be assigned. Preventive medicine counseling can also be coded depending on the length of the visit (AMA, 2002).

When considering office management, another aspect of reimbursement is often ignored. In general, a registered nurse can manage level 1 visits for an established patient. Monthly vitamin B_{12} injections are an example. This visit can be billed under the physician or nurse practitioner provider number as long as the provider is present on site at the time of the delivered service.

A research project that surveyed 53 family nurse practitioners to determine the CPT codes most often used revealed that telephone calls for consultation or medical management (99013) were performed the most (92.5% of respondents). Next in frequency (87% of respondents) was adult history taking (90750). Also included in the list were adolescent history taking (90751) by 81 percent of respondents, office medical service with an established patient (90040) by 77 percent of respondents, removal of impacted cerumen (69210) by 76 percent of respondents, dressings or débridement (16020) by 70 percent of respondents, cytopathology smears (88150) by 66 percent of respondents, and various diagnostic tests. This study reflected the wide range of activities performed by nurse practitioners in family practice (Robinson & Griffith, 1997).

))) MEDICARE BILLING AND DOCUMENTATION

Medicare is a government program that was established in 1965 to provide payment for hospital care (Part A) and physicians' and other providers' services (optional Part B) for United States residents over age 65, and for younger people with kidney failure or other major disability. Medicaid was established at the same time to provide medical care to the medically indigent. Because Medicaid is administered with matching money from the states, it can vary in its programs and payment systems from state to state. Medicaid uses documentation guidelines consistent with Medicare requirements.

For many years, Medicare paid providers on a fee-for-service basis with rates set as being "customary and reasonable." Over the years, the cost of such a system soared, and the federal government devised a different system of payment to standardize and control costs. In 1988, the Centers for Medicare and Medicaid Services (CMS) (formerly Health Care Financing Administration) and the American Medical Association developed a resource-based relative value scale (RBRVS) based on a research technique reported by Hsaio and colleagues (Hsaio, Braun, Yntema, & Becker, 1988). The relative value unit is a calculation based on provider productivity, cost of malpractice, and cost of overhead (including staff and equipment). A geographic factor is also built in because it is more expensive to provide service in certain areas of the country (e.g., Harlem) than in others (e.g., rural Alabama). Licensed physicians are paid at a higher rate than nurse practitioners, reflecting the greater educational and training costs required for the physician. The RBRVS is used by health maintenance organizations (HMOs) as well as other third-party payors.

Documentation guidelines for Medicare have been revised over the years. The most recent set of regulations are dated June 2000 and are available at the CMS website *http://cms.hhs.gov/*. The 2000 revision is less strict in how history information can be recorded. For example, in the review of systems, a specific system (e.g., pulmonary) with no abnormal data can be recorded as "Pulmonary—negative." In previous versions, specific data were required to be reported, such as "Pulmonary—denies cough or wheeze, no history of asthma, tuberculosis, or pneumonia." One cannot report "ROS negative," however, because this does not indicate which systems were explored. Carolyn Buppert, a nurse practitioner and attorney, suggests that nurse practitioners learn and use one version of the HCFA/CMS guidelines for documentation, either the 1995 or 1997 guidelines. Both are acceptable to auditors (2000b).

Nurse practitioners have fought for direct reimbursement for their services since the inception of the role. Beginning in the 1990s, nurse practitioner reimbursement by Medicare was limited to services provided to patients in nursing homes and in rural and underserved areas. But with passage of the Balanced Budget Act of 1997, direct reimbursement of nurse practitioner services was no longer limited to certain areas. The level of reimbursement for specific procedures is determined by resource-based relative value units (RBRVUs).

The federal government delegates the oversight of payments to providers through designated local carriers. Over the years, nurse practitioners have gained access to Medicare reimbursement for their services, and with the passage of Public Law 105-33 as part of the Balanced Budget Act of 1997, nurse practitioners can now bill directly for their services using their own unique personal identification number (Richmond, Thompson, & Sullivan-Marx, 2000). Formerly, the activities of nurse practitioners, physician assistants, and registered nurses were all recorded as the activities of the physician, making health-care manpower studies impossible to conduct.

There are two systems of nurse practitioner reimbursement: either 80 percent of the fee charged by the practice for the service or 85 percent of the physician fee, whichever is lower. To illustrate the former, if a nurse practitioner bills 80 percent for a service for which the practice charges $100, which includes a $20 patient co-pay, the nurse practitioner can be paid the full $80 by Medicare as long as the care is provided "incident to" the care of a physician. The "incident to" guidelines require that, at the time of the service, the physician was present and the service was provided based on a plan already devised by the physician. For example, if the nurse practitioner does diabetic teaching for a patient for whom diabetes has already been diagnosed, the full amount can be reimbursed. The physician need not be directly involved in the care, but must be present. This can be documented by a note in the chart or by time logs that document presence. Incident-to billing can result in higher payments to a practice, but it prevents the nurse practitioner's contribution to patient care from being identified individually because the visit is coded under the physician's provider number. If the problem is newly diagnosed by the nurse practitioner, billing at 85 percent of the physician's fee is required (Rapsilber & Anderson, 2000). The incident-to rule does not apply to nurse practitioner services provided in hospitals. These services must be billed under the nurse practitioner's provider number (Buppert, 1999b).

Research using the Hsaio method to compare RBRVUs assigned by nurse practitioners and family physicians shows that no significant differences in time with patients or time spent in making decisions were found between the two groups for three commonly used CPT codes. Nurse practitioners reported higher intraservice or face time, whereas physicians reported higher pre- and post-service time usually used in studying records, following up with consultations, and documentation (Sullivan-Marx & Maislin, 2000). Nurse practitioners can obtain their own provider number by applying to the Medicare Carriers contracted for their geographic area. The CMS website lists the authorized Medicare carriers at *http://cms.hhs.gov*. In order to obtain a provider number, nurse practitioners must meet current requirements. For example, as of January 1, 2001, a nurse practitioner must be a registered professional nurse authorized to practice as a nurse practitioner by the state in which he or she practices and must have passed a national certifying examination. After January 1, 2003, a nurse practitioner applying for the first time for a Medicare provider number must meet this requirement and hold a master's degree in nursing (Havens & Williams, 1999). Holders of Medicare provider numbers who are considered "inactive" because of the lack of claims filed by them directly can have their provider number dropped. It can appear that a nurse practitioner provider has been inactive if all that nurse practitioner's services are billed as incident to a physician's care (Mazzocco, 2000).

Ensuring Compliance and Avoiding Fraud

The cost of providing services through Medicare is increasing. One way to control costs is for Medicare to pay only for services rendered. When a provider submits a claim at a level higher than what was truly delivered, he or she is billing for services not rendered. This is fraud. The Office of the Inspector General (OIG) of the United States is charged with the responsibility to investigate fraudulent claims for payment made to the federal government. In 2002 the OIG enacted a more stringent program of detecting fraud and abuse (Starr, 2003). Even if an honest error in coding is discovered, there can be negative ramifications. Denial of payment, fines, prosecution resulting in jail time, loss of license, or prohibition from filing future claims are all possible.

The government reports that in 1999 it paid out $12.6 billion for claims that were erroneous or fraudulent, and that in 1999, 8 percent of claims were submitted in error (Buppert, 2001). Fraud is the knowing submission of false claims, but as in other legal matters, ignorance of the practices used by an office's billing department or of the details of coding rules is no defense. Patterns of filings are important when auditors look for fraud. High rates of level 5 billing might trigger an audit. Another trigger might be a provider who bills all visits at the same code level. In real life, patients vary in the complexity of their cases. Documentation should reflect that. On the other hand, underbilling "just to be safe" results in lost revenues to a practice, so it is not recommended.

Buppert (2000a) provides an example of a 99214 visit billed as a 99213. The difference in payment for nurse practitioner services is about $21. That seems small until you multiply the number of such cases a nurse practitioner might see in a year. Five such visits a day, 5 days a week, for 50 weeks in the year would result in lost revenue of $26,250. This is a costly and unnecessary error.

RULE OF THUMB: By knowing the coding guidelines and using them consistently, you protect yourself and your practice revenue.

The OIG has set up recommendations for compliance plans for individual and group practices. At this time, compliance plans are voluntary, but they are a good idea and will help a practice minimize the risk of being charged with fraudulent billing. The full guidelines are available on the Worldwide Web at *http://www.access.gpo.gov*. Generally, a successful compliance plan includes the following features:

- ◎ Written policies stating a commitment to truthful billing practices
- ◎ A designated compliance officer who is responsible to coordinate the compliance program
- ◎ Training opportunities so that clinicians and office staff members are clear about guidelines and rules
- ◎ Designated lines of communication to deal with questions and disputes
- ◎ A plan for internal monitoring and audits to detect errors
- ◎ Documented responses to detected errors

Consultants are available to practices so that they can appropriately code for services delivered. Attendance at annual update conferences on billing and coding can assist the nurse practitioner in staying current with rules and regulations.

Special Situations

Acute-care nurse practitioners (ACNPs) have a unique set of issues related to billing. If the ACNP is employed by a hospital and the service that is provided is considered part of hospital care, Medicare is paying for that service under Medicare Part A, and billing under Part B provisions as described previously is not allowed. If, on the other hand, an independent practice group employs the ACNP, services provided to patients at clinics attached to hospitals can be considered billable with certain restrictions.

For example, in a private surgical practice that employs an ACNP, that ACNP manages all patients who require postoperative wound care. The ACNP must bill at 85 percent of the physician rate under the ACNP's provider number in the morning while the surgeon is in the operating room. For patients seen by the ACNP in the office later that day, when the surgeon is seeing patients in the same office, the ACNP's services could be billed under the physician's provider number at the higher rate under the incident-to regulations (Richmond, Thompson, & Sullivan-Marx, 2000, p. 54).

Not all patient care is reimbursed on a fee-for-service basis. Capitated systems pay an annual rate to a practice or group to provide care to the person covered by that system. The system pays by "head count"; hence the term "capitation." Some capitated systems, however, pay a practice for an event of care, such as the provision of coronary artery bypass surgery. Ambulatory wound care following that surgery might be considered part of that care and therefore not be billable separately (Richmond, Thompson, & Sullivan-Marx, 2000).

Pediatric nurse practitioners may not consider it desirable to obtain a Medicare number, but services provided to some of their patients might be reimbursed under Medicare provisions, such as those pertaining to the disabled or those with chronic renal disease. No provider can submit claims to Medicare without a provider number; therefore someone in a pediatric practice will need to maintain a Medicare provider number (Havens & Williams, 1999).

Home evaluation and management by nurse practitioners are billable to Medicare if the patient is homebound. The nurse practitioner cannot bill for physician-level services if the care is really home nursing care. If the nurse practitioner works for a home-care agency and provides nursing-care services, the agency can bill for the nurse practitioner's nursing services using the prospective payment system. The differences between activities that can be carried out by the nurse practitioner are that to have them count as nursing services, the nurse practitioner would do a nursing assessment, develop a plan of care, carry out medical orders, and coordinate care, performing all these activities as a registered nurse. The nursing services must have been ordered by a physician. To bill for physician services, the nurse practitioner would perform functions different from that of the registered nurse, such as conducting a comprehensive history and physical examination, developing medical diagnoses, and coordinating care. The visit to provide physician services must be justified by an ICD-9 code (Buppert, 2002b).

Billing and coding for specific settings will have unique requirements, and these requirements, as in the primary-care setting, will continue to evolve. It is the responsibility of the nurse practitioner in any setting to learn about and stay current in billing and coding mechanisms appropriate to the setting.

)) PRIVACY OF HEALTH CARE RECORDS

Congress enacted the Health Insurance Portability and Accountability Act (HIPAA) in 1996. It contained provisions to improve the efficiency and effectiveness of health care by regulating the transmittal of electronic health information. Beginning April 14, 2003, any health-care entity that conveys information electronically, in order to receive reimbursement for care or to make referrals, was required to ensure privacy of patient health-care records. The United States Department of Health and Human Services Office of Civil Rights (OCR) will enforce these regulations and can impose sanctions including fines and jail terms. Access to individual patient information is limited to the purposes of patient care, payment, or operations. Health-care operations include quality improvement and guidelines assessment for use by the practice. The act also prohibits sharing information such as selling patient information to drug or marketing companies. Individual practitioners are obligated to follow these rules and to have compliance plans in place for the practice (Buppert, 2002a).

The regulations require that each practice formulate policies and procedures for protecting the privacy of patient information. Be aware that individual states can promulgate their own privacy rules, which can be more stringent than the federal rules and which must also be followed. According to HIPAA, practices need to designate a privacy officer who is responsible for overseeing compliance activities. Patients need to be provided with information about how their health-care data will be used and protected, and patient records need to be secure at all times. Cabinets must be locked and computer systems must be password protected. Any service, such as a clinical laboratory with which a practice has a contract, must also follow the guidelines. The act prohibits providers and practices from sharing patient information with third parties for marketing or promotion, or for research purposes without specific written authorization. Any paper records with identifiable data must be shredded to prevent unauthorized access to patient information. Individual practices can design systems appropriate to their settings as part of the compliance plan and must show that they have educated all employees and monitor their own compliance.

Several common activities in a primary-care practice are allowable. These include having a patient sign-in sheet as long as there is no recording of "reason for visit." Patients can be called to the examination room by name in the waiting room. Charts can be placed in a rack by the patient door and providers can discuss patient information in common areas as long as reasonable care to prevent general hearing is taken. Faxing of information to other providers is allowed, but care must be taken to ensure that a fax that contains patient information goes only to intended audiences. Telephone messages must be left carefully to prevent information about the patient from being heard by family members. Patients should authorize in writing what information can go to which family members. Patients can choose to restrict health information from being shared with anyone, including family members. Postcard reminders for appointments could be a problem. Practices can have patients fill out their own reminder card or letter while at the office so that they assume responsibility for address accuracy. Patients have access to their record for the purpose of their interest and to correct any errors. The practice can charge a reasonable copying fee for preparing records to give to the patient (Herrin, 2003).

The rules for enforcing HIPAA have been adjusted several times as the implementation date approached. Two websites that provide HIPAA related information are *http://www.hhs.gov/ocr/hipaa/* and *http://www.aspe. dhhs.gov/admnsimp/index.shtml.*

⟩⟩ COMPUTERIZED RECORDS

Many independent practices, as well as integrated health systems such as large HMOs or the Veterans Administration, make use of computerized medical records. The advantages of the computerized systems are many. One powerful advantage is that providers have immediate access to patients' records at any location that provides access to the system. This benefit can be appreciated by anyone who has tried to deliver care to an ill patient whose medical record could not be located at the time of the visit. Another advantage is the availability of audits, which can help practitioners examine coding and billing as well as conduct peer reviews. In addition, computerized records guarantee legibility and offer prompts, which ensure completeness of the record.

Computerized records also have disadvantages, however. Learning such systems can be time consuming. The predetermined fields can limit the recording of such data as functional health-pattern information, which is useful to nurses but might not be appreciated by other members of the team.

Computerized systems can be as simple as dictated or voice recognition notes that make use of templates for visits. This can standardize documentation and support care that adheres to nationally recognized care guidelines if the system is set up with these in mind. More involved systems include linkages to pharmacies, laboratories, and specialists as well as digitized images from radiology or dermatology settings. In some cases, the provider who is consulted is distant from the patient and reviews images and data that are transferred over the Internet, closed circuit television, or fiber optic cable. Other systems provide decision support by suggesting diagnoses or further tests.

The specific information needs of advanced-practice nurses were investigated by an informatics team using focus-group methodology. The team determined that the most important information needed by nurse practitioners and other advanced-practice nurses was up-to-date clinical data about the patient. This information included recent observations, plans, medications, and consultations with other care providers. The specific content needed differed by specialty of the advanced-practice nurse, but clinical data was the most important category. The research team recommended that information systems be designed with the users' needs in mind and that advanced-practice nurses need both clinical as well as economic and policy guideline linkages. The system should facilitate the face-to-face patient encounter and should not require more attention than the patient receives. It would also be useful for the computerized system to include reference resources, such as pharmacy formularies and drug-interaction data, and to support the unique contribution of nurse practitioners in linking patients with community resources. Because productivity is a concern in every practice, the computerized system should support nurse practitioner productivity (Brennan & Daly, 1996).

Another use of computerized systems is to track student nurse progress in clinical practice. One school tracked over 4000 client encounters over 3 semesters and was able to determine the patient type, diagnoses using ICD-9, CPT codes, and medications prescribed. This allowed faculty members to ensure a broad range of experiences for students and to revise their curriculum to cover frequent primary-care issues (Longworth & Lesh, 2000).

A study designed to survey the use of computer technologies in one western state showed that of the 104 respondents working in public clinics, private practice, and HMOs, nurse practitioners in HMOs were most likely (94%) to use computers in their daily practice with still substantial use in public clinics (77%) and private practice (71%). Computers were used to obtain records from other departments, for word processing, and for e-mail. Less than half of the respondents reported using computers for Internet searches (Dumas, Dietz, & Connolly, 2002). In the future, computer usage for obtaining guidelines and resources and the use of hand-held computers to track patient information will grow. Nurse practitioners need to be active in shaping the systems that support their practice.

))) SUMMARY

Documentation is an important aspect of nurse practitioner practice. It reflects the process of clinical judgment and supports quality care. The practice of recording data that supports problem solving and that reflects a

---

Box 5–4 Words of Wisdom

Don't let reimbursement drive your care. Follow these principles:
1. Practice your best care.
2. Document that care clearly.
3. Check the codes that are being submitted by your practice for reimbursement periodically.
4. Pay attention to updates in documentation and reimbursement guidelines.

---

patient's health status requires attention and time, but even in today's busy practice environment, it is essential for quality care. This chapter has shown an organized approach to documenting care in such a way as to support reasonable reimbursement for that care in a variety of settings (Box 5–4). Just as practice continually evolves, the system used to document that care and to be reimbursed will continue to evolve. Part of professional practice is to keep one's knowledge of documentation guidelines current. Nurse practitioners need to use documentation of care as a means of demonstrating the uniqueness and value of their care.

REFERENCES

American Medical Association/Health Care Financing Administration (1997). *Documentation guidelines for evaluation and management services.* Chicago: Author.

American Medical Association (2002). *Current Procedural Terminology 2003.* Chicago: Author.

Brennan, P. F., & Daly, B. J. (1996). Information requirements of advanced practice nurses. *Advanced Practice Nurse Quarterly, 2*(3), 54–57.

Buppert, C. (1999a). *Nurse practitioners' business practice and legal guide.* Gaithersburg, MD: Aspen.

Buppert, C. (1999b). When NPs need attorneys. *Nurse Practitioner World News, 4*(3), 1, 15.

Buppert, C. (2000a). Why be picky about CPT codes? *Nurse Practitioner World News, 5*(2), 1, 6.

Buppert, C. (2000b). Two recent developments in reimbursement. *Nurse Practitioner World News, 5*(4), 1, 14.

Buppert, C. (2000c). Two frequently asked questions concerning coding. *Nurse Practitioner World News, 5*(1), 1, 22.

Buppert, C. (2000d). How to make sure your CPT codes match your notes. *Green Sheet 2*(6), 1–4. Annapolis, MD: Author

Buppert, C. (2001). Avoiding Medicare fraud part 1. *Nurse Practitioner, 26*(1), 70, 72–27.

Buppert, C. (2002a). Complying with patient privacy requirements. *The Nurse Practitioner, 27*(5), 12, 14–15, 19–20, 23–24, 26, 29, 32.

Buppert, C. (2002b). Home visits: Keeping clear the distinction between physician services and nursing services. *Nurse Practitioner World News, 7*(5), 1, 18.

Castillo, S. A., Hopkins, C. A., & Aaron, W. S. (Eds.). (1998). *St. Anthony's ICD-9-CM Codebook for physician compliance* Vol. 1 & 2. Reston, VA: St. Anthony Publishing.

Chase, S. K., & Leuner, J. D. (2000). Documentation of nurse practitioner practice: Challenges and opportunities. In M. J. Rantz & P. Lemone (Eds.). *Classification of Nursing Diagnoses: Proceedings of the Thirteenth Conference of the North American Nursing Diagnosis Association* (pp. 299–304). Glendale, CA: CINAHL Information Systems.

Davis, A. L., Holman, E. J., & Sousa, K. H. (2000). Documentation of care outcomes in an academic nursing clinic: An assessment. *Journal of the American Academy of Nursing Practitioners, 12*, 497–502.

Dumas, J. A., Dietz, E. O., & Connolly, P. M. (2002). Nurse practitioner use of computer technologies in practice. *Computers in Nursing, 19*(1), 34–40.

Havens, D. H. & Williams, M. D. (1999). Medicare billing numbers: A necessity for PNPs. *Journal of Pediatric Health Care, 13*, 304–307.

Herrin, B. S. (2003). Practical considerations of HIPAA privacy rules compliance. *Clinician News, 7*(1), 8, 19–20.

Hsaio, W. C., Braun, P., Yntema, D., & Becker, E. R. (1988). Estimating physicians' work for a resource-based relative value scale. *New England Journal of Medicine, 319*, 835–841.

James, P. A. (2000). Managing patient information longitudinally. *The Journal of Family Practice, 49*, 716–717.

Leuner, J. D., & Chase, S. K. (1997). Nurse practitioners and nursing diagnosis: Is nursing practice visible? In M. J. Rantz & P. LeMone (Eds.). *Classification of Nursing Diagnoses: Proceedings of the Twelfth Conference of the North American Nursing Diagnosis Association* (pp. 306–313). Glendale, CA: Cinahl Information Systems.

Longworth, J. C. D., & Lesh, D. (2000). Development of a student nurse practitioner computerized clinical log. *Journal of the American Academy of Nurse Practitioners, 12*, 117–122.

Mazzocco, W. J. (2000). Nurse practitioners and incident-to billing: The indirect billing method. Medscape Nursing. *http://www.medscape.com/viewarticle/408391*.

Powers, J., Gillett, P., & Goldblum, K. (2000). Forms facilitating primary care documentation. *Nurse Practitioner: The American Journal of Primary Health Care, 25*(11), 40–44, 49.

Rapsilber, L. M., & Anderson, E. H. (2000). Understanding the reimbursement process. *Nurse Practitioner: The American Journal of Primary Health Care, 25*(5), 36, 43, 46, 51–52, 54–56.

Richmond, T. S., Thompson, H. J., & Sullivan-Marx, E. M. (2000). Reimbursement for acute care nurse practitioner services. *American Journal of Critical Care, 9*(1), 52–61.

Robinson, K. R., & Griffith, H. M. (1997). Identification of current procedural terminology-coded services provided by family nurse practitioners. *Clinical Excellence for Nurse Practitioners, 1*, 397–404.

Sheahan, S. L. (2000). Documentation of health risks and health promotion counseling by emergency department nurse practitioners and physicians. *Journal of Nursing Scholarship, 32*, 245–250.

Starr, D. S. (1999). Medicolegal charting. *The Clinical Advisor for Nurse Practitioners, 2*(5), 65.

Starr, D. S. (2003). Fraud prevention gets tougher. *The Clinical Advisor for Nurse Practitioners, 6*(5), 9.

Sullivan-Marx, E. M., & Maislin, G. (2000). Comparison of nurse practitioner and family physician relative work values. *Journal of Nursing Scholarship, 32*(1), 71–76.

Weed, L. L. (1971). *Medical records, medical education and patient care: The problem-oriented record as a basic teaching tool.* Chicago: Mosby.

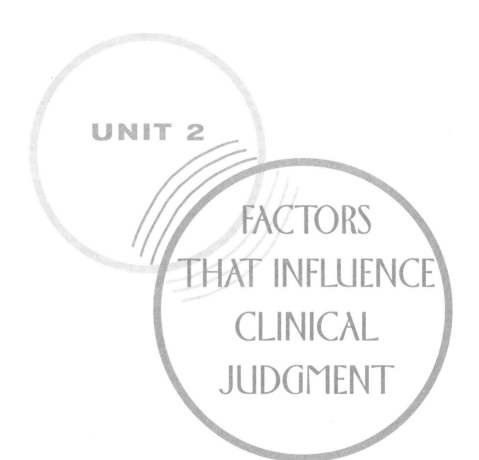

UNIT 2

FACTORS THAT INFLUENCE CLINICAL JUDGMENT

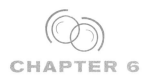

CHAPTER 6

Clinical Judgment for Special Populations

CHAPTER OUTLINE

Nurse practitioners can approach primary care in two ways. The first approach treats each individual as he or she appears to the practice. Good history taking and physical examination techniques support accuracy in diagnostic formulation and interventions selection. Each problem is dealt with appropriately, but something is missing in this approach. The second approach includes anticipating problems based on understanding patterns of risk that are associated with membership in various population subgroups. For example, young adults have different probabilities for illness than adolescents. Life issues that cause stress also vary by age group. Immigrants have unique access and illness problems. In some ways, knowing the population groups to which an individual patient belongs, for example, Central American immigrant, young adult, female, married, with rich extended family and limited English skills, living in poverty is one way of knowing the patient. Primary care should include preventive care, and knowing relative risk patterns as well as common predictable issues that affect health supports this aspect of care. The best care goes beyond problem-driven responses.

This chapter supports the use of the relationship-centered care model presented in Chapter 1. It provides information about what the patient brings to the clinical encounter. It encourages nurse practitioners to expand their knowledge about human development, culture, and family dynamics, among other things, and supports skill acquisition in clinical judgment. Further, it supports the development of an attitude of openness, acceptance, and respect for all of the human lives that nurse practitioners touch. All these topics help the nurse practitioner to recognize the unique health problems and health preferences that occur with different groups of patients so that clinical judgment can help nurse practitioners to efficiently diagnose problems and effectively assist patients in preventing health problems in the future.

SPECIAL POPULATIONS

When caring for patients who are members of special populations, nurse practitioners face a threefold challenge in applying clinical judgment. First, working with a member of a unique population requires special skill in establishing a therapeutic relationship. Members of vulnerable populations may have experienced impersonal care in the past. Immigrants may have been persecuted by "officials" in their home country or after coming to the United States. Adolescents may fear disclosure of private information about their behavior to their parents. Nurse practitioners must work to demonstrate that they are trustworthy and respectful by communicating clearly, keeping promises, and understanding that patients may experience barriers in maintaining their health because of their particular life situations. Nurse practitioners use the nurse-patient relationship for all patients, but special group status can affect the way in which relationships-centered care is enacted.

Second, nurse practitioners need to recognize that the range of diagnostic possibilities is affected by the patient's age and sociocultural or ethnic background. For example, if three young men present with fatigue, weight loss, and night sweats and one man is native-born white, one is native-born African-American, and one is a Central American immigrant, the likelihood of a tuberculosis infection is greater for the African-American and the Central American. Other differential diagnoses would include lymphoma. Considering incidence and prevalence data for subpopulations will support accuracy in forming clinical judgments.

Finally, nurse practitioners must understand that treatment goals and therapeutic choices vary by age group, culture and ethnicity group, and socioeconomic group. Building a knowledge base of various risks and strengths for each patient population discussed in this chapter requires years of experience, but it is very rewarding. The challenge for novice clinicians is to transcend their insecurities and focus on the person and the situation at hand to effectively guide health-related decision making. This chapter focuses on several special populations commonly encountered in clinical practice and offers a perspective that supports high-quality clinical judgments for all of these patients.

﹚ CULTURAL COMPETENCE

Culture encompasses many ways of being in the world. Social norms determine communication patterns, hierarchies of power, family and gender roles, values in relationships, health values, cleanliness beliefs, nutritional preference and laws, religious practices, and many other aspects of life. The National Organization of Nurse Practitioner Faculties (NONPF) has developed a set of competencies for graduates of nurse practitioner programs in the United States (DHHS, 2002). The NONPF based its initial set on domains described by Brykczynski (1989), which were the result of qualitative research with nurse practitioners. Box 6–1 lists the nurse

---

Box 6–1 Nurse Practitioner Competency Domains Identified by the National Organization of Nurse Practitioner Faculties (NONPF)

Domain
Management of patient health/illness status
The nurse practitioner-patient relationship
The teaching-coaching function
Professional role
Managing and negotiating health-care delivery systems
Monitoring and ensuring the quality of health-care practice
Cultural competencies

---

practitioner domains. The NONPF guidelines recommend that principles of epidemiology and demography be applied when determining populations at risk. NONPF guidelines include a domain of cultural competence, and elements of that domain are reflected in Box 6–2. American culture is becoming increasingly diverse. A global economy and economic and political forces bring people from all over the world to the shores of North America.

Educating new nurse practitioners for culturally competent care requires several phases (Chase & Hunter, 2002). First the novice nurse practitioner must *develop cultural sensitivity*. This phase raises awareness that cultural influences affect many aspects of life. It forces the nurse practitioner to recognize that people from other cultures are not just different from "us," but that each culture has a coherence of its own. One begins to develop cultural sensitivity by exploring one's own cultural values and suspending one's own cultural beliefs. This can be difficult because so much of culture is learned as a child, and much is taken for granted and

---

Box 6–2 Competencies of Cultural Competence as Identified by the National Organization of Nurse Practitioner Faculties

1. Shows respect for the inherent dignity of every human being, whatever his or her age, gender, religion, socioeconomic class, sexual orientation, or ethnicity
2. Accepts the rights of individuals to choose their care provider, participate in care, and refuse care.
3. Acknowledges personal biases and prevents these from interfering with the delivery of quality care to persons of differing beliefs and lifestyles.
4. Recognizes cultural issues and interacts with patients from other cultures in culturally sensitive ways.
5. Incorporates cultural preferences, health beliefs and behaviors, and traditional practices into the management plan.
6. Develops patient-appropriate educational materials that address the language and cultural beliefs of the patient.
7. Accesses culturally appropriate resources to deliver care to patients from other cultures.
8. Assists patients to access quality care within a dominant culture.
9. Develops and applies a process for assessing differing beliefs and preferences and takes this diversity into account when planning and delivering care.

left unexamined. It is often challenging to one's own values to realize that many cultures have values that may have advantages that do not exist in dominant western culture. For example, in many cultures older adults are respected and valued for the wisdom that they contribute to the family and to society. In contrast, western societies tend to value economic productivity and therefore marginalize older adults. This can lead to the problem of depression, which is a particularly western problem. When assessing an older client who may have decreased concentration abilities and decreased appetite and energy levels, several diagnostic hypotheses come to mind, including hypothyroidism and early dementia. Depression should be included on the differential diagnosis list for every elder presenting with these symptoms, but particularly for native-born Americans.

The second phase of developing cultural competence is to *gain knowledge of particular cultures*. One could choose to start with the cultures that are predominant in one's own area. For example, a California city might have large populations of Pacific island natives and Mexican-Americans who have newly immigrated or people whose families have been there for several generations. A Plains state might have more exposure to Native American people, whereas a nurse practitioner working in Miami will need to be familiar with several Latin-American cultures. One danger at this stage of learning is to resort to stereotyping. To say that all Latino males are motivated by machismo is a stereotypic thought. To understand how machismo operates in the Latino family in general can help one be sensitive to the variations of Latino family life that one might encounter in clinical practice, but individual persons and families maintain their own uniqueness.

Anthropology researchers who are studying a particular culture use a person who helps them understand called the key informant. The key informant is a person from the culture of interest who has the ability to reflect on the practices and customs of the culture and to describe them to an outsider. Extended conversations with a member of the cultural group allow for exploring such concepts as explanatory models of illness and particular health beliefs such as hot versus cold foods in some cultures. Explanatory models of illness are the beliefs about how and why illnesses occur. In Western culture we tend to use the germ theory to describe infectious diseases or a biomechanical model to describe such conditions as coronary artery disease. Eastern cultures use explanatory models that involve the balance of energy called yin and yang. Some illnesses are cold conditions and should be treated with special foods. Latino cultures also use the concept of hot and cold to describe illness.

Another reason why it is important to understand particular cultural practices is that it is easy to offend people from other cultures by simply being ignorant of different cultural practices. For example, many cultures see it as a sign of disrespect to engage in direct eye contact, but Westerners may misinterpret this behavior as lack of attention or interest. This kind of assumption can prevent a mutually trusting relationship from developing. Spending time in a specific community, attending community events, and sharing in community life can be ways in which student or even experienced clinicians can gain cultural knowledge.

Finally, the third phase of cultural competence enables one to *understand the person's experience of health from his or her own point of view*. This requires all the other levels, including suspending one's own cultural beliefs, in trying to understand the values and practices of the patient and family in one's care. It also requires individualizing the approach to the client. In a way, these are questions that one should consider when developing a relationship with anyone, but the issues are more variable and more powerful for people from another culture.

> RULE OF THUMB: Nurse practitioners can gain cultural competence by considering such questions as: "What is the theory of illness in use by this person, or how does the patient think that he or she got sick?" "What issues of acceptance must be negotiated in developing an intervention plan?" "What cultural practices already valued by this person will assist his or her health promotion and maintenance?" "Are there healers or practitioners from this person's culture whom he or she will also see, and how can a treatment plan be developed that is mutually compatible?"

This phase goes beyond the previous one in that the nurse practitioner does not rely on general assumptions about cultural values and practices, but goes on to use that knowledge to individualize care.

In order to establish care settings that are welcoming to people from other cultures, one can develop a community advisory board with membership from cultural groups who use the services of the practice. Some practices intentionally employ members of ethnic groups in order to have representation in the practice setting. Physical structure and decoration of the practice setting can establish a welcoming environment for care.

Language and Interpreters

In many settings, nurse practitioners who care for immigrants or foreign visitors need to use interpreters. However, there are limitations to using interpreters because they act as a filter between the nurse practitioner's words and the patient's words. Skilled medical interpreters understand the major health-related concepts that are of interest to the nurse practitioner and can approach the patient in a culturally competent manner. Issues of interpreter gender can be problematic sometimes. If the only Arabic interpreter available is male when taking a history from a Muslim woman, one can expect that the full range of information might not be available. It may seem ideal to have the interpreter be a member of the same cultural community as the patient, but issues of trust and confidentiality are important. The interpreter must understand these values and maintain strict confidentiality. When the nurse practitioner can gain skill in the language of the predominant cultural groups through formal language instruction, and informally through repeated exposure to the language through translation, this can increase the effectiveness of the communication. However, real translation requires deep understanding of patients' cultural ways; simply speaking the language may not be sufficient. One of the true joys of working with diverse groups of patients is the richness of learning about new cultures from the patients themselves. By taking time to try to learn the values and ways, we honor the people who present themselves to us for care.

)) FAMILY-FOCUSED CARE FOR ALL NURSE PRACTITIONERS

Family-focused care is not limited to family nurse practitioners. All nurse practitioners must take into account the individual's living situation, and family constellation is an important element of this context. Family constellation is important to the care of older adults as well as the care of children. Nurse theorists debate the importance and centrality of family as a concept necessary for care. Some argue that the family itself is the client and that individuals are important in relation to the way in which they contribute to the family function. Others argue that the family should be taken in context. This is an issue that individual nurse practitioners can decide based on what works in their practice and what values they hold. In any case, the family is important to consider in assessing, planning, and evaluating care.

Growth and Development

Growth and development are concepts that apply to every life stage. Psychological theorists of growth and development, such as Erikson (1986), have described stages of healthy growth for every age group. Healthy growth and development is a process that requires energy and can cause disequilibrium during stage change. By applying knowledge of developmental theories to practice, the nurse practitioner can use anticipatory guidance to support patients of all ages and their families through the stress of developmental change. For example, the task of adolescence is to forge an identity that is individual. This requires separation from the family of origin and attachment to a peer group. Parents may have difficulty relinquishing control over their adolescent, which can result in acting out behaviors by the adolescent. Helping parents understand effective communication and limit setting can assist them and the entire family as the adolescent works through the developmental tasks of that stage.

The family itself can be seen as experiencing predictable developmental tasks. Specific milestones and stressors are associated with the various stages of family life. At the *couple* stage, the new family establishes the partnership and develops new relationships with kin networks. At the *childbearing family* stage, the family adjusts to role demands of parenting. The *family with preschoolers* must maintain energy levels and financial security while supporting the growth of the child. The *family with school-age children* now relates to the community in more ways as the child enters school. The *family with adolescents* must learn to help the adolescent to balance freedom and responsibility. The *family with young adult children* will release the offspring to the community and re-establish the couple relationship. The *grandparenting family* prepares for old age and forges relationships with the new generation. The *family with older adults* adjusts to retirement, loss of spouse or partner, and increasing risk of chronic illness (Mandle, 2002). Each of these stages presents stresses and opportunities for nurse practitioner support in order to reduce health risks and promote quality of life and family functioning.

Infants and Children

Patterns of family function and of temperament and personality are formed and shaped from the very beginning. Caring for pediatric patients is a case of caring for a moving target. The growth and development of a person from infancy to adulthood is a story of constant change in the physical, psychological, emotional, family, and social context of the child. Clinical judgment regarding the care of infants and children is focused on healthy development and health promotion. Screening for health problems and for developmental delays forms the basis for much of pediatric practice. Maintaining a longitudinal database is essential to pediatric care because it tracks changes over time. The database will maintain records of developmental milestone attainment, physical growth, immunizations, and screenings for such risks as lead poisoning. Recording each piece of data in an episodic SOAP note will make retrieval of information difficult to track. Flow sheets for each of the specific data elements such as growth charts can be filed in the patient record. This database serves as a basis for "knowing the patient" in ways that are appropriate for pediatrics. Areas that are required to be documented include those listed in Table 6–1.

Clinical judgment begins with taking a history. For infants and young children, this invariably requires getting the history from a family member. In using this intermediary, the nurse practitioner must be sensitive to issues of competence that parents might feel when being questioned about their child. Getting to know the pediatric patient requires getting to know the family, with its hopes and fears and special circumstances. Because the

TABLE 6–1

Elements of the Pediatric/Adolescent Chart

Chart Element	Content	Strategies for Data Tracking
Demographic data	Birth date, address, insurance, ethnicity	Baseline with updates as needed
Family history	Health and illness of relatives	
Problem list	Episodic and chronic problems being addressed, with dates	Running list ideally in front of chart
Drug allergies	Substances and type of reaction	Prominently displayed on cover and front of chart
Medication list	Medications, dosages, dates	Running list near front of chart
Visit notes		
Reason for visit	Scheduled checkup or problem focused in family terms, could be behavior or development related	"S" in SOAP format or other consistent system
History of present condition	Concise evaluation using OLDCART or other format	"S" in SOAP
Past history	Birth history: includes maternal health, birth	"S" in SOAP

(Continued)

TABLE 6-1

Elements of the Pediatric/Adolescent Chart *(Continued)*

Chart Element	Content	Strategies for Data Tracking
	weight, special care required, Apgar score	
Past medical history	Summarized as pertinent to problem or focus of visits	"S" in SOAP
Daily life	Feeding, sleep patterns, elimination milestones, general activity level, who lives at home	"S" in SOAP
Review of systems	Systematic review to fill in gaps in history	"S" in SOAP
Developmental screening	Tracking on national norms, e.g., Denver development	Tracking forms filed in chart
Screening data	Include vision or hearing screening	"O" in SOAP
Growth charts	Tracking height and weight	Tracking forms filed in chart
Immunization record	Dates, lot numbers of all immunizations	Tracking forms filed in chart

Source: Adapted from Lustig, J. V. (1995). Approaching the pediatric patient. In W. W. Hay, J. R. Groothuis, A. A . Hayward, & M. J. Levin (Eds.). *Current pediatric diagnosis & treatment* (pp. 1–8). Norwalk, CT: Appleton & Lange. Reproduced with permission of The McGraw-Hill Companies.

health of the infant is dependent on the health of the family unit, the history-taking time is a time to obtain information about the family's skills, strengths, and questions.

Care of the infant ideally begins with prenatal visits. These visits introduce the care team to the family and, particularly for the first child, introduce the concept of pediatric care. Newborn visits are designed to screen for congenital or birth injury problems, to assess and support family-infant bonding, and to offer guidance for feeding and general care. Physical examination of the newborn includes inspection of skin, head, eyes, ears, nose, mouth, musculoskeletal system, and external genitalia; auscultation of chest and abdomen; and neurological reflex evaluation (Hay, Groothuis, Hayward, & Levin, 1995). The leading causes of death for children from birth to 1 year of age are congenital anomalies and other birth defects, disorders related to premature birth, and sudden infant death syndrome (U.S. Department of Health and Human Services, 2000). Knowing these risks, the nurse practitioner focuses assessment activities to detect these problems, as well as teaching and support to avoid preventable causes of death, such as trauma. General screening guidelines from the U.S. Preventive Service Task Force (USPSTF, 2003) are listed in Table 6–2, with recommend special screening for special populations in Table 6–3. For example, preterm infants are at risk for anemia, so screening is recommended. Children with chronic cardiac conditions should be screened for tuberculosis and should have pneumococcal and influenza vaccines administered. In addition, the Task Force recommends that clinicians remain alert for certain conditions that can be improved if detected early, such as signs of ocular misalignment, hearing impairment, and dental problems.

Developmental assessment includes physical, language, behavioral, and emotional changes that occur across the ages and stages of childhood and adolescence. General assessments of the ways in which the child responds to the experience of coming to the health center or office is one way of doing an overall assessment. Standard screening instruments such as the Denver II development screen (Frankenburg & Dodds, 1991) and the Early Language Milestone Scale (ELM) (Coplan, 1987) can be used to track milestones. These forms can be filed in a section of the chart to be

---

TABLE 6–2

Screening and Prevention, Birth to 10 Years

Screening	Preventive Education
Height and weight	Child car seats and shoulder belts
Blood pressure	Bicycle helmets
Vision screening ages 3–4	Smoke detector
Phenylalanine (birth)	Hot water heater temperature
Hemoglobinopathy (birth)	Window, pool, stair guards
T4 or TSH (birth)	Safe storage of drugs and chemicals
	Poison control and ipecac
	CPR training
	Nutrition and activity
	Passive smoking effects
	Dental care importance
	Immunizations

Source: Adapted from United States Preventive Services Task Force, 2003.

TABLE 6–3

High Risk Screening for Children, Birth to 10 Years

High-Risk Populations	Screening
Preterm or low birth weight	Hemoglobin/hematocrit (Hgb/Hct)
Mother at risk for HIV	HIV testing, mother and child
Low income, immigrants	Hgb/Hct
TB contacts	PPD
Travelers to developing countries	Hepatitis A vaccine
Native Americans/Alaskan natives	Hgb/Hct; hepatitis A, pneumococcal vaccine
Residents of long-term care facilities	PPD
Chronic cardiac or pulmonary disease	PPD, pneumococcal, influenza vaccines
Community lead exposure	Blood lead level
Water not fluoridated	Daily fluoride supplements
Family history of skin cancer, fair skin	Avoid sun exposure

Source: Adapted from United States Preventive Services Task Force, 2003.

updated on routine visits. Tracking the information in one place will assist clinical judgment regarding progress in meeting developmental milestones and will help the nurse practitioner determine if consultation or intervention is required to assist development.

In the special setting of neonatal intensive care (NICU), clinical judgment encompasses principles of neonatal care and general critical care, which include establishment of hemodynamic stability and oxygenation. Constant assessment for signs of sepsis, necrotizing enterocolitis, and intracerebral bleeding and vigilance in energy conservation for the infant by minimizing environmental stimulation are the hallmarks of NICU nursing for all nurses in that setting. Nurse practitioners provide leadership in quality care in the NICU setting and support the activities of the staff nurses. Having a child in the NICU is a stressful time for parents. They need honest communication about the status of their child and need preparation for the time they will be able to spend with the child. Each child is a unique individual, and sensitivity to the response patterns of each child will support excellence in clinical judgment and management of the NICU experience. Other critical-care judgment concepts are covered in Chapter 8, Clinical Judgment and Acute-Care Nurse Practitioners.

Office visits for toddlers usually require modification of the environment of a family practice suite. The physical environment should provide visual distraction and safe, cleanable objects that allow the nurse practitioner to observe the child's attention, manipulation, and engagement with novelty. The first phase of clinical judgment, the history, will continue to come from the parent for younger children. Often in pediatric or family settings, more than one member of the family is examined in the same visit (Box 6–3). This requires some adjustment of the normal order of an examination and may require information management to sort out—for example, which child is having the third ear infection and which is having trouble sleeping. The order of the physical examination frequently needs to be adjusted for the toddler. Although many physical assessment courses teach a head-to-toe approach, the ear examination can be the most invasive for the toddler and should be saved for last. The nurse practitioner can auscultate the chest while the child is seated quietly on the parent's lap. The chief cause of death in children aged 1 to 4 years is unintentional injury, with birth defects and cancer in second and third place (USDHHS, 2000). The nurse practitioner should consider these risk patterns when screening and providing anticipatory guidance.

A greater portion of the history for the school-age child can come directly from the child. The child's uniqueness is an important facet of the history. For the school-age child who develops shyness about his or her body, the nurse practitioner begins the exam while the child is clothed and

---

Box 6–3 Words of Wisdom

Yesterday I had a father coming in with his two children; the one was eight months and the one was three years. The father was foreign born; the children were born in the US, and it was an intact family. Both children were on Medicaid. I saw they were scheduled to be my 4:15 and 4:30 patients, but they were there at 1 o'clock in the afternoon, which was the first thing that struck me as odd...

Dad was very frazzled. He was sitting with the eight-month-old baby in his lap while the three-year-old was tearing apart the exam room. It was hard to interview dad to get at the essence of the purpose of the visit because the three-year-old was just out of control. And dad made no attempt to discipline her... The eight-month-old was there for a well baby check and the three-year-old because of an upper respiratory infection and behavior problems. These are new patients. Talking to dad, it was clear to me that he didn't have any sense of how or that he should discipline this little girl. Come to find out in getting a history from him, someone had called him in to HRS for hitting the child, maybe a year prior to this, because in his country, you were disciplined by physically spanking.

(Continued)

Box 6–3 Words of Wisdom *(Continued)*

He is from Haiti. He was born and raised in Haiti, as was his wife, and they saved up their money and they were married in Haiti. They didn't have any children in Haiti, but they came over on one of these boats illegally and really worked hard, and they got their green cards…Both children were born in the United States, but after his three year old was born but before the eight month old was born, he disciplined this little girl, and then the HRS incident occurred. They had done no discipline since that time. They were very worried about being called into HRS again. So they went from disciplining the child with smacking her bottom as he describes it to no discipline, and the child is out of control. He describes to me that she is even more out of control since the birth of this eight month old. That she is just horribly jealous and just does everything she can to get attention.

So we had to go back and do a whole lot of learning about what is normal growth and development at each stage, how to intervene with this, what is appropriate, how to discipline, why you would want to discipline. They have this little three year-old in a day care center and she is being asked to leave the day care because she is pushing children down. Both he and his wife work two jobs and they try to switch off in child care, and he has worked twelve hours by the time he picks this child up from day care and takes care of the eight month old as well. And, he has absolutely, positively no energy to discipline this child. So he does nothing, but he hates her because she is awful. He said to me, "I can't stand her." So you never know if that's something you want to go into; I mean this is basic stuff, but this is Advanced Practice. But, you know, are you going to write this kid off as a brat, or are you going to help this child and this family?…

So what did you do with this guy?

We got the history. He was there for a well baby visit and the three-year-old had an upper respiratory infection. Nothing horrible. Also she was not sleeping at night. I am not sure if it was just pure lack of discipline, but someone who is not sleeping at night is, you know in this age group where they are starting to dream about monsters. She had been immunized because she was in daycare, but not the baby. The baby has not had any immunizations because the baby is cared for by a relative, because I guess they can't afford two kids in day care. But this three-year-old is such a handful the relative won't take her.

The first thing we did was address the need for the little girl and I got the history, did the physical exam, and he held the baby. It was obvious he didn't want to interact with their little girl at all. So, I took care of her and I had to physically sit her on my lap and restrain her, and she cried and screamed the

(Continued)

Box 6–3 Words of Wisdom

whole time. It was a blood-curdling scream. I had to get a medical assistant to hold her to look in her ears and to look in her throat, and she chomped down on the stick, and she was very difficult to examine. But after about ten minutes, she settled down and she just sat down in my lap. I asked her to throw things out for me in the garbage and then come back, and she did.

She threw things out and she came back to me and was just the cutest little thing. Part of my education to the father was, "She really wants discipline, dad; she wants to please you. And it is OK to discipline her; it's OK to take her by the arms and sit her down, you know. Not jerking her arms, or shaking her, but just 'sit down here' and putting her in her room." And he said, "but she bangs on the door." I said, "It's OK. She can bang on the door."

She'll get angry and she will not eat for him; then she will just sit and scream. We had to talk about some education, that neurologically intact children don't starve themselves. From every aspect that I could see, this was a neurologically intact child who was actually quite pleasant when she understood that pulling things off the wall, taking everything out of cabinets was not going to be acceptable. She learned that there was a lollipop at the end of this rainbow; that there was a trip to the treasure chest and in this deal for her. I mean is that a typical thing in primary care? No, it's not. Most parents already have a clue that they have to discipline their children, but this guy was too frightened to discipline this child.

I treated the respiratory infection. We just treated her with a little antihistamine, a little Motrin; nasal drainage was clear and everything, and the baby's exam was normal, and the child seems to meet the mental milestones. But we talked about the importance of immunizations and education. But this gentleman just physically doesn't have the time.

What were your thought and feelings during the encounter?

I could identify with the man. I was first of all very impressed because we don't get a whole lot of fathers that come in. I was impressed by his diligence in getting to the United States, wanting better for himself and his wife. He had a very heavy accent, but he was very understandable if you took time with him. He was very understandable and made good sense. I could identify with the gentleman, you know, not the foreign born piece of it, but in working very hard, and raising a child and going to school and everything. I could really identify with this gentleman's frustration, and truthfully I know where he was at, because it is true, it would be easier to let the child run than to do some discipline. Discipline is a lot of work, a lot of work, after you have had a full day and you are tired yourself. It's not the first thing you want to do.

(Continued)

Box 6–3 Words of Wisdom *(Continued)*

The satisfying piece was when the little girl waved bye-bye to me at the end of the interview. You know, I almost felt like maybe I did make a difference in this child's life. Maybe this child won't be shunned by society because she behaves so horribly. Advocacy is not a new role, but my level of accountability is. I am willing to see that kid. I am willing to provide the medical care. So yeah, I see there is a higher degree of accountability, but I can say that I am willing to accept that accountability for the benefit of the child.

Source: Dunphy, L. (1999)The wisdom of advanced practice nurses: Approaches to diagnosis and treatment. Unpublished raw interview data. Used with permission.

proceeds to genital examination at the end of the assessment. The chief causes of death in children aged 5 to 14 years are unintentional injury, cancer, and homicide (USDHHS, 2000). Including the child in discussion of risk factors and safety is important for this age group. See Tables 6–2 and 6–3 for specific screening suggestions for children through age 10 (USPSTF, 2003). Children with chronic diseases such as asthma or diabetes need to learn principles of self-management. Concrete reinforcement of health progress through peak flow meter charts or blood glucose readings can be managed by the child in most cases. Nurse practitioners can develop a niche practice by specializing in care of chronically ill children (Lindeke, Krajicek & Patterson, 2001).

Adolescents

Adolescents grow and change tremendously during the teenage years. This is often a turbulent time in the family when adolescents test their independence and the capacity of home and school to limit their behavior. The office environment will need adjustment for the comfort of the adolescent. Ideally in a pediatric practice, an adolescent area can be developed, or scheduling can allow for young children in the morning and older children in the afternoon. A 15-year-old will not appreciate being interviewed and examined in a room with cartoon figures on the walls. In a family practice environment, adolescents can be seen in adult examining rooms.

Depending on state laws, adolescents are still minors and need consent for treatment by a responsible adult. Many adolescents are reluctant to have their entire history taken in the presence of a parent, so having the parent present for part, but not all, of the visit is an option. However, some families and cultures will find this approach unacceptable.

The nurse practitioner should discuss the visit with the adolescent and the parent and decide together how to proceed. For reluctant parents, the nurse practitioner can explain that adolescents will get more complete care if they feel free to ask any questions; however, the nurse practitioner should also recognize the importance of honoring the family's preference. This discussion can be affected by laws that allow adolescents to receive care independently under circumstances that allow them to be declared emancipated minors. Nurse practitioners need to be aware of federal, state, and local laws that govern consent and privacy (Maradiegue, 2003).

Clinical judgments about the health and the health risks for adolescents are affected by the risk patterns for the group. As with any age group, reducing the risk of injury and death requires knowing the greatest risk for a person of that age. The chief causes of death in young people aged 15 to 24 years are unintentional injury, homicide, and suicide (USDHHS, 2000). These are preventable deaths. Helping adolescents to be realistic about the risks that their new freedom entails is an important task for nurse practitioners working with adolescents in settings such as clinics, schools, or community centers.

Adolescents are at risk for death by trauma because they typically feel proud of their physical strength and engage in risk-taking behavior as a celebration of their strength and freedom. The tragedy of traumatic death or disability is a real threat to the lives and health of adolescents. The nurse practitioner should question each adolescent patient about seat belt and helmet use, sexual activity, drug and alcohol use, and peer group or school violence risk. Human immunodeficiency virus (HIV) infection is most often identified in the young adult age group. This means that many people are exposed to HIV during the adolescent years. The nurse practitioner can reduce risks of sexually transmitted diseases (STDs) and HIV infection by openly communicating about safe sex techniques before and after adolescents become sexually active. Cigarette smoking remains a risk factor for cardiovascular disease in later life. Patterns established during childhood and adolescence are hard to break in later life. Active smoking cessation programs for adolescents need to take into account the special needs of this age group to be accepted by peers. Group programs in settings that are accessible could make a difference in adolescent smoking patterns.

Adolescents are establishing health patterns that will affect their entire lives. Nurse practitioners can help adolescents to learn to make decisions that will protect their health in the present and the future. Table 6–4 reflects screening and prevention guidelines for young people aged 11 to 24

TABLE 6–4	
Screening and Prevention for Ages 11 to 24 Years	
Screening	Prevention
Height and weight	Patient education includes instruction about:
Blood pressure	◎ Seat belt use
Pap test for women (sexually active)	◎ Bicycle/motorcycle safety
Chlamydia screen (sexually active)	◎ Smoke detector
Rubella serology or vaccination	◎ Safe storage or removal of firearms
Assess for problem drinking	◎ Tobacco avoidance
	◎ Avoid underage drinking of alcohol
	◎ Avoid alcohol while driving, boating, swimming
	◎ STD prevention
	◎ Nutrition and exercise
	◎ Calcium intake (women)
	Dental care
	Immunizations
	Multivitamins with folic acid (women planning pregnancy)

Source: Adapted from United States Preventive Services Task Force, 2003.

years. Table 6–5 shows recommendations for high-risk populations in that age group.

Young Adults

Young adults aged 18 to 24 years are the least likely group of Americans to report having a regular source of primary care (USDHHS, 2000). Young adult women receive health care often for menstrual difficulties or for contraception. It is less likely for young adult men to receive regular preventive care. Kudzma (2002) cites government statistics that men are 66 percent less likely to receive primary care than women in matched age groups. Many entry-level jobs do not offer health insurance, so young people, even though they are working, may not have access to health care, and at the same time, their incomes may prevent them from receiving free care programs. Clinical judgment about health risks and problems from this age group is likely to be affected by limited access to the population.

TABLE 6–5

High-Risk Populations Ages 11 to 24 Years

Population	Potential Screening and Prevention
High-risk sexual behavior	RPR/VDRL, gonorrhea, *Chlamydia,* hepatitis A and B vaccine, HIV testing
Injection or street drug use	RPR, HIV, hepatitis A and B vaccine, PPD
TB contacts	PPD
Native Americans/Alaskan natives	PPD, hepatitis A, pneumococcal vaccine
Travelers	Hepatitis A vaccine
Chronic medical conditions	PPD; pneumococcal, influenza vaccine
Blood transfusion between 1975 and 1985	HIV screen
Institutionalized persons, health-care or lab workers	Hepatitis A, influenza vaccine
Family history of skin cancer, fair skin	Sun exposure prevention
Previous pregnancy with neural tube defect	Folic acid 4.0 mg daily
Inadequate water fluoridation	Fluoride supplement

Source: Adapted from United States Preventive Services Task Force, 2003.

The most likely places to see young adults are college or occupational health settings. As a group, young adults are relatively healthy and have few chronic health problems. However, when nurse practitioners identify health risks and engage in discussions supporting health promotion with young adults, lifelong patterns of health can be supported. The leading causes of death in young people aged 25 to 44 years are unintentional injury, cancer, and heart disease (USDHHS, 2000). Screening for cardiac risk factors, teaching breast and testicular self-examination, and maintaining an index of suspicion for testicular cancer and lymphomas, common young adult cancers, can improve diagnostic accuracy in this age group. Hypertension in this age group increases risk for cardiovascular disease in later life and should be identified and managed. Suicide is a health risk for young adults also. Primary care nurse practitioners need to be attentive to suggestions of depression and suicidal thoughts. Young people are accomplishing developmental tasks of finding a life mate and establishing a family. People in this age group are able to participate in their own care and make decisions that will affect their health in the years to come. The young adult years are the main childbearing years. Young adults of both genders may encounter issues related to their own or their offspring's genetic makeup. Understanding of possibly complicated transmission patterns can be supported by direct teaching by the nurse practitioner. Table 6–6 reflects screening and prevention guidelines for adults aged 25 to 64 years. Table 6–7 shows recommended screenings for special high-risk groups.

Middle-Aged Adults

Middle-aged adults have established their families and careers. They are frequently considered to be the "sandwich" generation with responsibilities for the care of their children and of their aging parents. Stress is high

TABLE 6–6	
Screening and Prevention for Ages 25 to 64 Years	
Screening	**Prevention**
Blood pressure	Tobacco cessation
Height and weight	Patient education includes instruction about:
Total blood cholesterol, men age 35+, women age 45+	◎ Avoid alcohol ingestion while driving, swimming, boating
Pap test for women	◎ Diet and exercise
Fecal occult blood test annually age >=50	◎ Calcium intake (women)
Sigmoidoscopy age 50+, every 5 years	◎ Seat-belt use
Mammogram for women age 50–69	◎ Motorcycle, bicycle helmets
Problem drinking	◎ Smoke detector
Rubella (women of childbearing age)	◎ Firearm safety
	◎ STD prevention
	◎ Unintended pregnancy prevention
	Dental care
	Immunizations
	Multivitamin with folic acid (women planning pregnancy)
	Discuss hormone replacement (perimenopausal women)

Source: Adapted from United States Preventive Services Task Force, 2003.

for this segment of the population because they are in their peak earning years, planning for retirement and beginning to see the effects of aging on their own health. There is a wide range of health issues for this age group. Many are as healthy as they ever were and maintain active lifestyles with balanced work and recreational life. Many others, however, are beginning to develop type 2 diabetes mellitus, heart disease, arthritis, menopause-related symptoms, and cancer. People in this age group are able to participate in their own care, but they may be overwhelmed with responsibilities and find it difficult to take on exercise programs or to change their diet. Economic differences take their toll, and there can be disparity in access to health care.

TABLE 6–7

High-Risk Populations Ages 25 to 64 Years

High-Risk Group	Potential Screening and Prevention
High-risk sexual behavior	RPR/VDRL, gonorrhea, *Chlamydia* screen, hepatitis A/B vaccine
Injection or street drug use	RPR/VDRL, HIV screen, hepatitis A/B vaccine, advice to reduce infection risk
Low income; TB contacts; immigrants; alcoholics	PPD
Native Americans/Alaskan natives	Pneumococcal, hepatitis A vaccine, PPD
Travelers to developing countries	Hepatitis A/B vaccine
Chronic medical conditions	PPD, pneumococcal, influenza vaccine
Blood product recipient	HIV screen, hepatitis B vaccine
Susceptible to measles, mumps, rubella, varicella	MMR, Varicella immunization
Institutionalized persons	PPD, hepatitis A, pneumococcal, influenza vaccine
Health-care workers, lab technicians	Hepatitis A/B influenza vaccines, PPD
Family with skin cancer, fair skin	Sun exposure prevention
Previous pregnancy with neural tube defect	Folic acid 4.0 mg daily

Source: Adapted from United States Preventive Services Task Force, 2003.

The leading causes of death in people aged 45 to 64 years are malignant neoplasms, heart disease, motor vehicle and other unintentional injuries, HIV infection, suicide, and homicide (USPSTF, 2003). These patterns form the basis for recommendations for screening and counseling. As a person ages, the likelihood of developing a chronic illness increases. Clinical judgment for middle-aged adults requires recognition of the likely causes of disease for that age group. Diagnostic hypotheses are affected by understanding risk factors and subpopulation membership. For example, subpopulations such as Hispanics and African-Americans are more likely to develop type 2 diabetes mellitus. Nurse practitioners should also be alert for symptoms of arterial disease in smokers and diabetics, skin lesions that could be malignant, and signs of oral cancer in tobacco users or heavy alcohol users. Thyroid disease has subtle signs and symptoms and should be assessed in middle-aged persons. Changes in functional status can be signs of early dementia or of reversible causes. Depression and suicide should be routinely screened for, as should evidence of family violence. See Table 6–6 for general screening and Table 6–7 for screening for special populations for people aged 25 to 64 years (USPSTF, 2003).

Older Adults

Older adults are the fastest-growing segment of our population in North America. This fact and the fact that people in this age group tend to have multiple chronic conditions result in their being a large percentage of primary-care patients. Gerontological nurse practitioners specialize in the complex management of older adults, but adult, family, women's health, and psychiatric nurse practitioners all see older people in their practices. Clinical judgment for this age group is affected in several ways. First, the complexity of the patient's history can lead the novice nurse practitioner to information overload. It can be difficult to sort out the most important or underlying problem from a long list of positive findings. One strategy for sorting out issues is to focus first on the problem that the patient identifies as the most troubling. Setting up subsequent regular appointments that will address health promotion and screening supports that strategy. Documentation for one visit can set an agenda for health issues for the next visit. For example, a patient might make an appointment for evaluation of troubling joint pain. The nurse practitioner can focus on evaluation and management of osteoarthritis on that visit and set up an appointment for a cardiac risk assessment at the next appointment. Of course, if the blood pressure is high on the osteoarthritis visit, that finding cannot be ignored and must be addressed.

Another reason that caring for older adults can be complicated is that altered homeostatic patterns cause altered compensatory mechanisms and a diminished margin of reserve. A problem that should be minor in young or middle-aged people can throw off a wide range of homeostatic mechanisms for older adults. Altered physiology also results in different presentation of common problems. For example, older adults may not demonstrate elevated temperatures, even with severe infections. The way in which these problems become apparent might be a change in affect or mentation.

Finally, dementia or cognitive decline can diminish the older person's ability to give an accurate history or describe symptoms. Noting subtle changes in behavior patterns for patients who may be demented takes an understanding of the patient's baseline patterns. Here, as in other areas of diagnosis and judgment, knowing the patient is key to accurate and timely diagnosis. When a patient is well known by the nurse practitioner, a new vagueness in response would be noted that would not necessarily be recognized by a practitioner meeting the patient for the first time. When doing an initial evaluation of an older client, the nurse practitioner may need to rely on the report of family members to determine if the patient is behaving at his or her usual level of alertness.

Another feature essential to the assessment of elder health is a focus on function. Activities of daily living (ADLs) include eating, toileting, dressing, bathing, transferring, and continence. Toileting is distinct from continence in that it involves recognizing the need to toilet, moving to the toilet, adjusting clothing to allow elimination, and cleaning and redressing. Difficulties in sensation or mobility can impair toileting ability. Instrumental activities of daily living (IADLs) include tasks that support independent living, such as meal preparation, shopping, home maintenance, laundry, using the telephone, managing medications, and handling finances (Sehy & Williams, 1999). Preserving the ability to perform ADLs and IADLs can be the best contribution the nurse practitioner can make. Geriatric care is always best provided by a team of caregivers who can offer the individual patient the support that he or she most needs. Some patients need physical therapy to maintain strength of ADLs; others need help from social services to manage financial and living arrangements.

RULE OF THUMB: Do not rely on patient report for functional checks.

◎ Perform such tests as the "up-and-go" test. Ask the patient to rise from a sitting position (ideally from a chair without arms), walk 10 feet, turn, and return to sit in the chair. The time it takes the patient to complete the test is recorded. Longer time indicates lower functional ability (Podsiadlo & Richardson, 1991).

◎ Ask patients to demonstrate the basics of ADLs to detect apraxias.

Some aspects of life for older adults can be difficult to assess and manage. Elders fear being seen as incompetent and may cover or deny their real needs for support. All-or-nothing thinking leads to this fear. All-or-nothing thinking means that many older adults feel that accepting help in one area of their lives indicates a decline or weakness that will result in institutionalization. For example, some may fear that if they need help in getting proper nutrition, they will be placed in a nursing home. Individually tailored supports are more humane and more economical for society. Changing our thinking about aging as a society can decrease fear of discussing the need for support. The nurse practitioner can be a catalyst for educating patients and their families about support options that are minimally invasive. For example, home delivery of food or home health aide care can obviate the need for moving to an assisted-living facility if the elder wishes to remain at home.

The US Preventive Services Task Force (2003) has recommendations for screening based on mortality and morbidity figures for this age group. Leading causes of death are heart disease, malignant neoplasms, cerebrovascular diseases, chronic obstructive pulmonary disease, pneumonia, and influenza. Clinical judgments about immunization are tailored for older adults. Maintaining tetanus immunization requires boosters every 10 years, and the pneumococcal vaccine is recommended for all patients over age 65 and for those who have chronic conditions such as cancer or splenectomy. Pneumococcal vaccine may need to be repeated every 7 years. Annual flu shots are recommended. Table 6–8 lists general screening recommendations for persons ages 65 and older and Table 6–9 lists screening recommendations for special populations in that age group (USPSTF, 2003).

Polypharmacy, the use of multiple prescription medications, is a major problem for older adults and contributes to loss of function and disability. Patients may have several health-care providers who prescribe without knowing what other medications the patient is taking. By having patients bring all medications, including eyedrops (which can have systemic effects) and supplements, to annual health screenings, the nurse practitioner can check for drug interactions and inappropriate dosages. Complicated medication regimens can be simplified by developing a written schedule or making a medication sheet with time boxes such those used in acute care. Pharmacists can prepare medication boxes or sheets that clarify the schedule for the drugs (Ramsdell, 2000). Figure 6–1 shows a medication sched-

TABLE 6–8

Screening and Prevention for Ages 65 Years and Older

Screening	Prevention
Blood pressure	Tobacco cessation
Height and weight	Avoid alcohol use with driving, swimming,
Fecal occult blood test annually	boating
Sigmoidoscopy	Diet and exercise
Mammogram	Calcium intake (women)
Pap smear (women with a	Seat belt use
cervix who have been sexually	Motorcycle/bicycle helmets
active)	
Vision screening	Fall prevention
Hearing screening	Firearm safety
Assess problem drinking	Smoke detector
	Hot water heater <120–130°F
	CPR for household members

Source: Adapted from United States Preventive Services Task Force, 2003.

ule organized by medication. Figure 6–2 shows a medication schedule organized by time, which might be easier for a person to follow in the home.

RULE OF THUMB: Make every effort to determine if patients are actually taking all of their medications. Are they skipping their diuretic on days when they have social engagements in the morning? Are they taking only half of expensive medications? Are they taking medications whose only purpose is to control side effects of other medications?

Cognitive assessment using a standard mental status examination can detect and follow changes. After age 75, cognitive declines are more common, so a screening might be indicated for all 75-year-olds, with focused screening for younger patients who express fear of losing memory or whose functional screening indicates potential problems. The issue of continuing to drive in the later years can cause family conflict. A spouse or child may believe that the elder is not a safe driver. Vision, hearing, and cognitive changes can make driving more hazardous. Even such things as limited range of motion can contribute to diminished ability to manage a car. The nurse practitioner can support frank conversations about driving because safety is a health issue. Driving evaluation tests can be performed

TABLE 6-9

High-Risk Populations Ages 65 Years and Over

Population	Potential Screening and Prevention
Institutionalized persons	PPD, hepatitis A, amantadine/rimantadine
Chronic medical conditions, TB contacts, low income, immigrants, alcoholics	PPD
Persons >75 at risk for falls	Fall prevention intervention
Cardiovascular disease risk factors	Cholesterol screening
Family with skin cancer, fair skin	Sun exposure prevention
Native Americans/Alaskan natives	Hepatitis A vaccine, PPD
Travelers to developing countries	Hepatitis A/B vaccine
Blood product recipients	HIV, hepatitis B screen
High-risk sexual behavior	RPR/VDRL, gonorrhea, chlamydia, HIV screen, hepatitis A/B vaccine
Injection or street drug use	PPD/RPR/VDRL, HIV screen, hepatitis A/B vaccine, advice to reduce infection risk
Susceptible to varicella	Varicella immunization
Health-care workers, lab technicians	Hepatitis A/B influenza vaccines, PPD, amantadine/rimantadine

Source: Adapted from United States Preventive Services Task Force, 2003.

in real or simulated situations. If a patient who is obviously impaired insists on continuing to drive, reporting his or her condition to the motor vehicle department may become necessary for his or her safety and for the safety of the public. At times such as these, the patient's judgment may be too limited to make good decisions. This is a paternalistic stance, but it may be justified. Open, clear communication with the patient may avoid such a standoff.

Finally, **clinical judgment** regarding older adults involves a shift in planning for outcomes. For the young or middle-aged patient, screening and treatment decisions are made to cure disease and prolong life. For older patients, maintaining function and enhancing quality of life may be the goal even if length of life cannot be prolonged. This requires a broader base of assessment and more intricate communication with the patient and family members.

Optimal treatment plans are based on research evidence. One difficulty in applying research findings to older adults is that many drug studies

Figure 6-1

MEDICATION SCHEDULE BY MEDICATION

Medication		Sun	Mon	Tues	Wed	Thur	Fri	Sat
Fosamax 10 mg	7 AM	x	x					
Lasix 40 mg	8 AM	x	x					
Captopril 12.5 mg	8 AM	x	x					
Captopril 12.5 mg	4 PM	x						
Captopril 12.5 mg	Bedtime	x						
Tylenol 650 mg, two tabs	8 AM	x	x					
Tylenol 650 mg, two tabs	4 PM	x						
Tylenol 650 mg, two tabs	Bedtime	x						
Aspirin 83 mg	8 AM	x	x					
Timoptic 0.25%, 1 drop	8 AM	x	x					

are conducted on young or middle-aged patients. Older patients may have side or therapeutic effects to medications that differ from those of younger people. Another issue for nurse practitioners is that, when assessing new patients for the first time, they may find that patients are not on optimal therapy. For example, beta blockers have been demonstrated to reduce the risk of reinfarction and death after myocardial infarction. Research shows, however, that only 21 percent of older patients who would have benefited from beta-blocker therapy had received even a trial dose of the medication. (Soumeri, et al. 1997). Physicians are reluctant to prescribe beta blockers because of perceived negative effects, yet other studies show that older

Figure 6-2

MEDICATION SCHEDULE BY TIME

Medication		Sun	Mon	Tues	Wed	Thur	Fri	Sat
Fosamax 10 mg	7 AM	x	x					
Lasix 40 mg	8 AM	x	x					
Captopril 12.5 mg	8 AM	x	x					
Tylenol 650 mg, two tabs	8 AM	x	x					
Aspirin 83 mg	8 AM	x	x					
Timoptic 0.25%, 1 drop	8 AM	x	x					
Captopril 12.5 mg	4 PM	x						
Tylenol 650 mg, two tabs	4 PM	x						
Captopril 12.5 mg	Bedtime	x						
Tylenol 650 mg, two tabs	Bedtime	x						

people benefit from low doses of beta blockers and have minimal negative effects (Chorzempa & Tabloski, 2001). In general, practitioners should review their own treatment practices and evaluate whether such "conventional wisdom" is justification for treatment practices. Consider in case review whether a patient 20 years younger would be managed differently in the practice simply because of the age factor. Research studies need to be completed with older subjects to support treatment guidelines that are appropriate for the group.

Older adults are not all alike. For independently living elders, the rates of malnutrition are low, but for those living in nursing homes, the rates of malnutrition range from 23 to 85 percent. Even hospitalization puts them at risk for malnutrition. One might expect that institutional care would provide a greater support for nutrition, but selection bias probably contributes to these findings. The most debilitated are those who live in nursing homes. Even though homes should provide adequate nutrition, many do not. The nurse practitioner should be vigilant in detecting malnutrition. Indicators of malnutrition include such simple observations as body weight and 24-hour calorie count. Physical findings include dehydration, skin breakdown, edema, muscle weakness, and swallowing problems. Poor dentition also contributes to malnutrition in older adults. Poverty and social isolation contribute to nutrition problems (Ennis, Saffel-Shrier, & Verson, 2001).

In general, caring for older adults in primary care or other settings is complex but very rewarding. People who have lived to be 80 or more are generally resilient and can recover, albeit more slowly, from many health-care insults. Western culture would be enhanced by valuing more openly the resilience and perspective of age.

⟫ END-OF-LIFE CARE

Death occurs to people of all ages. In the United States, health-care providers and patients alike support active, aggressive treatment of diseases. The values of aggressive treatment are laudable in that patients are provided with modern technology and a range of supports to lengthen life. The difficulty with an aggressive treatment model comes when these treatments are futile. Medical futility means that the likelihood of a particular treatment resulting in length or quality of life is low. Judgment about changing the focus of care from treatment to comfort measures is one of the most crucial that any patient, family, or provider can face. Palliative care is care that supports comfort in body, mind, and spirit, and it becomes the focus when a person has a terminal illness. The World Health Organization (WHO) has described palliative care as having several facets. These include defining dying as a normal process while at the same time affirming the value of life. The WHO recommends that caregivers should neither hasten nor postpone death, but should rather be concerned with pain and other symptom management, and integrate spiritual and psychological support into the care delivered. Families should be a focus of care and should be supported in giving care themselves. Palliative care should include bereavement preparation and support (White, Coyne, & Patel, 2001).

Palliative care involves a planned approach to the person who is dying, and that planning involves clinical judgment at several levels. One usually considers palliative care to be home or hospice based. End-of-life care is a broader term and can include patients who die in acute-care settings. Similar to palliative care, end-of-life care is concerned with supporting the person through the natural process of dying while actively controlling symptoms. Judgments about how best to provide end-of-life care include a relationship-centered care model similar to that discussed in Chapter 1 of this book. Relationships form the basis of the dialogue that supports judgment. The knowledge of the nurse practitioner about health and illness and about the dying process is supported by knowing the patient's and family's wishes so that they can work together to develop an optimal treatment plan. Symptom management, especially pain management and clarification of what the patient values as quality of life, can occur at any phase of treatment. End-of-life care includes care for the family and loved ones of the dying person. Psychological and spiritual care is particularly important for patients and families at the end of life. Depression is one of the facets of the grieving process. Family members may report somatic complaints during and after the dying process. Spiritual concerns often center on the meaning of life and of the suffering that the person is experiencing. Finding meaning in suffering can help the dying person and family transcend the pain of dying and loss. Encouraging patients and families to express love, gratitude, and forgiveness may ease the pain of loss.

End-of-life issues are affected by cultural and religious practices. Some cultures value life and want all possible measures used to preserve it. Others have a strong belief in an afterlife and accept palliative care for the dying. The nurse practitioner can help patients and families to clarify their values and can advocate as a member of the care team for the patient's wishes to be honored.

⏵)) VULNERABLE POPULATIONS

Patients who are members of vulnerable populations face an increased risk for morbidity or mortality. Examples of vulnerability include lack of access to care, decreased resources for self-care, and increased risk for health problems. Examples of members of vulnerable populations include immigrants, poor people, and homeless people, who have limited access to health care. Whatever the cause, these people, because of their status, gender, or age, may be disadvantaged by having aspects of their care ignored or negatively sanctioned. Some people, such as gay men and lesbians, have reported receiving care that is insensitive to their special concerns. Many patients have multiple reasons for vulnerability, and these problems can exacerbate their inability to obtain quality health care. For example, a person can be a member of a minority and be poor, which would make care difficult because medications and office visits are expensive, or be homeless and alcoholic and have no resources for receiving regular health care. Nurse practitioners often work in settings that have large numbers of vulnerable clients, partly because of employment and partly out of a commitment to provide for unmet needs of society. Developing skill in working with vulnerable clients is a rewarding aspect of nurse practitioner practice.

Racial Minorities

Racial minorities experience health disparities. Research repeatedly shows that African-Americans experience a disproportionately high rate of cardiovascular disease. These rates of disease may be related to lower socioeconomic and educational levels as well as poverty. One recent study showed that African-American women have higher rates of hypertension, angina, and diabetes mellitus. Contextual risk factors were found to affect health status and include health beliefs, educational level, financial status, and access to health care (Appel, Harrell, & Deng, 2002). Nurse practitioners can use epidemiologic and demographic data as they evaluate diagnostic information.

Studies continue to show disparities in treatments provided to members of racial minorities. African-Americans are less likely than whites to receive angiography or revascularization when presenting to the health-care system with chest pain (Funk, Ostfeld, Chang, & Lee, 2002). Treatment options vary depending on patient resources, which may vary by racial group. Nurse practitioners can advocate for equal treatment by educating patients about what to expect from the health-care system and by remaining an active member of the health-care team when patients are admitted to the hospital.

Homosexuals

Gay and lesbian patients can be found in any practice, and recent articles have challenged the health-care system to be sensitive to the special needs and concerns of this group (Bernhard, 2001; Lee, 2000). Many homosexual patients distrust the health-care system because they may have been ridiculed, threatened, or ostracized in the past. They are at increased risk of suicide, eating disorders, and substance abuse (Lee, 2000). The literature on whether lesbians are at increased risk for breast cancer is mixed (Bernhard, 2001). Nurse practitioners who adopt an open and accepting attitude can foster open communication, thus enabling more sensitive care. Human sexuality is part of each of our lives, so choosing not to discuss sexuality results in an incomplete assessment. Nurse practitioners should not assume that their views of sexuality are the same as their patients'. The range of human behaviors is wide, and personal identity is not as simple as "straight" or "gay." Sexual orientation refers to "adult stable sexual attractions, desires, fantasies, and expressions towards other adult men and women" (Ross, Channon-Little, & Rosser, p.162). A useful way of understanding sexual identity involves several aspects, including assignment at birth as male or female based on genitalia, gender identity, or the sense of being a man or woman, which may not correspond to genital expression, and social sex role, which is expressed as masculinity or femininity, often culturally determined, and which may not be related to sexual orientation (Ross et al., 2000).

> RULE OF THUMB: When taking a sexual history, ask each patient, "Do you have sex with men, women, or both?" This opens the conversation and lets everyone know that all possibilities can be discussed. If a person seems offended by the question, you can simply reply that it is your custom to ask everyone the same question.

Homosexual adolescents are particularly anxious about their sexuality and about fears of rejection by gay and straight peers. Homeless adolescents are often homosexual, having been forced out of their homes and spending time prostituting themselves on the street to survive (Lee, 2000). Homosexual behaviors change the risk pattern for sexually transmitted diseases. Keep in mind, too, that oral sex and anal intercourse can be engaged in by same- or opposite-sex couples, so decisions about screening for sexually transmitted disease and culture samples to be taken depend more on individual sexual practices than on sexual orientation.

As with any patient, good clinical judgment with homosexuals requires obtaining an accurate history to provide for accurate risk assessments. Maintaining an open and accepting attitude will increase the likelihood that you will be trusted by patients and will obtain a complete history. When working with homosexual patients, be sensitive to the words used in describing family. Many homosexuals are offended when the system assumes that they are either married or single. Their partners may be excluded from important health-related conversations or from family visiting hours. Partners and friends will be an important part of the support network for gay and lesbian patients. They should be included in the planning process if the patient requests this.

Homeless People

Homeless patients have tremendous medical, dental, and mental health needs. Although they may have access to clinics associated with homeless shelters or local medical centers, these patients often face difficulties using the health-care system. For example, they may have trouble making appointments, arranging transportation to and from appointments, maintaining health insurance cards, and obtaining and maintaining prescriptions. Homeless patients are often labeled noncompliant by health-care providers because they miss appointments and are often unable to follow treatment recommendations, but in many cases, these individuals are doing the best they can against insurmountable odds.

Caring for the homeless can be extremely rewarding when the system supports their efforts in obtaining care. Homeless people are often appreciative of the simplest recognition of their humanity. They report that on the streets, most people try not to look at them, denying their existence in the world. Dealing with this existential pain simply and directly can make a difference in a homeless person's life. One typically considers the homeless person to be a young to middle-aged man. In fact, families with children and older adults are growing segments of the homeless population (Gillis & Singer, 1997). Costs of living in urban areas and the growing disparity between rich and poor have contributed to increasing homelessness. Special considerations in clinical judgment for the homeless include what parts of the health-care system they are connected with, drug and alcohol history, medications prescribed and taken, nutritional problems, and foot and skin problems. Knowing community resources for referrals will increase your effectiveness with the homeless.

An innovative nurse practitioner-managed clinic for homeless women and children provides episodic care on a walk-in basis and histories and physicals by appointment. To encourage immunizations, the clinic gives a toy to the child at the time of the immunization. To encourage returns for tuberculin test readings, each woman who comes during the correct time window for the reading is given free perfume. The clinic is associated with a substance-abuse treatment facility and shelter on the site of a former church. The center also provides health education and over-the-counter medications (Behler, 1998).

Substance Abusers

Patients who abuse drugs or alcohol require particular clinical judgment activities. These patients are often reluctant to admit their habits because they fear disapproval or legal ramifications. A matter-of-fact approach to asking patients about their use of tobacco, alcohol, and other substances opens the door to communication. If the conversation reveals that the patient needs help with substance abuse, the nurse practitioner's nonjudgmental attitude increases the likelihood that the patient will feel comfortable discussing rehabilitation or other supportive treatment, such as 12-step programs. Even if such a discussion is not possible, the nurse practitioner is less likely to prescribe drugs that have abuse potential or can interact with the drugs patients are using. People who have used injectable drugs are at increased risk for hepatitis B and C and for HIV infection. Screening can lead to early treatment.

Drug-seeking patients pose other challenges to clinical judgment. Some have a verifiable chronic pain syndrome; others do not. Drug-seeking patients typically have many providers. They may telephone for medication refills when they know their regular provider will not be available, requiring a provider who does not know them to respond. Patients who request specific drugs or have a list of drugs that have been tried and found unsuccessful should be referred to a chronic pain service. Nurse practitioners need to respond to real pain, but by prescribing drugs of abuse to patients, they can perpetuate dangerous habits. Practitioners who become known in the community as "easy marks" for medications will see patients who are dependent on medications finding their practice. Brykczynski (1989) described the wisdom of nurse practitioners in recognizing drug-seeking behavior. Drug seekers are organized and intentional. On the other hand, some patients with difficult problems to solve are mistakenly thought to be drug seeking. Nurse practitioners, in describing the drug-seeking patient, related that "affect and tone are not consistent with their stories" (1989,

p. 84). After an initial attempt to meet the patient's need, open communication about your reservation in prescribing drugs that can be abused can help to build a bridge between you and the patient.

Patients with Disabilities

Disabled people are considered a vulnerable population because they have problems with access to health care and often receive care that is fragmented and focused on their disability. Disabled persons have need for the full range of primary-care services. The particular disability becomes the context for health-care services, but it should not be the only focus. For example, persons with Down syndrome experience increased risks for cardiac disease, frequent ear infections, leukemia, musculoskeletal problems, depression, and developmental delays. Regular health maintenance activities can promote function and quality of life for the Down syndrome patient and his or her family (Bosch, 2003).

Severe mental illness (SMI) puts individuals at risk for maintaining other aspects of their health. Persons with schizophrenia, bipolar disorder, major depression, and major personality disorders experience a higher rate of circulatory, respiratory, and endocrine problems than the general population. Many persons with SMI have obesity and associated hypertension and diabetes. Substance abuse and anxiety-related disorders are also associated with SMI. Antipsychotic medications cause their own group of side effects, including weight gain, menstrual irregularities, and immune disorders. Preventive health care is an important feature of care that nurse practitioners can provide to this population. Nurse practitioners need to support compensatory strategies such as reminders for medications that use pictures or reminder telephone calls (Perese & Perese, 2003).

⟩⟩ SUMMARY

The clinical-judgment process for members of special populations remains essentially the same, but the filters through which data is processed may be different for different populations of patients. Paying attention to membership in special populations assists clinical judgment in several ways. First, it changes the probability of specific conditions being present, increasing the likelihood of some and ruling others out. This simplifies the process to a certain extent. Second, by paying attention to values and culture, the nurse practitioner is able to form a relationship that is genuine and considers the experience of the whole person. Clinical effectiveness is enhanced by this relationship because it increases the likelihood of trust and communication. This will enhance the quality of assessment data gathered and increase the patient's participation in treatment decision making. Finally, by being competent in understanding the worldview of various populations of patients, the nurse practitioner will choose management strategies that have a likelihood of working. Depending on the area in which nurse practitioners work, they will develop experience and filters of their own that help them establish working relationships with patients and families. This will help them determine the issues and problems that need to be addressed and will help them to make appropriate intervention selections for the specific population with which they work.

Nurse practitioner organizations have committed themselves to a reduction in health disparities—that is, the differences in health status that different groups experience. Health disparities reflect differences in health status between advantaged and disadvantaged groups. Research into differential access to health care and the societal responses to the health of populations will support a reduction of health disparities in the future (Flaskerud, 2002). Nurse practitioners may be called on to advocate for access to health-care availability to all populations of their community.

REFERENCES

Appel, S. J., Harrell, J. S., & Deng, S. (2002). Racial and socioeconomic differences in risk factors for cardiovascular disease among southern rural women. *Nursing Research, 51*, 140–147.

Behler, S. (1998). NP-run clinic provides health care and education for the homeless. *Nurse Practitioner World News, 3*(7), 1, 6, 8.

Bernhard, L. A. (2001). Lesbian health and health care. In J. J. Fitzpatrick, D. Taylor, & N. F. Woods (Eds.). *Annual Review of Nursing Research: Vol. 19. Women's health research* (pp. 145–77). New York: Springer.

Bosch, J. J. (2003). Health maintenance throughout the life span for individuals with Down syndrome. *Journal of the American Academy of Nurse Practitioners, 15*(1), 5–17.

Brykczynski, K. A. (1989). An interpretative study describing the clinical judgment of nurse practitioners. *Scholarly Inquiry for Nursing Practice, 3*, 113–120.

Chase, S. K., & Hunter, A. (2002). Cultural and spiritual competence: Curricular guidelines. In M. K. Crabtree & R. Pruitt (Eds.). Advanced nursing practice: Building curriculum for quality nurse practitioner education (pp. 10–28). Washington, D.C.: National Organization for Nurse Practitioner Faculties.

Chorzempa, A., & Tabloski, P. (2001). Post myocardial infarction treatment in the older adult. *The Nurse Practitioner: The American Journal of Primary Health Care, 26*(3), 36, 39–40, 42, 45–46, 49.

Coplan, J. (1987). *Early Language Milestone Scale.* Austin, TX: Pro Ed.

Department of Health and Human Services. (2002). Nurse practitioner primary care competencies in specialty areas: Adult, family gerontological, pediatric and women's health. Rockville, MD: Author.

Ennis, B. W., Saffel-Shrier, S., & Verson, H. (2001). Diagnosing malnutrition in the elderly. *The Nurse Practitioner: The American Journal of Primary Health Care, 26*(3). 52–54, 56, 61–62, 65.

Erikson, E. (1986). *Childhood and society.* New York: Norton.

Flaskerud, J. H. (2002). New paradigm for health disparities needed. *Nursing Research, 51,* 139.

Frankenburg, W. K., Dodds, J., Archer, P., Shapiro, H., & Bresnick, B. (1991). The Denver II: A major revision and restandardization of the Denver Developmental Screening Test. *Pediatrics, 89,* 91.

Funk, M., Ostfeld, A. M., Chang, V. M., & Lee, F. A. (2002). Racial differences in the use of cardiac procedures in patients with acute myocardial infarction. *Nursing Research, 51,* 148–157.

Gillis, L. M., & Singer, J. (1997). Breaking through the barriers: Healthcare for the homeless. *Journal of Nursing Administration, 27*(6), 30–34.

Hay, W. W., Groothuis, J. R., Hayward, A. A., & Levin, M. J. (Eds.). (1995). *Current pediatric diagnosis & treatment.* Norwalk, CT: Appleton & Lange.

Kudzma, E. C. (2002). Young adult. In C. L. Edelman & C. L. Mandle (Eds.). *Health promotion throughout the lifespan* (5th ed., pp. 649–680). St. Louis: Mosby.

Lee, R. (2000). Health care problems of lesbian, gay, bisexual and transgender patients. *Western Journal of Medicine, 172,* 403–408.

Lindeke, L. L., Krajicek, M., & Patterson, D. L. (2001). PNP roles and interventions with children with special needs and their families. *Journal of Pediatric Health Care, 15,* 138–143.

Lustig, J. V. (1995). Approaching the pediatric patient. In W. W. Hay, J. R. Groothuis, A. A. Hayward, & M. J. Levin (Eds.). *Current pediatric diagnosis & treatment* (pp. 1–8). Norwalk, CT: Appleton & Lange.

Mandle, C. L. (2002). Health promotion and the family. In C. L. Edelman & C. L. Mandle (Eds.). *Health promotion throughout the lifespan* (5th ed., pp. 169–198). St. Louis: Mosby.

Maradiegue, A. (2003). Minor's rights versus parental rights: Review of legal issues in adolescent health care. *Journal of Midwifery and Women's Health, 48,* 170–177.

Perese, E. F., & Perese, K. (2003). Health problems of women with severe mental illness. *Journal of the Academy of Nurse Practitioners, 15,* 212–219.

Podsiadlo, D., & Richardson, S. (1991). The timed "Up & Go": A test of basic functional mobility for frail elderly persons. *Journal of the American Geriatrics Society, 39*, 142–148.

Ramsdell, J. (2000). Taking better care of our elderly patients. *Consultant, 40,* 1725–1728.

Ross, M. W., Channon-Little, L. D., & Rosser, B. R. (2000). *Sexual health concerns: Interviewing and history taking for health practitioners*, 2nd ed. Philadelphia: F. A. Davis Company.

Sehy, Y. B., & Williams, M. P. (1999). Functional assessment. In J. T. Stone, J. F. Wyman, & S. A. Salisbury (Eds). *Clinical gerontological nursing: A guide to advanced practice* (2nd ed., pp. 175–202). Philadelphia: W.B. Saunders Company.

Soumeri, S. B., McLaughlin, T. J., Spigelman, D., et al. (1997). Adverse outcomes of underuse of beta-blockers in elderly survivors of acute myocardial infarction. *Journal of the American Medical Association, 277*(2), 115–121.

United States Department of Health and Human Services. (2000). Healthy People 2010 (Conference Edition, in Two volumes). Washington, DC: Author.

United States Preventive Services Task Force, (2003). *Put prevention into practice.* Rockville, MD: Agency for Healthcare Research and Quality. *http://www.ahrq.gov/clinic/ppipix.html.* Downloaded June 28, 2003.

White, K. R., Coyne, P. J., & Patel, U. B. (2001). Are nurses adequately prepared for end-of-life care? *Journal of Nursing Scholarship, 33*, 147–151.

CHAPTER 7

Special Settings

CHAPTER OUTLINE

)) INTRODUCTION

Expertise in clinical judgment results from day-to-day experience in a specific practice setting. That experience also shapes the particular knowledge of individual nurse practitioners. Skill in clinical judgment requires application not only of a general process, but also of particular, situated knowledge (Benner, 1984). Nurse practitioners were first prepared to function in primary-care settings, but they quickly adapted their skills to other settings. Although many early nurse practitioners valued the freedom of primary care as compared to hospital-based employment, roles for advanced practice nurses also developed in acute care. Nurse practitioners are now found in virtually every aspect of health care. This chapter focuses on how the setting in which the nurse practitioner delivers care can affect the process of clinical judgment.

The previous chapter showed that, when using clinical judgment for special populations, nurse practitioners can narrow the diagnostic focus and the treatment options by incorporating their knowledge of risks and preferences for specific groups. Special settings affect clinical judgment not so much by altering diagnostic probabilities as by shaping the goals of therapy. For example, treatment goals during emergency care of an asthmatic patient would differ from those established during a routine primary care visit. In the former case, the nurse practitioner focuses on stabilizing respiratory function and determining the cause for exacerbation. In the latter case, the goal is long-term management. Special settings might alter the depth and breadth of data that are collected because of the focused goals of therapy. In all clinical judgment situations, the nurse practitioner is searching for an explanation of the findings and an appropriate response. The range of both diagnoses and interventions can be considered a "search field." The search field is adapted for appropriateness to the specific setting. New nurse practitioners and students may be surprised that the standard history and physical can be performed in different ways in different settings. The depth of the history, the order of the physical examination procedures, and the difference in treatment plans can vary by situation and setting. What does not change, regardless of the setting, is the essential nature of the nurse practitioner-patient relationship, which forms the basis for good history taking and creative intervention selection.

The American Nurses Association has responded to the need to differentiate practice for various populations and settings by approving a range of Standards and Scope of Practice Statements. Box 7–1 lists those that are related to clinical practice. Most of these standards apply to registered nurse practice and are not specific to nurse practitioner practice, but they

---

Box 7–1   *American Nurses Association Available Clinical Standards of Practice*

Scope and Standards of Advanced Practice Registered Nursing
Scope and Standards of College Health Nursing Practice
Scope and Standards of Diabetes Nursing
Scope and Standards of Forensic Nursing Practice
Scope and Standards of Home Health Nursing Practice
Scope and Standards of Nursing Practice in Correctional Facilities
Scope and Standards of Parish Nursing Practice
Scope and Standards of Pediatric Oncology Nursing
Standards and Scope of Gerontological Nursing Practice
Standards of Addictions Nursing Practice with Selected Diagnoses and Criteria
Standards of Clinical Nursing Practice
Standards of Clinical Practice and Scope of Practice for the Acute Care Nurse Practitioner
Statement on the Scope and Standards for the Nurse Who Specializes in Developmental Disabilities and/or Mental Retardation
Statement on the Scope and Standards of Genetics Clinical Nursing Practice
Statement on the Scope and Standards of Oncology Nursing Practice
Statement on the Scope and Standards of Otorhinolaryngology Clinical Nursing Practice
Statement on the Scope and Standards of Pediatric Clinical Nursing Practice
Statement on the Scope and Standards of Psychiatric Mental Health Clinical Nursing Practice
The Scope and Standards of Public Health Nursing Practice
Statement on the Scope and Standards of Respiratory Nursing Practice

---

nevertheless apply to nurses who practice in the expanded role. Nurse practitioners are nurses first, and standards apply across both practice levels. These standard statements can guide the new nurse practitioner in establishing safe practice in new settings.

)) HOSPITAL-BASED CARE

Nurse practitioners who work in hospitals bring advanced-practice knowledge to patients in settings other than primary care. An important consideration for nurse practitioners who work in hospital settings is what part of the organization they report to. Do they work within a department of nursing or a specialty medical department? Do their responsibilities include some of those traditionally associated with the clinical nurse specialist role, which is working with and through other nursing staff, or do they provide direct patient care only? The answers to these questions will determine the responsibilities and outcomes for which the nurse practitioner is accountable and the nature of the relationship the nurse practitioner has with patients and other providers. For example, if nurse practitioners are employed by a specialty practice outside the hospital, the primary responsibility will be to the patients and to the practice that employs them. These nurse practitioners will not be involved in the committee structure or the policy setting or orientation aspects of the hospital. The relationship with other nurses will be less direct, and success will be determined by patient outcomes and economics. On the other hand, nurse practitioners employed by the hospital will have more responsibility for overall functioning of the unit and hospital, with a more direct relationship with other nurses in the system. Success in this setting will depend on improving the quality of care for the unit and may require working through others.

Nurse practitioners who are employed by hospitals and who perform "physician services" will find that it is safer to be a revenue generator than an expense. Once the appropriate accounting system is devised, nurse practitioners can easily document the amount of revenue they generate and then use the numbers to negotiate salary and other aspects of employment (Buppert, 2001, p. 16)

Economic impact will be demonstrated by reducing costs of delivering care, for example, through decreasing lengths of stay and preventing readmissions. Clinical judgments are part of either of the arrangements described previously. In the first case, individual patients are more the focus. In the second, groups of patients are more the focus. Some of these issues were addressed in Chapter 5, entitled Documentation, and others will be addressed in Chapter 9, entitled Issues in Primary Care.

Acute and Critical Care

Nurse practitioners are increasingly employed in acute-care settings for their skills in managing the varied aspects of patient care, including assessment, diagnosis, intervention selection, and evaluation. Despite the different types of treatment options available in acute care, the process of clinical judgment is similar to that used in primary care. For example, the nurse practitioner attempts to understand the situation from the patient's point of view in order to devise the most appropriate treatment plan. Patients who need to be admitted to acute-care settings usually require such interventions as sophisticated monitoring, intravenous medications, and possibly surgical intervention and follow-through. Understanding patient responses to acute illness is the basis for acute-care nurse practitioner judgment. (See Chapter 8 for a full discussion of clinical judgment by acute-care nurse practitioners.)

Emergency Care

The emergency care system is set up to triage patients so that the most urgent cases are seen in a timely fashion and an appropriate-level health-care provider manages the less urgent cases. In the emergency setting, the nurse practitioner can take on several roles. A study by Frank and Ramirez (2000) reported a survey of 72 nurse practitioners in emergency settings that showed that common skills included fluorescein staining, removal of foreign body from the eye, interpreting a 12-lead electrocardiogram, and single-layer suturing. Digital nerve blocks, splinting, and wound management were also rated as skills frequently performed. These nurse practitioners reported learning some of these skills during formal educational preparation, but most were learned on the job or through continuing education. For less seriously ill patients, the nurse practitioner with acute-care skills can manage lacerations, fractures, or common medical complaints such as asthma attacks. Providing this level of care is ideally suited to nurse practitioners because of their skill in patient teaching and in establishing a relationship that serves as the basis for full assessments. For example, a nurse practitioner may notice a patient's increasing frequency of visits for asthma exacerbations. This is an opportunity to discuss the effectiveness of the management plan and to determine if the patient is having difficulty following it. Referral back to community services so that improved asthma management results in fewer acute attacks is important. Emergency rooms are the bridge between the community and the acute-care system. Nurse practitioners can be effective in treating acute problems and in referring patients to community resources.

Many emergency centers have established specialty areas to streamline care and provide the highest levels of service. Examples of this include acute psychiatric care and sexual assault teams. Specialized services in the emergency context can be provided by nurse practitioners. Female nurse practitioners can establish a bond with female patients who may be victims of domestic abuse and may be more effective in screening for this cause of traumatic injuries. Sexual assault teams provide care to the traumatized victim and maintain a chain of evidence that will be useful to the criminal justice system.

Emergency rooms are used more often for nonacute problems by low-income patients than by those in higher socioeconomic groups. A study (Sheahan, 2000) was conducted to compare documentation of health risks and health-risk counseling by physicians and nurse practitioners in an emergency room. Charts for low-acuity patients were audited and showed that physicians documented more health risks, but that nurse practitioners were more likely to document smoke cessation counseling. The emergency room provides a good opportunity for nurse practitioners to offer health screening and counseling to patients who may not have access to primary-care services.

For more acutely ill patients, nurse practitioners with acute-care skills not only can assist with procedures such as line placement and chest tube insertion, but can also establish supportive relationships with patients and families to help reduce the stress of dealing with trauma or medical emergencies. Again, the benefit of having a nurse practitioner present is the breadth of background and the ability to establish relationships that are supportive, which can do much to ameliorate the stress for patients and families that a trauma or medical emergency can engender. Important decisions are made regarding the diagnosis, the appropriate treatment plan, and the necessity for hospital admission and follow-up care. The nurse practitioner who specializes in trauma can initiate a coordinated effort that will follow the patient from acute or critical care through to rehabilitation.

As in other settings, the emergency nurse practitioner must consider relative risks for health problems. Knowledge of unique patterns of disease presentation can improve diagnostic accuracy. Certain emergency clinical judgments have more attendant risk than others, especially those involving cardiac care. Every year, 5 million Americans go to an emergency department with a complaint of chest pain. One million of these will rule in for myocardial infarction. Between 2 and 8 percent of patients with acute myocardial infarction are misdiagnosed and sent home, resulting in increased risk of death. (Pope, Aufderheide, & Ruthazer, 2000). Unrecognized ischemia often occurs with female patients, particularly those under age 55, who often describe symptom patterns different from those seen in men, and with nonwhites, who are more likely to be discharged with ischemia and myocardial infarction. A national conference on emergency cardiac care suggested goals for management of emergency cardiac patients, as follows:

◎ Distinguish coronary causes from other conditions such as aortic dissection.

◎ Assess the risk of early complications of myocardial ischemia.

◎ Initiate treatment promptly (Ewy & Omato, 1999).

Unrecognized acute illnesses result in poor patient outcomes and an increased risk for litigation. Triage staffs make the most critical of clinical judgments in this case. On the other hand, exposing patients to expensive and risky diagnostic procedures unnecessarily is neither cost effective nor desirable for the patient. Nurse practitioner judgments that are sensitive to context and personal situations can support accurate assessment in the emergency setting.

Preanesthesia Screening

One setting where nurse practitioners with either an acute- or a primary-care background can have an important impact is in preanesthesia screening. Two-thirds of all surgical procedures now occur on either an outpatient or same-day admission basis (Brockway, 1997). Consequently, all necessary testing and screening must occur before the day of surgery. This setting allows for history and physical examination to assess anesthesia risk, blood work, and electrocardiogram and radiography testing as appropriate, and serves to develop a database for the anesthesia and perioperative plan of care.

The role of the nurse practitioner in this setting is to provide an assessment of anesthesia risk and to assist the patient in preparing for the procedure. The chief risks of anesthesia are the rare malignant hyperthermia and the unexpected myocardial infarction or cerebrovascular accident. Airway difficulties are another concern of the anesthesia team. These might include unusual pharyngeal anatomy, a history of asthma, or gastroesophageal reflux that can predispose the patient to aspiration. The history and physical examination are focused on previous surgical and anesthesia experiences, particularly negative experiences such as life-threatening malignant hyperthermia or other problems such as with general regional or spinal anesthesia. In this setting, nurse practitioner judgment is used with a focus on anesthesia risk, but even here, the entire patient situation must be considered. Patients who face surgery for cancer or debilitating conditions need emotional support. They need to know that the health-care system they are entering understands their particular needs. Even in this setting, emotional or spiritual care can be at least a part of the visit.

◉)) SPECIALTY SETTINGS

Women's Health

Nurse practitioners have had a subspecialty in women's health for many years. The focus of women's health practice is truly one of health promotion. Women's health can extend from adolescence through old age, although fertility-related care is often seen as a focus of the practice. Clinical judgment in the women's health setting will begin with a detailed menstrual and pregnancy history, which is an important basis for women's health care. Additional information to consider includes disease and sexually transmitted infection (STI) history, number of sexual partners, risk factors for STIs, fertility issues, risk for domestic violence, preferences for family planning, and, if appropriate, menopause management. Screening for breast, cervical, and other gynecologic cancers is an important aspect of ongoing care. Although management of vaginal discharges, contraception, and menopause is a vital feature of the practice, in recent years women's health nurse practitioners have expanded to the management of common health concerns such as hypertension. As always, a warm, supportive relationship serves to improve the quality of data assessment and to assist the nurse practitioner in planning follow-up care.

The setting in which care is delivered to women can be made warm and inviting. This recognizes the importance of the environment in establishing the tone of the visit. When women feel safe and well cared for, they can form relaxed and personal relationships with their health-care providers. One practice that included a female physician and female nurse practitioner was in a homelike setting and had each room decorated in a different pattern by a familiar designer. The entire atmosphere supported personal, feminine care.

Pediatric Health

Pediatric nurse practitioners frequently work in community-based settings, but a survey of hospitals in the National Association of Children's Hospitals and Related Institutions (Pitts & Seimer, 1998) showed that of the 49 hospitals responding, 88 percent employed nurse practitioners. They worked most often in neonatology, hematology/oncology, and primary care. It is interesting to note that only 22 percent of hospitals reported that the nurse practitioners had prescriptive authority. Perhaps the coordination of care aspects of the advanced practice role were more important in the hospital setting. Another study of data from the national Hospital Ambulatory Medical Care Survey (Mills, McSweeney, & Lavin, 1998) reported that nurse practitioner practice was distinguished by offering more health promotion and counseling and offering services to women and children. Nurse practitioners can develop practices in a variety of settings, including hospital outpatient departments. Clinical judgment in these settings is supported by knowledge and experience that the nurse practitioner has in the particular context.

Medical Subspecialties

Nurse practitioners are active members of subspecialty settings, in either private practices or institution-based clinics. Orthopedic nurse practitioners manage acute and follow-up care for patients with fractures and for those with chronic conditions such as orthopedic oncology. They can also have a subspecialty in sports medicine. Oncologic nurse practitioners are involved with symptom management and family support. Cardiologic nurse practitioners manage interventional cardiology patients in the cardiac catheterization laboratory and in the recovery setting. Nurse practitioners are involved as team members on transplant teams and in gastrointestinal practices, where they perform routine screening examinations and manage complex chronic clinics for such conditions as Crohn's disease.

Board-certified physicians usually head the clinic or practice, and residents in training may rotate through the practice, but the nurse practitioner functions as a stable member of the team who comes to know patients over time and who can provide continuity of care. Of course, as in other settings, the nurse practitioner uses the skills of relationship building as the basis for clinical judgment. What is unique in the subspecialty setting is the focus on the range of conditions that are likely for that specialty. Some critics question whether nurse practitioners are practicing medicine when they engage in any advanced practice. It is the nurse practitioner who controls the breadth and depth of patient involvement, and that is what determines whether the nurse practitioner is including nursing in his or her practice. A focus on the patient's response to his or her condition and the treatment plan is what distinguishes the practice of a nurse practitioner from that of a physician. Nurse practitioners are also skilled in patient education and health promotion, which are important in specialty settings. Nurse practitioners can manage aspects of specialty practice, such as managing patients who are on anticoagulants, independently. When nurse practitioners assume responsibility for this aspect of a practice, care is optimized and more patients can be managed by the practice as a whole. The nurse practitioner can be a representative for all of nursing by demonstrating the positive effect of the nursing perspective on patient outcome and cost-effective care.

Subspecialty settings can benefit in several ways from the perspective of the advanced-practice nurse. Nurse practitioner assessment of patients tends to be broad and to include data from all aspects of a person's life. When the full picture of a person's life is assembled, diagnostic accuracy is supported. Resisting the narrow focus can lead to important findings.

In a study by the Cardiovascular Health Study Collaborative Research Group (Ariyo et al., 2000), patients at risk for developing coronary heart disease (CHD) were followed and their risk factors were evaluated. More than 4000 patients who had no cardiovascular disease at the start of the study were followed for 6 years, noting whether they developed CHD or died. Assessment data included depression scores. After controlling for age, race, sex, education, and chronic health problems such as diabetes, hypertension, smoking, and cholesterol levels, the risk for developing CHD was elevated for those with higher depression scores. Those with the highest depression scores had an increased risk of CHD of 40 percent and an increased risk of death of 60 percent. In applying the findings of this study, the nurse practitioner who includes a full patient history, including functional status and satisfaction with life, will be more likely to include all the demonstrated risk factors for cardiovascular disease than a provider who focuses on physiologic function. This study did not evaluate whether improving depression scores with medication or counseling would reduce the risk of death, but every nurse practitioner should include depression evaluation when considering risk of CHD.

Developing guides for the management of chronic health problems has been a focus of advanced-practice nurses. One group devised a tool that evaluated congestive heart failure patients' ability to manage their own health concerns (Riegel, Carlson, & Glaser, 2000). Each patient's response to the tool becomes the basis for teaching and deciding how much support the patient needs. The nursing perspective brought a conceptual framework based on self-management principles and patient decision-making theory. The patient's decision-making strategies to support health include attention to symptoms, ability to make inferences about the meaning of symptoms, and choice to take action. Nurse practitioners in other medical subspecialties could adapt this tool for their own patient population.

Another subspecialty that has used the nurse practitioner as a member of the health-care team is vascular surgery. The nurse practitioner collaborates with surgeons in both ambulatory and hospital-based care to reduce fragmentation of care, shorten length of hospital stay, and prevent hospital readmissions. Direct-care activities are supported by indirect activities such as coordination of ancillary services and patient conferences (Knaus, Davis, Burton, Felton, & Fobes, 1996).

Oncologic nurse practitioners work increasingly in ambulatory settings (Bush & Watters, 2001). Oncologic services, including chemotherapy and radiation therapy, are delivered in ambulatory centers that are either attached to hospitals or freestanding centers. Oncologic nurse practitioners work in collaboration with oncologists to manage symptoms, offer palliative care, and provide education and support to patients and families. Clinical judgment is key to all these as well as to monitoring the patient's responses to the therapies. Oncologic nurse practitioners include skills in primary care as they monitor and manage holistically the patient's response to the disease, along with acute-care skills as they manage complex patient problems and provide specialized technical skills such as bone marrow aspiration and line placement (Bush & Watters, 2001). One oncologic nurse practitioner has conducted research in such a setting on the response of patients' families at the time of cancer recurrence. Based on this research, new modes of supporting family members are being applied (Creamer, 2002).

Just as with the specialty of oncology, the first advanced-practice role in psychiatry was the clinical nurse specialist. Unlike medical subspecialty clinical nurse specialists, however, psychiatric clinical nurse specialists often worked independently with clients in the outpatient setting. The role of nurse practitioner is now finding a place in the psychiatric setting (Dyer, Hammill, Regan-Kubinski, Yurick, & Kobert, 1997). Nurse practitioners can provide full primary care in psychiatric settings. They use specialized knowledge of psychotropic drugs and their side effects and the ability to form therapeutic alliances with patients to provide primary care to psychiatric patients. Additionally, psychiatric nurse practitioners can focus on the psychiatric problems that present themselves in the primary-care setting. Some psychiatric nurse practitioners prepare with subspecialty knowledge such as care of children and adolescents or older patients.

Clinical judgment in specialty practice areas is tailored to focus on conditions related to the specialty of interest, but the nurse practitioner offers whole-person care, which enhances the effectiveness of the practice. Nurse practitioners become expert in the specialty practice, but they can also base their practice on a holistic model that adds a unique perspective to the care management team.

Public Health Settings

Nurse practitioners can be found in many public health settings, including travel clinics, infectious disease clinics, and STI clinics. In these settings, the focus is on the health of a population and often involves such practices as epidemiological study of disease transmission and incidence patterns. Nurse practitioners have the research-based skills that promote a true population-focused approach. For example, nurse practitioners working in STI clinics serve the health interests of the person being treated as well as the health of the population as a whole. Counseling to reduce risks of exposure and to get treatment for sexual partners is important. Frequently, recipients of care in public health settings are immigrants and those with limited access to primary care for reasons of poverty, language barriers, and lack of education. The nurse practitioner's sensitivity to cultural issues can enhance the effectiveness of the clinic. Clinical judgment in these settings includes use of both individual and population-based data to increase the precision of the judgments made. For example, knowing the drug resistance pattern of tuberculosis in a particular community can assist the nurse practitioner in selecting an appropriate drug regimen.

)) INSTITUTION-BASED CARE

Institutions such as schools, colleges, and work sites or factories have responsibilities for the health of their key constituencies. When providing care in schools, workplaces, residential facilities, or prisons, nurse practitioners manage the health of those institutions' key constituencies, which might include students, employees, or residents. Nurse practitioners are frequently employed in such settings because of their focus on health promotion, risk reduction, and cost-effective care. Institution-based care has many features of community-based care in that the "client" is not necessarily the individual, but is thought of as the community as a whole. Principles of community health promotion need to be used. These include assessment and monitoring of the health of the whole population rather than of individuals alone. Population-based interventions are implemented and evaluated. The North American Nursing Diagnosis Association (NANDA) recently included diagnoses for communities in its revised taxonomy (NANDA, 2001). Assessment data for communities may include incidence patterns for accidents or diseases. Interventions such as educational programs or safety campaigns involve the community as a whole.

When nurse practitioners work in settings that are communities, they are often agents of the institution, which can affect the nature of the nurse practitioner-patient relationship. Ethical principles require that the nurse practitioner act in the best interest of the patient, and usually that is also in the best interest of the setting. Clear policies and procedures can guide the nurse practitioner when these interests may seem to conflict. For example, an employee health clinic is not only concerned about the total health of an employee but also about safety in the workplace and the employee's fitness for duty. True comprehensive care may be better delivered in a primary-care setting. On the other hand, settings such as those described in this section can promote the health of students, residents, and employees by providing wellness programming and screening with a frequency not usually offered in standard primary care.

School Health

Nurse practitioners in school-based health clinics provide access to primary-care services that many students might otherwise miss. Some school-based clinics focus on risk reduction, with an emphasis on sexuality, alcohol, and drugs as well as violence. Providing a message that is counter to the many messages of violence in our culture is a task that school-based nurse practitioners manage. Reducing the spread of infectious diseases and infestations and tracking immunizations are also functions of school-based nurse practitioner care. Nurse practitioners who work in elementary schools teach about healthy lifestyle issues and screen for high-risk conditions such as hearing and vision impairment, scoliosis, and cognitive disorders. Because of policies of inclusion, most schools are also places of learning for chronically ill children, so school-based health centers may provide complex care for students with developmental and congenital disorders and chronic diseases such as seizure disorders, asthma, and diabetes. Nurse practitioners work with school nurses, families, pediatricians, and pediatric nurse practitioners to provide comprehensive care.

As in the primary-care setting, the nurse practitioner in the school setting must be alert for evidence of child abuse and neglect. Reporting of suspected cases is mandatory. In 2000 there were 1200 child fatalities associated with child abuse or neglect, with 85 percent of victims being younger than age 6 years (Koschel, 2003). School nurse practitioners can detect patterns of bruising or injuries in different stages of healing. The most frequent perpetrator is a family member or person living in the home. A focus on the perpetrators of abuse and neglect has shown that many were victims themselves (Nester, 1998).

In middle and high schools, nurse practitioners work with students who are facing the challenge of body image changes, which can lead to eating disorders. Substance abuse, including tobacco use, often begins during the middle school years. Students who are intent on a sports scholarship or career may overtrain or indulge in anabolic steroid use. Many high schools today have day-care centers attached for the care of children born to students. The opportunities for health-risk reduction are many. Programs to teach parenting skills can help to break the cycle of abuse and neglect among young, inexperienced parents. Sexuality issues are dealt with by students with or without the guidance of teachers and health-care providers. Because 3 million American teenagers are diagnosed with an STI annually, the *Clinicians Handbook of Preventive Services* recommends counseling to reduce these risks (United States Public Health Service, 1998). All these pressures will serve to shape the practice of the school-based nurse practitioner. Nurse practitioners in the secondary school setting must consider the risk factors appropriate to the age group of the students as well as the context of the community in establishing health programming for the school.

In all school settings, the nurse's office can be a haven for students who have school-related stress. Uncovering the reasons behind a visit may reveal adjustment problems, learning disabilities, and self-esteem issues that, if dealt with early, can change the trajectory of a student's life.

Schools are complex political structures as well as places of learning. The scope of practice for school-based health clinics must be developed by nurse practitioners in conjunction with superintendents, school boards, and public health boards. Some states require special certification for school nurses, and these requirements may extend to nurse practitioners working in school settings. Guidelines such as the United States Preventive Service Task Force (USPSTF) for screening can be a guide for the nurse practitioner developing a health program (USPSTF, 2003). Using such well-accepted guidelines can provide support for programs that require budgetary approval and funding.

College Health

College health settings are key places for the delivery of health-care services and for supporting healthy lifestyle choices. The college years may be the first time the student lives away from home and has real freedom in decision making. College dormitories put students in close proximity, and infectious diseases such as mononucleosis and hepatitis have high frequency. Substance abuse, particularly of alcohol, can escalate to life-threatening proportions. Many colleges have programs or student affairs officers with a responsibility for developing alcohol-use policies. Nurse practitioners can contribute to such policy development by participating in the School Life or Residence Hall advisory committees. College nurse practitioners develop expertise in immunization recommendations by maintaining currency in guidelines from federal, state, and local public health departments. In addition, body image issues are powerful, and many students may develop eating disorders. Student athletes' health may be an issue, with pressure for performance in highly competitive programs. In addition, the college health setting provides primary-care services to the entire college or university community.

Many college-age students, including international students, have no health insurance, and their main source of health care is the college health setting. In addition, faculty and staff members are often served in the college health setting. Even for faculty and staff members who have their own primary-care providers, the college health nurse practitioner can establish worksite health programs that target high-risk areas. Health fairs, stress reduction, and cardiovascular risk reduction are health programs that are suited to the college setting. Nurse practitioners who enjoy working predominantly with young people will be able to apply their clinical judgment skills to the promotion of health for the college or university community. Clinical-judgment skills are needed to treat the individuals who are seen in the health setting as well as to monitor the health of the entire college community.

Employee Health

In this setting, the nurse practitioner provides workplace health promotion programs, screens employees to ensure they are able to return to work after injury, and recognizes the health risks at the particular settings. For example, the nurse practitioner must know what chemicals workers are exposed to in an assembly area, or whether radioactive materials are used in research areas. Occupational Safety and Health Administration (OSHA) guidelines must be made available and followed, and records must be kept. The nurse practitioner may be involved with implementation plans. For example, responses to fire or chemical-spill emergencies can be improved through the use of drills that the nurse practitioner can support. Noting patterns of illness can help to identify ventilation problems or sick building syndrome. Clinical judgments in this area and in other institutional settings are made regarding the health of the entire community.

One area of concern for nurse practitioners in employee health involves the ethical issue of accountability. The nurse is, of course, accountable to the patient for providing care according to standards and guidelines. On the other hand, as an agent of the employer, the nurse practitioner should clearly understand who has access to patient records and how that information might be used. Employee-health nurse practitioners are involved with workers' compensation cases and therefore need to become familiar with the state's regulations regarding these issues.

People spend many hours a week at their work site, and the employee-health nurse practitioner is in a perfect position to establish wellness programs that can make a real difference in employees' overall health. For example, a worksite weight loss program could reduce cardiovascular risk factors. Employee assistance programs can bring health promotion activities and stress reduction to the location where people spend many of their waking hours, and can offer support that many patients are reluctant to seek from their primary-care provider.

Assisted-Living Facilities

Assisted-living facilities are expanding as the population ages. Residents of these facilities require assistance in one or more of the activities of daily living in order to maintain an independence of life that they value. Most such facilities provide congregate meals and housekeeping and laundry service, and contract for certain hours per day of assistance with such activities as bathing, grooming, and dressing. Some facilities also provide medication management. Many settings have activity programs that help promote quality of life. Because the purpose of such facilities is to maintain independence of function for as long as possible, a health promotion model works particularly well here. Nurse practitioners are ideal providers to oversee and manage health issues before they become serious and necessitate transfer to acute- or long-term care facilities. Clinical judgment in assisted-living facilities involves supporting residents' overall function and quality of life and minimizing the effects of aging and chronic illness.

Nursing Homes: Extended- and Chronic-Care Facilities

More than 1.5 million Americans live in nursing homes (Brozovic & Wold, 2000). Because of the vulnerability of nursing-home residents, and partly because of abuses in the past, the nursing-home industry is heavily regulated. Clinical judgment in extended-care facilities is partly determined by those regulations. For example, mandated data sets, which include data that nurse practitioners use in forming clinical judgments, are required in the nursing-home industry. The Minimum Data Set (MDS) for Resident Assessment and Care Screening was developed as a result of the Omnibus Reconciliation Act of 1987. This act required a standardized resident assessment that included functional, medical, mental, and psychosocial status with regular reassessment (Sehy & Williams, 1999). Nurse practitioners, of course, are not limited to the data collected in these data sets, but the data and required reports are part of the context of clinical judgment in the nursing-home setting.

Many patients in nursing homes, such as those with Alzheimer's disease and other dementing illnesses, have lost their ability to express their own concerns. Screening assessments that rely on objective data are necessary in these settings because the patient may not be able to contribute subjective data. Staff members, including the nurse practitioner, must be vigilant for high-risk problems. Families and staff members who spend extended time with nursing home residents, even those with Alzheimer's disease, note behavior patterns that have meaning and can detect when a change in behavior has occurred. Behavior change can be a sign of new problems, such as infection, or metabolic changes, including glucose abnormalities and other physiological problems. Clinical judgment for residents of nursing homes is unique in that the goals of care are most likely to be comfort and preservation of function. Invasive diagnostic and treatment methods are often avoided, and issues related to end-of-life care take prominence. Assisting patients and their families through this phase of life requires an ongoing commitment from the nurse practitioner, especially when caring for patients who have Alzheimer's disease or other forms of dementia and who are unable to convey their wishes regarding end-of-life care. One way in which nurse practitioners can assist both patients and families is to support advanced directives decisions. Making end-of-life decisions requires time for all parties, particularly family members, to examine their values. Nurse practitioner clinical judgment is involved in several ways. First, recognizing an appropriate time to initiate and continue discussions about treatment preferences requires judgment. Second, once preferences are made known, the nurse practitioner must honor the provisions of the advanced directives and establish systems so that the directives are followed.

One qualitative study (Forbes, Bern-Klug, & Gessert, 2000) of family decision making about end-of-life issues for their loved ones with Alzheimer's disease showed that these family members need emotional support as they negotiate the multiple decisions related to end-of-life care. Families need help in understanding the trajectory of the disease process. "Family members need to communicate with a consistent provider, a provider who is educated in end-of-life decision-making in a culture where multiethnic values, old age, and Western medicine are likely to clash" (Forbes et al., 2000, p. 257). One of the common clinical judgments that must be made regarding nursing-home residents is whether to transfer them to the hospital when their conditions worsen. More than 25 percent of the 1.5 million people who live in nursing homes are hospitalized each year. The most frequent causes of hospitalization are urinary tract and lower respiratory tract infections. One study (Brooks, Warshaw, Hasse, & Kues, 1994) that examined the decision by physicians of whether to treat in place or admit to the hospital found that the factors most predictive of hospital admission were confusion and agitation for urinary tract infections and decreased blood pressure for respiratory infections. Patients' families were involved in only 5.6 percent of decisions. Several factors predicted hospital admission. For example, patients who functioned independently and had been hospitalized in the previous 6 months were more likely to be hospitalized. Nursing homes at that time had the capability of providing intravenous medication as well as inhaled bronchodilator therapy, but may not have had sufficient nursing staff to provide such care (Brooks, et al., 1994).

Gerontologic nurse practitioners have developed models that provide for management in place for many nursing home patients. Some nurse practitioners are employed by the nursing home itself, and some by a physician practice. In a third model, nursing home residents are managed by a health maintenance organization (HMO) called EverCare, which provides services to nursing-home residents that include intravenous medications and on-site laboratory testing so that costs of hospitalization can be avoided and continuity of care maintained. These services are funded by Medicare on a contract, not a fee-for-service basis. An evaluation of this model found that EverCare patients and, even more so, their family members were more satisfied with their access to the nurse practitioner and with the level of information they had about care (Kane, Flood, Keckhafer, Bershadsky, & Lum, 2002). Care in which the patient is known and comfortable can result in better continuity and reduced trauma to patients, many of whom have dementia.

Because a nursing home is a residential facility, patient problems with activities of daily living (ADLs) are an important aspect of care. Nurse practitioners have direct access to the living situation of the residents and will form judgments about function and behavior. A common problem in nursing homes is depression. Diagnosing depression requires attention to subtle cues (see Rule of Thumb in Box 7–2).

Nurse practitioner judgments in the nursing-home setting can provide individualized, compassionate care for vulnerable members of society. The setting provides an opportunity for nurse practitioners to improve the daily life of nursing-home residents.

Box 7–2 RULE OF THUMB:
Diagnosing Depression

(SIG E CAPS = Take Energy **Caps**ule)
Look for change in the following:
Sleep
Interest in activities
Guilt
Energy
Concentration
Appetite
Psychomotor (loss or agitation)
Suicidal (ideation)

Source: Modified from Brozovic, B., & Wold, K. (2000). Managing depression in nursing home elderly. *The Clinical Advisor for Nurse Practitioners, 3*(11/12), 45.

Psychiatric and Mental Health Settings

Nurse practitioners are now preparing for practice in an arena that was formerly led by psychiatric clinical nurse specialists. Psychiatric nurse practitioners provide whole-person care for patients with chronic psychiatric conditions. These patients are vulnerable for two reasons. First, they are on complicated medical regimens with medications that cause troubling and sometimes dangerous side effects. Second, the psychiatric patient may be less able to manage the complexities of the current health-care system independently. A provider who can manage a wide range of psychiatric and primary-care issues can make a difference in a psychiatric patient's life. Furthermore, primary-care practitioners provide the bulk of psychiatric care provided in the United States. Although self-limited and mild forms of psychiatric illnesses can be successfully managed in primary-care settings, the more complicated or extended forms of the illnesses should be referred to providers with special knowledge and experience. Psychiatric nurse practitioners can fill this need.

Assessment by psychiatric nurse practitioners focuses on psychiatric problems and treatments. Clinical judgment in the psychiatric setting includes judgment about mental health promotion, mental illness prevention, management of severe mental illness, various mental disorders, and psychosocial problems as well as support in coping (Oakley & Potter, 1997). Forging a therapeutic alliance with patients who have psychiatric disturbances takes the special care of psychiatrically trained personnel. In addition to taking a psychiatric history, the psychiatric nurse practitioner also focuses on functional areas and physiologic side effects and complaints, and considers co-occurring health problems such as hypertension, diabetes, and other chronic conditions. Psychiatric nurse practitioner programs often prepare students in both standard pharmacology and psychopharmacology. Goals of therapy include return to function, protection from harm, optimizing the pharmacological treatment plan, and support in developing relationships.

Assessment of the psychiatric patient occurs in both psychiatric and primary-care settings. The reason why the psychiatric nurse practitioner is key to excellent care is that patients frequently have co-morbidities that include physical health problems and side effects from complicated medication regimens. Clinical judgments are effective when they include the whole person. Care that ignores important conditions is inefficient and costly. The challenge for primary care generalists and for psychiatric nurse practitioners is to maintain openness to both psychiatric and physical causes for patient distress. Often, general questions that would be part of any health history can alert the nurse practitioner to mental health problems. Such questions might include the following: "Have you felt sad, blue, or down? Have you had trouble sleeping or concentrating? Has your appetite changed? Are you having difficulty with work or home responsibilities?" Responses to these questions may lead the nurse practitioner to consider a more formal psychiatric evaluation. Any fear of suicidal intentions or the possibility for harming others must be reported and care and advice documented (Book, Kates, & Strauss, 1999). The safety of the nurse practitioner is a concern as well. Agitated patients can do harm, whether intentional or not. Practitioners must take care to avoid becoming trapped in treatment rooms or isolated areas. The physical examination for the psychiatric patient must include evaluation of key areas. Table 7–1 indicates the areas of focus during physical examination.

Psychiatric care in community settings has supported good outcomes for patients. In one study (Hunkeler, Meresman, et al., 2000), specially trained primary-care nurses provided regular telephone follow-up to patients with depression. For 6 months, the treatment group received standard medication therapy as well as regular telephone calls, whereas the control group received medication therapy alone. At the end of that time, 58 percent of patients in the treatment group had fewer depression symptoms, compared with only 37 percent of patients in the control group. During the calls, nurses provided emotional support, offered advice about resuming normal physical activities, and suggested strategies for medication management. Nurse practitioners offer leadership in providing holistic care in psychiatric settings (Box 7–3).

TABLE 7-1

Physical Examination for the Psychiatric Patient

Examination	Considerations
Neurological	Headache can be caused by, or a sign of, depression or anxiety, brain tumor, or temporal arteritis.
Cardiovascular	Chest pain, tachycardia. and palpitations can be caused by, or a sign of, anxiety, coronary artery disease, or dysrhythmia.
Respiratory	Shortness of breath can be caused by anxiety, asthma, or chronic obstructive pulmonary disease.
Gastrointestinal	Constipation can be caused by depression, or be a medication side effect. Diarrhea can be caused by anxiety or irritable bowel disease.
Genitourinary	Menstrual disorders can arise from anxiety and depression. Sexual function may be affected by post-traumatic stress disorders or premenstrual dysthymic disorder.
Musculoskeletal	Pain can be associated with anxiety, depression, substance disorders, or chronic fatigue with trigger points.

Source: Modified from Book, S. W., Kates, N., & Strauss, G. (1999). A form-free psychiatric evaluation. *Patient Care for the Nurse Practitioner, 2*(8), 17–24, 27–28, 31.

Box 7-3 Words of Wisdom

Early in my career I was nurse practitioner of a sixty bed locked dementia unit and the patient was a patient that historically had ... been labeled a problem patient. And had a lot of negative staff feelings attached to this individual. She had failed on all the other floors in the nursing home and I heard various bits and pieces...We met as a team and looked at the problem and tried to develop strategies as to how to prevent the problem from occurring on my unit. She was bipolar and she had a personality disorder. At the time I got her she was totally dependent. She had been institutionalized for the last twenty years of her life. She was incontinent, had a Foley, she could not walk, she had contractures of both hands and a seizure disorder. She had been abused by her father as a child....   *(Continued)*

Box 7–3 Words of Wisdom (Continued)

So I met with the patient and said, you know, these are what the rules are, and I'll do the best for you, but you've got to do the best for me. She had many medical problems, but the most significant one that came to mind was, because of her psychiatric history she would have seizures, grand mal seizures. [The psychiatrist believed the seizures were fabricated by the patient] So I negotiated with the Chief of Psychiatry and the Chief of Neurology to sit down with me and review the lady's case. I finally co-opted the Chief of Neurology to really listen to me that this lady needed to have her medication management changed, and once they were able to unblock their view of this woman as a psychiatric patient, they could truly see that she needed more aggressive neurology management, and her medication profile was changed so that her seizures were then under control. I had to fight not only one discipline, I had to fight the history of the patient.

[So once her seizures were better controlled, her behavior became the issue.] I went and I said, "You know something Louise, you keep saying to me that you want the staff to treat you better. You need to think about how you treat the staff and the problems that you cause that are really preventable problems. You want people to treat you with respect, yet you don't respect them. You want to be able to leave this place some day, yet you don't act like you really want to. If you really want to leave, then you're going to have to take responsibility for your health. You are going to have to stop smoking cigarettes, you're going to have to start acting like you want to get rehabilitated, and actually do it. I'll work with you if you work with me." And that was like …like the turning point for our relationship and the way I treated her. I treated her from that point on like she could be rehabilitated, not like her historical medical record. I got her Foley out, I got her walking with a walker, and I got her to be discharged. She even ended up having a boyfriend. She got engaged; she drove a car.

I knew I had to go through a lot of [hard work] to get the patient taken care of. And at the end of a hard day, you really don't want to have to go through all that and just like it was much easier for them to just throw up their hands and say "Oh, well, she's in the nursing home: and forget about it. But I just couldn't forget about it. I would go home and read up about seizures and about medications and think that maybe I missed something.

Source: Dunphy, L. (1999). The wisdom of advanced practice: Approaches to diagnosis and treatment. Unpublished interview data. Used with permission.

Prisons

Clinical judgment in prison settings is affected by setting constraints and by unique disease prevalence patterns. Many inmates are in prison because of drug abuse-related charges. Consequently, the prevalence of HIV and hepatitis among inmates is high. There are concerns that unprotected sex in prisons actually contributes to higher incidence rates of those diseases. Nurse practitioners who practice in prison settings will become expert at managing these diseases as well as providing primary care to the inmate population, which includes young adults through older adults. In the prison setting, the nurse practitioner is the employee or contractor for the corrections system and will be responsible for knowing and enforcing policies specific to that setting. Having a rich network of referrals available for consultation will help the nurse practitioner deal with restrictions that prevent patients from traveling to outside evaluations. Supervising inmate caregivers may also be an aspect of the advanced-practice nurse's responsibilities.

⟫ COMMUNITY-BASED CARE

Clinical judgment in community settings differs from that used in specific institutions in that the community and its resources become part of the assessment and intervention phase of the process. For example, when considering the health of the community, such issues as clean air and water, transportation, and service agencies are important considerations. Nurse practitioners in community settings can advocate for the health of the community by connecting to policy level groups and informing them of health patterns and needs for the patients served in that community. Nurse practitioners can become members of health boards and influence community health directly.

Urgent Care

Urgent-care settings provide walk-in care for patients who do not consider their condition to constitute an emergency but for one reason or another cannot wait for an appointment with a primary-care provider. There are two goals of treatment for the urgent-care nurse practitioner. First, the history and physical examination are focused on the patient's chief complaint. Most likely, the nurse practitioner will not be familiar with the patient. In some cases, an old record may be available, but most likely it will not. Sorting through a history to determine underlying conditions beyond the problem that the patient is currently having may affect treatment options. For example, a history of ulcers will limit the choice of painkillers that can be recommended. Many nonsteroidal anti-inflammatory medications irritate the stomach lining. The second aspect of care should be to determine whether the patient has access to a primary-care provider and therefore to routine screening and health promotion. Referral to appropriate community care for primary care is an important contribution that the nurse practitioner can make that offers more to the patient than simple symptom management.

Faith Communities

Faith communities are community-based institutions where members come together to practice elements of their faith. Health issues and faith have been linked since prerecorded times. Parish nurses provide body-mind-spirit care and offer health promotion opportunities and health teaching (Solari-Twadell & McDermott, 1999). The scope of practice for registered nurses as well as nurse practitioners is regulated by state nurse practice acts and guidance is offered by the Scope and Standards of Parish Nursing Practice (ANA, 1998). Parish nurses can be paid or volunteers, and they can work in a congregational setting or be connected to a health-care facility or network with outreach to specific congregations. Faith communities are good locations for health promotion because clients are known in the context of family and community, people in a wide range of age groupings can be served, and facilities are available for meetings.

The spiritual dimension of health care is frequently overlooked in other health-care settings, but spiritual aspects of illness, such as bereavement and life transition, affect a person's overall health and can be addressed particularly well in the faith community settings. Clinical judgment in the faith community context includes spiritual assessment in a particular framework, which can be more direct. For example, the nurse practitioner can assist families with progressive decline in function of an older family member in the context of the belief in God's love and care for all. The spiritual dimension adds support to assessment and referrals that might be part of routine care. Nurses in the faith community context see people regularly over time and therefore are sensitive to subtle changes in function or energy level. Because of this extended contact, the nurse practitioner can detect conditions that require intervention and referral. Registered nurses can manage simple screening such as regular blood pressure clinics, but nurse practitioners can provide program guidelines, incorporate evidence-based practice, and evaluate program effectiveness.

A survey of parish nurses working in urban and rural settings (Chase-Ziolek & Striepe, 1999) showed that of the 58 who responded, the rural parish nurses were older, valued the support of the clergy member, and made more contacts to their patients in homes and nursing homes and through telephone than urban parish nurses, who were younger, better educated, and more likely to see patients in the church itself. Parish nurses in both urban and rural settings reported setting up health maintenance programs, health screenings, and support to patients that allowed them to remain at home and avoid institutionalization. These services were not provided by the parish nurses alone, but through coordination of volunteers. Advanced-practice nurses were more likely to function in the urban setting.

Nurse-Managed Centers

Nurse-managed centers or academic nursing centers provide a setting that supports nursing models of health-care delivery. These centers are not necessarily organized around a medical model of service delivery. Some nurse-managed centers provide health services to college populations, housing developments, or other community-based settings. Holistic assessments and a wide range of therapeutic options can be offered. Clinical judgments in the nurse-managed setting include diagnosis and treatment as well as health promotion and illness prevention. Because they are based in the community, nurse-managed centers use rich referral networks to provide care in the local context.

Funding for program development often comes from grant support, but contracts with government agencies or residential facilities can support nurse-managed centers. The concerns of managing a practice include funding and fiscal concerns; human resource issues including hiring, credentialing, and evaluating staff; and policy development for the practice. Nurse practitioners can be active in the communities in which their practice exists by advocating for environmental and social structure that support health.

Academic nursing centers provide opportunities for faculty and student practice and provide settings where evidence-based practice and services based in theoretic models can be tested. Faculty members who spend part of their work week in the nurse-managed clinic will need to arrange for follow-up and coverage for days when they are not present in the clinic. They will be able to be role models for students learning to be nurse practitioners, and can use the setting as a research site after obtaining approval by research review boards.

Homeless Shelters

Nurse practitioners provide services to clients in homeless shelters. Clinical judgments in this setting require an understanding of the health problems and risks that the homeless population is likely to experience and also knowledge of local community resources that are available to residents of the shelter. Services such as a nurse's clinic in a shelter can provide foot and wound care, health screening, and facilities for homeless people to keep their medications safely. Many medical centers provide comprehensive medical care to homeless people, but medical care is not all that the homeless require. Some shelters specialize in care of subpopulations such as homeless adolescents, families with children, and individuals with psychiatric and substance-abuse disorders, as well as rehabilitation support for persons in work training programs.

Migrant Health

Care for migrant populations may include settings such as migrant workers' camps. Community health principles regarding water supply, sanitation, and access to food and refuse disposal may be key to ensuring the health of a group of workers. Clinics can be established at migrant camps or through mobile facilities such as trailers that are outfitted for primary-care services. Migrant workers frequently engage in farm work, which has many hazards, including power machinery and chemical exposure. They frequently have no evidence of immunization for communicable diseases. Nurse practitioners use knowledge of health risks and cultural practices for specific migrant groups in forming clinical judgments about diagnoses and interventions. Immigrant families are often young families, so fertility care and care of young children are an important aspect of services that need to be provided.

Rural Health Clinics

Care in many rural areas requires creativity and independence on the part of the nurse practitioner. In many rural areas, particular ethnic or cultural groups predominate, so the nurse practitioner must become familiar with local folkways of health and treatment. Rural health nurse practitioners must deliver care often in the absence of high-tech equipment such as magnetic resonance imaging (MRI) or angiography, so clinical judgments will be made based on excellent history taking and physical diagnosis. An evaluation (Alexy & Elnitsky, 1998) of a rural mobile health unit in a mid-Atlantic state compared two service delivery models, one based on home visits and another on service delivered by nurse practitioners in community settings such as senior centers or post offices. The project was designed to increase access of rural elders to nursing services, to improve or maintain functional status and to increase health promotion activities, to evaluate health service utilization such as hospitalization and emergency room usage, and to provide a practice setting for graduate students. The study found that 222 patients participated over 5 to 28 months and had 1773 encounters with nurse practitioners. Compared with baseline, breast and cervical cancer screenings were increased, emergency room visits were decreased, and immunization rates were increased. Functional status was not significantly changed.

Poverty and lack of transportation, which affect access to care, and methods of follow-up affect clinical judgment in rural settings. Patients are less likely to see a provider for preventive care or even for minor health problems. Therefore problems are often seen in later stages of development and may be more refractory to treatment and unique treatment options and constraints in specific settings.

Home Care

Because of the high cost of inpatient care, many patients are receiving health care in home settings. The advantages of home care include helping patients recover in their family and community context, assisting them in acquiring self-management skills for chronic conditions in real-world settings, and reducing overall health-care costs. The disadvantages include reduced monitoring of changes in health status and reduced efficiency in providing a range of services. In addition, family members may need to take time from their own work to provide care to patients at home.

Because of the increase in home care, nurse practitioners may include home visits in their range of services. Clinical judgment in the home setting involves assessment of functional status and safety in the setting. Blood tests and even portable x rays can be obtained in the home setting to assist decision making. Decisions about the need to transfer patients to health-care facilities may be required, but will increase the cost of care.

Hospice Care

Hospice care offers a way to provide palliative care for patients for whom aggressive care is no longer effective or desirable. Hospice care occurs primarily in the home setting, with a designated lay caregiver providing much of the direct care with support from hospice staff and volunteers. Some hospice care is delivered in special palliative care units that are connected to acute-care institutions or located in extended-care facilities or in free-standing hospice residences. No matter what the setting, the aim of the hospice is family-based personal care with a goal of controlling symptoms. Hospice programs include many caregivers, such as nurses, physicians, social workers, and clergy. Nurse practitioners with expertise in palliative care can promote team coordination and, in most states, manage medication adjustments and minimize side effects. Clinical judgments in the hospice setting are focused on symptom management and emotional support for the dying person and the family. The range of diagnostic possibilities is affected by the processes of dying as well as by a shift in the goals of care.

Some visiting nurse associations that also provide hospice care offer "bridge" or transitional care to assist patients who need palliative care but may not choose a hospice or may not qualify because of ongoing active treatment. One problem with hospice care is that patients are often referred late in their course of illness, and therefore miss the support that hospice care could have provided. From an agency standpoint, having a patient on a hospice benefit for only a matter of days requires expensive care that is not effective in long-term symptom control. As primary-care providers, nurse practitioners can encourage patients and families to consider hospice care early in the course of a terminal illness. Hospice care could also be offered as an alternative as patients complete advance directives or living wills. Although hospice care is often seen as an option only for cancer patients, it also works for patients with congestive heart failure, chronic lung disease, and chronic progressive neuromuscular conditions. Some patients fear that a hospice means that the health-care team is giving up on them. A hospice can be a more acceptable option to patients and families with education about the active support that a hospice entails and the services that it can provide to family members as well as patients.

⟩⟩ VIRTUAL-CARE SETTINGS

Telehealth

With the improvement and widespread availability of technology, more care is being delivered using methods other than simple face-to-face encounters. Telephones have been a source of direct communication for years, but newer methods, including e-mail communication, websites that provide general health information and peer support networks, and two-way video or photo imaging, are augmenting care in many settings. Many patients want 24-hour access to primary-care providers to schedule appointments and to receive test results, and this may be a factor in their choosing a provider. Care delivery modes such as telehealth or telemedicine promise health-care delivery that is more efficient and better coordinated, and that is able to surmount barriers such as a patient's geographic distance from a health-care facility or inability to be transported (as is the case with homebound, institutionalized, or incarcerated patients).

Current applications of telehealth include three major areas. First, health-related information is available via the Worldwide Web. This has been a real advantage to persons with rare diseases or to those who may have conditions that limit mobility. Widespread information capacities require that large numbers of patients have access to computers. This day is at hand. Even those with no computer in the home have access through public libraries and medical center health information facilities. The Internet can be a source of useful health information from reputable sources such as the National Institutes of Health or organizations such as the American Heart Association. It can also be a marketplace where products of unproven benefit to health can be sold to an uncritical audience. Patients may need guidance in interpreting the vast array of health-related information to which they have access. Not all information is of high quality or necessarily related to a particular patient. Nurse practitioners can encourage patients to bring printouts of health information that they have found so that it can be reviewed. The nurse practitioner can reinforce the use of reasonable health information and can screen out information that is not useful.

A second application of telehealth is in self-care and monitoring. Examples of this include home blood glucose monitors that store data, home electrocardiogram (EKG) monitoring that is delivered to a provider over a normal telephone line, and two-way photo or video communication that can assist monitoring of such conditions as wound care. Self-monitoring can be provided through algorithms and reminder systems that are computer based.

Finally, telehealth systems can enhance shared decision making. For example, patient data that can be digitized, such as MRI or computerized tomography (CT) scans, EKGs, or monitor tracings, can easily be transferred via telephone or cable connections between providers. Internet connections provide two-way communication of photographic or even moving images, allowing rural or remote providers to consult with specialists who may be far away. Care-providing networks will no longer require geographic proximity (Russo, 2001).

All the exciting promise of telehealth must be tempered with concern over several important issues (Andrews & Crane, 2001). These include privacy, confidentiality, and licensing concerns. The Health Insurance Portability and Accountability Act of 1996 was designed to provide increased access to health care, but its language concerning patient confidentiality affects all aspects of health care. Another issue raised by telehealth includes patients not being able to see or directly interact with their care providers. Several security issues arise at various points in the process of telehealth. Data capture requires unique participant identifiers. Data transfer involves linkages, storage, and the use of Internet connections, all of which need to be secure. Storage and retrieval of data is also an issue. Who owns the data? Who is responsible for its secure storage?

Provider licensure is another issue affecting telehealth. If nurse practitioners provide health information and advice to patients who live out of state, they may be in violation of state nurse practice laws. Providers at this time are required to hold separate licenses in each state in which they deliver care, even if they are not physically present at that site. A possible solution to this problem is mutual recognition by states that agree to recognize each other's licensees. With this approach, individual state boards of nursing recognize licensure from other states but require nurses practicing within their particular state to follow all of their state's regulations. To date, recognition of advanced practice designation on licenses has not occurred. National organizations are working with state licensing boards for all types of providers to work out these difficulties, so contact your local state board or that of any state in which patients are reached for details on current regulations (Borchers & Kee, 1999).

Principles of clinical judgment apply to health-care decision making, whether the patient encounter is conducted face to face, over the telephone, or via telehealth. A full assessment database appropriate to the situation is necessary. Documentation of judgments, decisions, and patient instructions is necessary for collaborative care as well as for reduced liability exposure. Telehealth offers the possibility of new means of collecting patient data with ongoing monitoring. It also offers a new way to provide ongoing support. Nurses are active in developing telehealth applications and need to advocate for the inclusion of the nursing perspective in telehealth. This would include maintaining respect for individual persons in a holistic environment. Sharing information freely with patients so that they can be active partners in decision making is an important advantage of many forms of telehealth.

)) SUMMARY

Nurse practitioners are found in virtually every segment of health care. Clinical judgment processes are affected by the setting in which the nurse

TABLE 7–2

Web Sites of Interest

Association	Web address
American Association of Critical Care Nurses	*http://www.aacn.org*
American Association of Occupational Health Nurses	*http://www.aaohn.org*
American Correctional Health Services Association	*http://www.corrections. com/achsa*
American Heart Association	*http://americanheart.org*
American Nursing Informatics Association	*http://www.ania.org*
American Telemedicine Association	*http://www.atmeda.org*
Association of Perioperative Registered Nurses	*http://www.aorn.org*
Association of Women's Health Obstetric and Neonatal Nurses	*http://www.awhonn.org*
American Psychiatric Nurses Association	*http://www.apna.org*
American Psychiatric Association clinical practice guidelines	*http://www.psych.org*
American Nurses Association	*http://www.nursingworld.org*
Emergency Nurses Association	*http://www.ena.org*
Migrant health:	
Agency for Toxic Substances and Disease Registry	*http://www.atsdr.cdc.gov/ HEC/natorg/mcn.html*
National Association of School Nurses	*http://nasn.org*
National Health Care for the Homeless Council	*http://www.nhchc.org*
National Hospice and Palliative Care Organization	*http://nhpco.org*
National Rural Health Association	*http://www.nrharural.org*
International Parish Nurse Resource Center	*http://ipnrc.parishnurses.org*
Telehealth: American Telemedicine Association	*http://www.atmeda.org/*
Visiting Nurses Association of America	*http://www.vnaa.org*

practitioner sees a patient. The practice setting primarily affects judgment by requiring nurse practitioners to shift their goals for expected outcomes of care. It also influences nurse practitioners' scope of concerns. Nurse practitioners are independent professionals who negotiate their scope of practice in multiple settings and adapt basic processes to fit each particular setting. Websites related to particular settings are listed in Table 7–2.

REFERENCES

Alexy, B. B., & Elnitsky, C. (1998). Rural mobile health unit: Outcomes. *Public Health Nursing, 15*, 3–11.

American Nurses Association. (1998). *Scope and standards of parish nursing practice*. Washington, DC: Author.

Andrews, A. D., & Crane, L. S. (2001). Recommended practices for protecting privacy in telehealth: Presented at the Sixth Annual Meeting of the American Telemedicine Association; June 3–6, 2001; Fort Lauderdale, FL.

Ariyo, A. A., Haan, M., Tangen, C. M., Rutledge, J. C., Cushman, M., Dobs, A., Furberg, C. D. (2000). Depressive symptoms and risks of coronary heart disease and mortality in elderly Americans. *Circulation, 102*(15), 1773–1779.

Benner, P. (1984). *From novice to expert: Excellence and power in clinical nursing practice*. Menlo Park, CA: Addison-Wesley.

Book, S. W., Kates, N., & Strauss, G. (1999). A form-free psychiatric evaluation. *Patient Care for the Nurse Practitioner, 2*(8), 17–24, 27–28, 31.

Borchers, L., & Kee, C. C. (1999). An experience in telenursing. *Clinical Nurse Specialist, 13*, 115–118.

Brockway, P. M. (1997). The ambulatory surgical nurse. *Nursing Clinics of North America, 32*, 387–394.

Brooks, S., Warshaw, G., Hasse, L., & Kues, J. R. (1994). The physician decision-making process in transferring nursing home patients to the hospital. *Archives of Internal Medicine, 154*, 902–908.

Brozovic, B., & Wold, K. (2000). Managing depression in nursing home elderly. *The Clinical Advisor for Nurse Practitioners, 3*(11/12), 42, 45–46, 49–51.

Buppert, C. (2001). How hospital NPs become revenue-generators rather than expenses. *Nurse Practitioner World News, 6*(1), 1, 16.

Bush, N. J., & Watters, T. (2001). The emerging role of the oncology nurse practitioner: A collaborative model within the private practice setting. *Oncology Nursing Forum, 28*, 1425–1431.

Chase-Ziolek, M., & Striepe, J. (1999). A comparison of urban versus rural experiences of nurses volunteering to promote health in churches. *Public Health Nursing, 16*, 270–279.

Creamer, S. (2002). *The lived experience of lay caregivers of cancer patients at the time of progression or recurrence*. Unpublished doctoral dissertation, Boston College.

Dyer, J. G., Hammill, K., Regan-Kubinski, M. J., Yurick, A., & Kobert, S. (1997). The psychiatric-primary care nurse practitioner: A futuristic model for advanced practice psychiatric-mental health nursing. *Archives of Psychiatric Nursing, 11*(1), 2–12.

Ewy, G. A., & Omato, J. P. (1999). 31st Bethesda Conference: Emergency cardiac care. *Journal of the American College of Cardiology, 35,* 825–880.

Forbes, S., Bern-Klug, M., & Gessert, C. (2000). End-of-life decision making for nursing home residents with dementia. *Journal of Nursing Scholarship, 32,* 251–258.

Frank, C. & Ramirez, E. (2000). Activities and procedures performed by nurse practitioners in emergency care settings. *Journal of Emergency Nursing, 26,* 455–463.

Hunkeler, E. M., Meresman, J. F., Hargreaves, W. A., Fireman, B., Berman, W. H., Kirsh, A. J., Groebe, J., Hiurt, S. W., Braden, P., Getzell, M., Feigenbaum, P. A., Peng, T. A., Salzer, M. (2000). Efficacy of nurse telehealth care and peer support in augmenting treatment of depression in primary care. *Archives of Family Medicine, 9,* 700–708.

Kane, R. L., Flood, S., Keckhafer, G., Bershadsky, B., & Lum, Y. (2002). Nursing home residents covered by Medicare risk contracts: Early findings from the EverCare evaluation project. *Journal of the American Geriatrics Society, 50,* 719–727.

Knaus, V. L., Davis, K., Burton, S., Felton, S., & Fobes, P. (1996). Vascular nurse practitioner: A collaborative practice role in the acute care setting. *Journal of Vascular Nursing, 14*(2), 40–44.

Koschel, M. J. (2003). Is it child abuse? *American Journal of Nursing, 103*(4), 45–46.

Mills, A. C., McSweeney, M., & Lavin, M. A. (1998). Characteristics of patient visits to nurse practitioners and physician assistants in hospital outpatient departments. *Journal of Professional Nursing, 14,* 335–343.

Nester, C. B. (1998). Prevention of child abuse and neglect in the primary care setting. *Nurse Practitioner: The American Journal of Primary Health Care, 23*(9), 61–62, 67–68, 70, 73.

North American Nursing Diagnosis Association. (2001). *Nursing diagnoses: Definitions and classification, 2001–2002.* Philadelphia: Author.

Oakley, L. D., & Potter, C. (1997). *Psychiatric primary care.* St. Louis: Mosby.

Pitts, J., & Seimer, B. (1998). The use of nurse practitioners in pediatric institutions. *Journal of Pediatric Health Care, 12*(2), 67–72.

Pope, J. H., Aufderheide, T. P., & Ruthazer, R. (2000). Missed diagnoses of acute cardiac ischemia in the emergency department. *New England Journal of Medicine, 342,* 1163–1170.

Riegel, B., Carlson, B., & Glaser, D. (2000). Development and testing of a clinical tool measuring self-management of heart failure. *Heart & Lung, 29,* 4–12.

Russo, H. E. (2001). Successful aging: Older adults and technology applications. Presented at the Sixth Annual Meeting of the American Telemedicine Association; June 3–6, 2001; Fort Lauderdale, FL.

Sehy, Y. B., & Williams, M. P. (1999). Functional assessment. In J. T. Stone, J. F. Wyman, & S. A. Salisbury (Eds). *Clinical gerontological nursing: A guide to advanced practice* (2nd ed., pp. 175–199). Philadelphia: W. B. Saunders Company.

Sheahan, S. L. (2000). Documentation of health risks and health promotion counseling by emergency department nurse practitioners and physicians. *Journal of Nursing Scholarship, 32,* 245–250.

Solari-Twadell, P. A., & McDermott, M. A. (1999). *Parish nursing: Promoting whole person health within faith communities.* Thousand Oaks, CA: Sage Publications.

United States Preventative Services Task Force, (2003). *Put prevention into practice.* Rockville, MD: Agency for Healthcare Research and Quality. *http://www.ahrq.gov/clinic/ppipix.htm* Downloaded June 28, 2003.

United States Public Health Service. (1998). *Put prevention into practice: Clinician's handbook of preventive services.* McLean, VA: International Medical Publishing.

CHAPTER 8

Clinical Judgment and Acute-Care Nurse Practitioners

Robin Whittemore, RN, PhD

The nurse practitioner role has been developing steadily in acute-care institutions over the past decades. Increased complexity of patient care, organizational changes in physician residency programs, and cost-containment efforts to expedite patients through the system has created opportunity for advanced-practice nursing in acute-care settings (Kleinpell, 1998; Knaus et al., 1997). Acute-care nurse practitioners (ACNPs) have evolved to become responsible for providing specialized patient care as well as ensuring continuity of care and patient advocacy as members of the health-care team.

ACNPs blend the clinical skills and accountability for treatment plans of the nurse practitioner role with the case management, knowledge of systems, and leadership potential of the clinical nurse specialist role (Ackerman et al., 1996; Moorhead & Huber, 1997). However, there are distinct role differences in current practice settings because nurse practitioners typically spend significantly more time in autonomous direct patient care, whereas clinical nurse specialists spend more time in education, consultation, research, and administration (Sechrist, 1998). Currently, in the acute-care institution, various practice models are seen. For example, some institutions promote collaborative clinical nurse specialist and ACNP practice, whereas others promote either a clinical nurse specialist practice model or an ACNP model of advanced-practice nursing.

In all practice models, ACNPs typically provide direct and comprehensive care to acutely ill patients with complex health problems, beginning with admittance to an acute-care setting and continuing until discharge to a home or community setting. ACNPs promote the stabilization of the acute illness, the prevention of complications, and the restoration of maximum health potential through the provision of physical and psychosocial support measures to patients with acute illnesses and their families (Morse & Brown, 1999). ACNPs can contribute expert specialized and holistic care to patients within a system fraught with fragmentation, multiple health-care providers, and an impersonalized environment (Keane & Richmond, 1993). Providing continuity of care and facilitating a smooth progression through the acute-care system are important elements to ACNP practice that contribute to both quality of care and improved efficiency.

Increasing numbers of ACNPs are demonstrating the benefits of this aspect of advanced nursing practice in critical care units, oncology units, emergency rooms, and acute-care units of extended-care facilities. Since 1995, more than 1400 advanced-practice nurses have sought certification as ACNPs (Kleinpell-Nowell, 1999). Although each acute-care specialty or practice setting may differ with regard to the specific clinical practice of ACNPs, clinical judgment, diagnostic reasoning, treatment decision making, and case management are essential elements to the role (Hravnak et al., 1998; Piano, Kleinpell, & Johnson, 1996). The process of clinical judgment is similar to that previously described in regard to nurse practitioners in primary care. However, setting and role differences of ACNP and nurse practitioner practice render an impact on this process that will be explored in this chapter. Practical strategies to enhance the process of clinical judgment of ACNP practice will subsequently be proposed.

)) SIMILARITIES AND DIFFERENCES OF NURSE PRACTITIONERS AND ACUTE-CARE NURSE PRACTITIONERS

Because the ACNP role evolved from the nurse practitioner role, there are many practice similarities. For example, both ACNPs and nurse practition-

TABLE 8–1

Similarities Between Nurse Practitioner and Acute-Care Nurse Practitioner Practice

Functions within a nursing model

Provides care that is holistic and encompasses family

Provides care that is person centered, not disease centered

Establishes relationships of mutuality with patients

Focuses on health restoration and health promotion

Practices within a collaborative care model

Is accountable and responsible for treatment plan, including nursing and medical measures

Performs decision making about diagnostic tests and therapeutic options

Requires critical thinking and astute clinical judgment

ers conduct histories and physical examinations, make decisions regarding diagnostic tests and therapeutic options, practice in collaboration with a physician, are accountable and responsible for nursing and specified medical measures, practice within a holistic nursing model, and provide person-centered, not disease-centered care (Table 8–1). However, the emphasis on acute care in contrast to primary care contributes to distinct differences between the nurse practitioner and ACNP roles (Table 8–2), all of which can affect clinical judgment. The clinical practice of caring for acutely ill patients in the inpatient setting involves communication and coordination with multiple specialty physicians, with departments of the health-care system such as radiology and pharmacy, and with outside community agencies. A large part of the ACNP role is coordinating this complex system (Kleinpell, 1998). This coordination factors into the ACNP's critical thinking and diagnostic reasoning related to particular patients.

Clinical Practice with Acutely Ill Population

ACNPs provide care to patients with complex, acute, and often life-threatening health problems that are vastly different from the health needs of primary-care patients. Life-threatening hemodynamic instability, pulmonary compromise, and nosocomial infections are frequent concerns related to acutely ill patients. Many hospitalized patients have multisystem diseases, which can contribute to an atypical presentation of symptoms. Acute complications of chronic illnesses can develop in response to thera-

TABLE 8–2
Uniqueness of Acute-Care Nurse Practitioner Role
Acutely Ill Patient Population
Different health problems of acutely ill patients
Physiologic instability of patients
Intensive relationship with patients over a shorter time frame
Potential for greater interaction with family and significant others
Inpatient Setting
Continual access to patients
Multiple and continuous sources of data
Increased use of technology
Role Response to System Inefficiency
More collaboration with health-care team, particularly with medical therapeutic options
Minimize risks inherent in acute-care institutions
Coordinate care and transitions

peutic treatments for other conditions (e.g., an acute exacerbation of congestive heart failure after blood transfusion). Complexity of health problems and clinical judgment is compounded by therapeutic interventions or technologic modalities that often obscure important physical assessment findings (e.g., central nervous system depressants, intubation, mechanical ventilation) (Szaflarski, 1997). The risks associated with the physiologic instability of patients and the potential of developing life-threatening complications require the ACNP to make clinical judgments rapidly in tense environments. Data can be simultaneously overwhelming and incomplete. These factors potentially challenge the diagnostic reasoning process, impeding hypotheses generation and evaluation, problem identification, and treatment decision making.

Relationships with patients are generally intense and of a shorter duration than those seen in primary care. In addition, the ACNP has the potential for greater interaction with family and significant others. Providing information, support, and referrals, as well as promoting coping strategies, is often extended beyond individual patients to their support network. Family members have identified the need for information as a top priority during critical illness of a loved one (Kleinpell, 1999); therefore, one feature that distinguishes the ACNP role from the nurse practitioner role is the intensity of services provided to family and significant others. Difficulties in clinical judgment can subsequently be encountered as a result of competing needs, requests, and priorities. Complex ethical issues are not uncommon. For example, members of the family may be in conflict about end-of-life decisions or patient transfer. Communication among multiple consulting physicians and multiple family members in addition to the patient can increase the complexity of decision making.

Inpatient Setting

The inpatient setting provides an advantage to ACNP clinical practice by virtue of the continual access to patients. Multiple and continuous sources of data and an increased use of technology provide multifaceted and intricate data about a patient's continually changing physiologic status. In the best of circumstances, this can facilitate knowing individual patients holistically and contribute to enhanced clinical judgment and decision-making. Knowing a patient has been identified as an important element of nursing practice. "Knowing a patient" consists of knowing the experiences, behaviors, feelings, perceptions, and patterns of responses of a particular patient (Radwin, 1995; Tanner, Benner, Chesla, & Gordan, 1993). Knowing patients causes certain data to stand out as salient and other data to recede in importance. In addition, the ACNP can make qualitative distinctions by comparing the particular patient to typical patients. By recognizing any relevant changes and early warnings of complications, the ACNP can make better informed clinical decisions that promote progress. (Tanner et al., 1993). Small changes that are often clinically insignificant in isolation take on new meaning when the patient is known (Minick, 1995). Knowing a patient can therefore guide the clinical judgment process and the selection of optimally therapeutic interventions (Radwin, 1996).

It is important to recognize that multiple and continual sources of data do not automatically yield a cohesive and holistic understanding of a particular patient. The sheer volume of data accrued on a patient in a critical-care unit over a 24-hour time frame can be overwhelming, especially to the novice practitioner. Data from multiple sources can be conflicting and even contradictory. The process of clinical judgment can be extremely challenging and fraught with error amid these circumstances. A systematic examination of discrepant data will help the ACNP avoid the diagnostic error of ignoring discrepant data. Furthermore, the ACNP can develop a sense of the wholeness of the situation by asking such questions as, "Are the patient data moving in an overall positive or negative direction?" The ACNP can also listen carefully to the impressions of the staff nurses who are in prolonged contact with the individual patient in making diagnostic and treatment decisions.

Role Response to System Inefficiency

The ACNP works in a complex care delivery system. The more complex a system is, the greater the potential for miscommunication. The ACNP strives to reduce fragmentation of services and thereby to reduce the risks inherent to the acute-care experience. In primary care, the majority of patient care needs are managed through independent nurse practitioner practice with physician consultation and referral. In contrast, critical and acute health problems typically require a greater number of health-care providers simultaneously caring for an individual patient. Acutely ill patients require ongoing collaboration and dialogue, not only between an ACNP and a physician, but also among a myriad of other specialists and health-care practitioners (Herman & Ziel, 1999). Collaboration is therefore essential to the ACNP role. This ultimately affects data collection and the overall process of clinical judgment as the breadth and depth of understanding about a particular patient are expanded. However, competing priorities or contraindicated therapeutic options can be proposed. ACNPs typically evaluate the impact of each treatment recommendation of medical specialists in the overall care trajectory of the patient. Concerns and issues are continually identified to more fully examine risk and benefit ratios. In addition, ACNPs keep key providers informed of important issues, changes in therapeutic treatments, and/or plans for the future.

Norsen et al. (1997) identified that coordination of care and continuity of care are two essential components of ACNP practice. The highly technological and specialized units within acute-care settings, along with the volume of health-care providers involved with any one particular patient, can lead to fragmentation of services and erroneous clinical judgment. ACNP role development was one response to circumventing these issues because ACNPs provide care across a range of services.

ACNPs provide patient advocacy as patients progress through the health-care system, from one level of care to the next. However, much of ACNP clinical judgment involves making the system work for patients, families, and significant others (Richmond, Dubendorf, & Monturo, 1999). Timing of procedures, recognizing stability, and determining the transition of patients from one treatment to another (i.e., weaning from ventilators) or from one unit to another require specialized knowledge of illness and recovery trajectories, knowing the patient, and leadership amid collaboration. ACNPs are integral to effective orchestration of care and astute decision-making of transitions (Richmond et al., 1999).

Last, the risks associated with acute-care therapeutic interventions contribute to differences in the health promotion focus of ACNPs and nurse practitioners. Hravnak (1998) identified that a unique feature of the ACNP role is minimizing the potential risks that are inherent within acute-care institutions. Understanding physiologic risks such as immobility and those occurring as complications of invasive procedures, psychological risks such as sleep deprivation and altered self-image, and the risks of multiple caregivers is crucial to developing expert knowledge of ACNP practice (Hravnak, 1998). Clinical judgment therefore involves the activation of therapeutic strategies that will involve care by a team of providers, such as when directing the weaning of a patient from mechanical ventilation to prevent risks and ultimately promote health.

Attention to continuing health needs related to other chronic illnesses or disabilities also factors into the ACNP's health-promoting decision-making. ACNPs participate in the identification of therapeutic options that not only contribute to the physiologic stability of patients, but also assist in restoring maximum health potential. Through thorough data collection and aggregation, continual identification of existing or potential health problems, education, consultation with other professionals, and knowing the patient, health promotion similar to that practiced in primary care can also be addressed in acutely ill patients.

⟫ CLINICAL JUDGMENT IN ACUTE-CARE NURSE PRACTITIONER PRACTICE

The practice, environment, and role differences of ACNP and nurse practitioner practice can affect critical thinking and diagnostic reasoning. Yet the overall process of clinical judgment is similar to that delineated in Chapter 2 (specifically Figure 2–1). Early generation of hypotheses is an important aspect of the reasoning process. The ACNP acquires data, narrows the search field, and then refines the data acquisition to yield a stronger hypothesis. Physical examination helps the ACNP to further refine the hypothesis under consideration, and appropriate laboratory and diagnostic testing is used to support or refute differing diagnostic possibilities. The ACNP then considers treatment options, taking into account patient and family preferences, co-morbidities, and capacities. In primary-care settings, encounters with patients are limited to short appointments (20 to 60 minutes), whereas in acute-care settings, the nurse practitioner has continual access to patients. This allows for continual observation of patient responses that facilitate the modification of hypotheses and treatment plans within the limits of the time required for caring for multiple patients. In the acute-care setting, follow-up reasoning often occurs simultaneously as part of data collection. In addition, potentially life-threatening health problems demand immediate data collection and treatment decisions.

Clinical judgment has been identified as a difficult aspect of role transition from an experienced nurse to an ACNP (Shah, Bruttomesso, Sullivan, & Lattanzio, 1997). Despite familiarity with the clinical setting and expertise with a specialized population, the complexity of clinical reasoning with acutely ill patients can be daunting. The need to consciously develop clinical judgment skills is an essential and ongoing component of ACNP practice.

Mechanisms to enhance clinical judgment in the ACNP role have been identified. Formal and informal education that involves case studies; think-aloud reasoning exercises, which involve reviewing the data considered and the impressions that are formed during the diagnostic process with another person; and supportive consultation with peers and mentors can provide practice and feedback to foster confidence associated with clinical judgment. In addition, enhancement of clinical judgment can occur through specialization, focused data collection, attention to patterns and trajectories, dealing with uncertainty, and collaboration. Specific techniques to improve clinical judgment are proposed in Table 8–3.

Education and Specialization

In addition to traditional nurse practitioner education, in-depth formal knowledge of the health problems, trajectories, and technology of specialized populations is required for ACNP practice. Opportunities to apply advanced clinical decision making through case studies and clinical practice during educational experiences can expose the complexities inherent in clinical judgment. Mentoring relationships ideally allow increasing independence in clinical judgment and diagnostic reasoning. Feedback from experienced practitioners can help novice ACNPs to gain confidence in their clinical judgments. Experience allows ACNPs to integrate the data from multiple sources more fluidly, contributing to improved clinical judgment (Benner, 1984; Hravnak et al., 1998).

Specialized knowledge helps ACNPs organize and retrieve pertinent information, which in turn helps them evaluate the meaning of presenting signs and symptoms, build lists of possible diagnoses, and identify treatment options for patients. Acute illnesses evolve over time. The condition of a patient in early shock is very different from that of a patient who is experiencing the sequelae of the shock experience. These evolutionary changes are commonly referred to as a trajectory because they reflect change over time. Knowing how specific illnesses evolve over time helps the ACNP to increase diagnostic accuracy. Experts typically have an astute knowledge of standards of care for the specialty population and the trajectory of acute illness experiences. This knowledge helps them recommend

TABLE 8–3
Techniques to Improve Clinical Judgment

Education and Specialization	Having specialized knowledge and experience in a particular clinical area
	Having knowledge of specific illnesses and recovery trajectories
	Learning the clinical judgment process in formal education
	Developing mentoring relationships
Data Collection	Providing a holistic approach to patient care
	Performing thorough initial assessments
	Performing frequent and vigilant assessments prn
	Considering multiple data sources
	Using assessment forms that assist in clustering data
	Maintaining an active problem list to monitor complex cases
Trend and Pattern Evaluation	Looking for patterns in data
	Paying attention to subtle changes in status
	Providing continuity of care
	Knowing the patient
	Using long-term flow sheets
Dealing with Uncertainty	Using protocols and practice guidelines as appropriate
	Generating hypotheses early in the diagnostic process
	Continually evaluating patient responses to treatment
Collaboration	Cultivating relationships with staff nurses and team members
	Demonstrating clinical competence
	Educating staff regarding ACNP role and responsibilities

appropriate treatment interventions based on their early recognition of deviations from expected outcomes. The ability to "chunk" or cluster data is enhanced through specialized experience. Specialized knowledge and expertise acquired through specialization also contribute to the ACNP's ability to recognize patterns and intuitively grasp the whole patient experience. Hypotheses generation and evaluation occur more rapidly and without a conscious deliberative process.

Data Collection

Holistic and thorough data collection can be considered a strength of the nurse practitioner role. Nursing in general is accustomed to having a myriad of data sources to sift through in order to determine a meaningful interpretation of a patient's current status. The need to acquire accurate and relevant data are amplified in the ACNP's decision-making process because of the potential risks to patients associated with errors or lapses in judgment and the speed at which a patient's condition can deteriorate.

Ruddy-Stein & Logan (1999) identified the types and purposes of assessments ACNPs typically perform: comprehensive, interim, and focused assessment. The comprehensive assessment is the initial history and physical examination that is performed with every new patient admitted to the hospital. This is similar to that performed by a nurse practitioner in the primary-care setting. The purpose is to evaluate the primary health problem in detail, determine presenting status, and identify other health conditions that pose risks to the patient or those caring for him or her. The interim assessment is performed at least daily to assess the patient's response to treatments and monitor for complications. For example, an interim assessment with a patient recovering from a complicated sigmoid resection would require a thorough abdominal assessment as well as an assessment of mental status, pain, fluid volume status, wound healing, nutrition, and mobility. Assessment of potential complications related to infection, pneumonia or atelectasis, cardiac output, skin breakdown, and coping would also be important to evaluate with this patient. Lastly, focused assessments are performed whenever there is a change in a patient's baseline status. These assessments are often critical to initiating therapeutic interventions related to life-threatening conditions and are guided by presenting symptoms and an understanding of the patient's current health status.

The acute-care environment allows dynamic and continuous assessment of patients over time. Subtle changes that reflect either progression or complications often steer the treatment decision-making process. Snapshots of stability represent desirable outcomes, and any deviation should alert the ACNP to a potential complication. By detecting complications early, the ACNP can help avert or minimize serious sequelae. Frequent assessments are the cornerstone to full actualization of the ACNP role in that they support detection of early changes so that treatments can be initiated in a timely fashion.

Assessment data are collected from a myriad of different sources. When generating and evaluating hypotheses, the ACNP considers data not only from the patient's history, physical examination, and laboratory/diagnostic test reports, but also from such sources as physiologic monitors, written and verbal progress reports from other health-care providers, and the patient's family. Although this provides a richer and more extensive database, conflicting reports and inundation of data must be appropriately considered.

As part of the ACNP's specialized knowledge base, knowledge of the accuracy and limitations of specific technology is required. It is imperative that ACNPs understand the current state of the science regarding diagnostic tests and technology so they can prioritize data generated from these sources. For example, inaccuracies in hemodynamic measurement can contribute to misinterpretation of hemodynamic values and inaccurate diagnostic impressions (Szaflarski, 1997).

Practicing within a conceptual framework, such as functional health patterns, helps reduce disparate pieces of data into meaningful clusters, allowing the ACNP to interpret and identify potential problem areas more easily. Mechanisms that contribute to data clustering ease the cognitive challenges of analyzing and integrating large databases. Using assessment forms that assist in clustering data (i.e., functional health patterns) and maintaining an active problem list of complex patients facilitate the thoroughness of this effort.

Trend and Pattern Evaluation

Because of the continuous nature of data collection, examining trends in data, in contrast to the results of an isolated test, facilitates clinical judgments. Specialized knowledge and a keen understanding of typical illness and recovery trajectories alert the ACNP to unexpected or divergent trends. Knowing the patient and continuity of care help the ACNP to identify subtle changes in patient responses and illness trajectories.

Clustering of signs and symptoms into patterns (e.g., long-term flow sheets) is an important aspect that facilitates the diagnostic reasoning process, allowing the ACNP to quickly identify the similarities between patterns exhibited in a patient that deviate from the anticipated trajectory. More frequent assessments or a change in the treatment plan may be warranted. Each individual patient experience contributes to the long-term clustering of data bits about particular diagnoses and complications. Any area of concern ideally causes the ACNP to generate hypotheses regarding diagnostic possibilities. Early and continual hypotheses generation facilitates the refinement of diagnostic reasoning as relevant data can then be examined to confirm or eliminate these hypotheses. As in primary care, early generation of hypotheses directs a more efficient approach to clinical judgment and the reasoning process (Szaflarski, 1997).

Dealing with Uncertainty

Diagnostic uncertainty is inherent to the process of clinical judgment. Ordering diagnostic tests and observing treatment effectiveness are measures that nurse practitioners take to reduce uncertainty. Clinicians must be prepared to approach issues of uncertainty as logically as possible, seeking the most reasonable conclusion (Kussmaul, 1999). At the same time, diagnostic reasoning may be viewed as an iterative process, a constant refinement that leads from hypotheses generation (uncertainty) to problem identification (increased certainty).

Uncertainty in diagnostic reasoning is accentuated while caring for critically ill patients. Physiologic instability and critical illness require rapid decision making, and interventions that exert a continuous effect (e.g., ventilators, pharmacologic paralysis) can often obscure symptoms. The treatment itself may conceal important diagnostic criteria (Szaflarski, 1997). For example, sedation after open-heart surgery may mask a subtle yet significant change in mental status. In addition, patients themselves may be poor historians while in pain, under the influence of pharmacologic agents, or overwhelmed by a critical illness.

Several mechanisms can assist in dealing with uncertainty in acute-care clinical judgment. Protocols, practice guidelines, and collaborative practice agreements assist in identifying the scope of provider services and therefore the decision making in clinical practice. Protocols provide an organized method for analyzing frequently observed symptoms or complications, generally for those aspects of care that require medical authorization (Paul, 1999). These practice guidelines usually do not include independent nursing judgments and primarily serve as recommendations that are adapted in order to individualize care, meeting specific needs of patients. Because the ACNP is an evolving role, many ACNPs are actively involved in developing protocols that affect their institutional practice. Practice guidelines (*http://www.guidelines.gov*) and decision trees are also helpful to novice practitioners, particularly when dealing with potentially life-threatening health problems and stressful situations.

Purposeful data collection through early hypotheses generation can also reduce uncertainty. Evaluating patient responses to treatment can clarify the reasoning process by providing expected or unanticipated responses (Szaflarski, 1997). For example, if a patient with a diagnosis of congestive heart failure develops dyspnea and crackles in the left lower lobe that do not respond to intravenous furosemide, an alternative diagnostic hypothesis of pneumonia should be considered. Lastly, the maxim of "When hearing hoofbeats, suspect horses, not zebras" is helpful when dealing with uncertainty, because when several competing hypotheses are being considered, the most commonly occurring one is often correct.

Uncertainty in the diagnostic process can be stressful, particularly with acutely ill patients. However, the opportunity for continuous data collection can validate the decision-making process, providing immediate feedback and ultimately decreasing uncertainty.

Collaboration

Collaborative practice affects the clinical judgment and decision-making process. For example, data collection does not consist solely of information collected by an individual ACNP. Data in acute-care institutions is generated from technology, staff nurses, and other health professionals. Strong collaboration yields positive communication that can enhance the concerted effort to care for an individual patient.

Collaborative practice agreements or job descriptions define the practice of an ACNP, delineating rights and responsibilities within a health-care environment with multiple caregivers. These agreements can serve as the foundation for clinical decision-making (Herman & Ziel, 1999). They can also provide essential information for staff nurses and other advanced-practice nurses (e.g., clinical nurse specialists) that clarify practice boundaries. Knaus et al. (1997) report that one of the greatest barriers to ACNP implementation has been with conflicting responsibilities between physicians and ACNPs and nurses and ACNPs. Clear role definition and staff education greatly influence the potential success of the ACNP role. For example, positive relationships with staff nurses will result in timely communication of patient problems. Cultivating relationships with staff and demonstrating competence will also help develop collaborative practice and informed decision making.

◯)) SUMMARY

The ACNP role has developed in response to highly complex and technological acute-care institutions, in which the ACNP provides direct and indirect patient care collaboratively with other health-care professionals. The increased emphasis on direct care by this advanced-practice nurse is one response to the challenge of placing the best-prepared nurses central to the delivery of patient care. This role requires the ACNP to integrate knowledge of a specialized population and the associated health care and technology with nursing's holistic view of patient-centered care (Keane & Richmond, 1993). For full actualization of this role, the ACNP must engage in critical analysis of complex patient care problems and creative collaboration with other health-care providers. Developing confidence and expertise in clinical judgment enhances role development and the quality of patient care provided.

REFERENCES

Ackerman, M. H., Norsen, L., Martin, B., Wiedrich, J., & Kitzman, H. J. (1996). Development of a model of advanced practice. *American Journal of Critical Care, 5,* 68–73.

Benner, P. (1984). From *novice to expert: Excellence and power in clinical nursing practice.* Menlo Park, CA: Addison-Wesley Company.

Herman, J., & Ziel, S. (1999). Collaborative practice agreements for advanced practice nurses: What you should know. *AACN Clinical Issues, 10,* 337–342.

Hravnak, M. (1998). Is there a health promotion and protection foundation to the practice of acute care nurse practitioners? *AACN Clinical Issues, 9,* 283–289.

Hravnak, M., Kobert, S. N., Risco, K. G., Baldisseri, M., Hoffman, L. A., Clochesy, J. M., Rudy, E. B., & Snyder, J. V. (1998). Acute care nurse practitioner curriculum: Content and development process. *American Journal of Critical Care, 4,* 179-183.

Keane, A., & Richmond, T. (1993). Tertiary nurse practitioners. *Image, 25,* 281–284.

Kleinpell, R. M. (1998). Acute care nurse practitioners: Reports from the practice setting. In R. M. Kleinpell & M. R. Piano (Eds.). *Practice issues for the acute care nurse practitioner* (pp. 1–9). New York: Springer Publishing Company.

Kleinpell, R. (1999). Approach to the hospitalized patient. In P. Logan (Ed.). *Principles of practice for the acute care nurse practitioner* (pp. 111–116). Stamford, CT: Appleton & Lange.

Kleinpell-Nowell, R. (1999). Longitudinal survey of acute care nurse practitioner practice. *AACN Clinical Issues, 10,* 515–520.

Knaus, V. L., Felter, S., Burton, S., Fobes, P., & Davis, K. (1997). The use of nurse practitioners in the acute care setting. *Journal of Nursing Administration, 27,* 20–27.

Kussmaul, N. G. (1999). Medical reasoning. In P. Logan (Ed.). *Principles of practice for the acute care nurse practitioner* (pp. 141–147). Stamford, CT: Appleton & Lange.

Minick, P. (1995). The power of human caring: Early recognition of patient problems. *Scholarly Inquiry of Nursing Practice, 9,* 303–315.

Moorhead, S., & Huber, D. G. (Eds.) (1997). *Nursing roles: Evolving or recycled?* Thousand Oaks, CA: Sage Publications.

Morse, C. J., & Brown, M. M. (1999). Collaborative practice in the acute care setting. *Critical Care Nursing Quarterly, 21,* 31–36.

Norsen, L., Fineout, E., Fitzgerald, D., Horst, D., Knight, R., Kunz, M. E., Lumb, E., Martin, B., Opladen, J., & Schmidt, E. (1997). The acute care nurse practitioner: Innovative practice for the 21st century. In S. Moorhead & D. G. Huber (Eds.). *Nursing roles: Evolving or recycled?* (pp.150–169). Thousand Oaks, CA: Sage Publications.

Paul, S. (1999). Developing practice protocols for advanced practice nursing. *AACN Clinical Issues, 10,* 343–355.

Piano, M. R., Kleinpell, R., & Johnson, J. A. (1996). The acute care nurse practitioner and management of common health problems: A proposal. *American Journal of Critical Care, 5,* 289–292.

Radwin, L. E. (1995). Knowing the patient: A process for individualized interventions. *Nursing Research, 44,* 364–370.

Radwin, L. E. (1996). Knowing the patient: A review of research on an emerging concept. *Journal of Advanced Nursing, 23,* 1142–1146.

Richmond, T. S., Dubendorf, P., & Monturo, C. (1999). Scope and standards of clinical practice. In P. Logan (Ed.). *Principles of practice for the acute care nurse practitioner* (pp. 11–23). Stamford, CT: Appleton & Lange.

Ruddy-Stein, Y. A., & Logan, P. (1999). The history and physical examination. In P. Logan (Ed.). *Principles of practice for the acute care nurse practitioner* (pp. 117–139). Stamford, CT: Appleton & Lange.

Sechrist, K. R. (1998). Role of the clinical nurse specialist: An integrative review of the literature. *AACN Clinical Issues, 9,* 306–324.

Shah, H. S., Brutomesso, K. A., Sullivan, D. T., & Lattanzio, J. (1997). An evaluation of the role and practices of the acute care nurse practitioner. *AACN Clinical Issues, 8,* 147–155.

Szaflarski, N. L. (1997). Diagnostic reasoning in acute and critical care. *AACN Clinical Issues, 8,* 291–302.

Tanner, C. A., Benner, P., Chesla, C., & Gordon, D. R. (1993). The phenomenology of knowing the patient. *Image, 25,* 273–280.

CHAPTER 9

Issues in Primary Care

CHAPTER OUTLINE

From the inception of the nurse practitioner role, nurse practitioners have been agents for change (Draye & Brown, 2000). Being effective as a nurse practitioner requires more than understanding patient care; it involves learning how to shape systems of care. Nurse practitioners face issues in the health-care system that affect their ability to engage in the full range of clinical judgments described in this book. Several issues, such as nursing model of practice versus the medical model of practice, legislative authority to practice, and the ability to be paid for one's work, affect nurse practitioner practice now and are anticipated to continue their influence into the future. This chapter focuses on the key issues that affect nurse practitioner judgment and therefore practice. After reading this chapter, new nurse practitioners will be able to engage in the active debate that surrounds and affects nurse practitioner practice. In addition, they will be able to engage in meaningful change in their practice settings that will increase nurse practitioner effectiveness and the quality of patient care into the future.

⟩⟩ COLLABORATION

Working collaboratively has been set as a goal for a redesigned health-care system (Hurtado, Swift, & Corrigan, 2001). Collaboration ensures that each member of the health-care team offers his or her particular expertise when caring for patients. Although collaboration should promote an environment of trust and respect, it also requires focused attention and repeated clear communication. Collaboration can occur within a local practice office or with referring practitioners, including physicians, other nurses or nurse practitioners, psychologists, pharmacists, nutritionists, and various types of therapists. When collaborating with consulting physicians, the nurse practitioner must be sure that the patient's situation is fully understood and communicated. Such communications should be documented. Another aspect of collaboration may involve interdisciplinary education and training. In all such cases, nurse practitioners can inform other disciplines of their unique perspective on clinical judgment, goal setting, and intervention selection.

Nurse practitioners can support collaborative practice by training new nurse practitioners and physicians in such a working model. Renegotiating practice arrangements to support innovative collaborative models can help the practice transcend old traditions and develop new ways of operating. These new models put patient needs at the center and allow for the provider with the most important skill set to take the lead in designing care. This model differs from the hierarchical system that was dominant for many years. Educational curricula need to provide interdisciplinary educational opportunities so that each new provider (nurse practitioner; physician; and others such as those involved in social work, pharmacy, physical or occupational therapy, and psychology) understands the perspective and values of others (American Association of Colleges of Nursing, 1995). Specific skills in teamwork, negotiating, conflict management, and systems design need to be included in curricula for all health providers. New models for doctoral education that are more interdisciplinary will help to prepare faculty members to teach using collaborative modes. Ryan (1999) points out that collaboration does not occur automatically, but that communication skills and attitudes must be learned.

A Canadian study that used direct observation of interdisciplinary practice patterns showed that responsibilities and roles shifted in response to specific patient needs. The group of health-care providers was able to process vast amounts of patient data and allowed individual expertise to be brought to bear on patient problems. Primary-care providers delivered continuous care with intermittent support by consultants as needed. The communication process was supported by teamwork and trust that reduced the burden of interactions (Patel, Cytryn, Shortliffe, & Safran, 2000).

Several studies have compared nurse practitioner and physician practice. One study showed that nurse practitioners offer unique models of care to a practice setting. It compared nurse practitioner practice patterns with a matched group of physician practices using a standardized survey, the National Ambulatory Medical Care Survey (NAMCS). The study showed that nurse practitioners cared for higher proportions of both younger patients and female patients. They performed fewer office surgical procedures and spent more time in teaching and counseling interventions than their physician counterparts (Moody, Smith, & Glenn, 1999). A different study using the same national survey showed patient demographics similar to those in the Moody and others study, but also showed that primary-care practices by nurse practitioners and physician assistants were more alike than either group as compared with physicians (Hooker & McCaig, 2001). Another study comparing nurse practitioner and physician practices using the NAMCS showed that setting variables were better predictors for practice pattern than educational preparation. The authors suggest that more collaborative models be used in the education of both groups (Mills & McSweeney, 2002).

Although collaborative models of practice allow appropriate contributions by all providers, one aspect of collaboration can be problematic. The problem is that "collaboration" has been made mandatory by some states' legislation or regulation, which really means oversight and control of nurse practitioner practice by a "collaborating" physician, which can limit the full exercise of nurse practitioner judgment (Lee & Pulcini, 1998). Safriet (quoted in Lee & Pulcini, 1998) points out the irony of a professional whose ability to practice has been recognized by national certifying bodies and by state authority being required to seek permission of an individual of a related but separate profession for permission to practice. If "collaboration" leads to economic control or limitation in access of patients to the services of nurse practitioners, that mandatory collaboration limits the scope of practice of nurse practitioners.

)) NURSING VERSUS MEDICAL PRACTICE MODEL

Is There a Place for Nursing Diagnosis?

To fully enact the clinical judgment model, the nurse practitioner must be able to assess the patient's situation fully, choose from a wide variety of interventions (based on both the nursing and biomedical models), and document the full range of assessment, intervention, and outcomes of the nurse-patient partnership. Many nurse practitioners work in settings that do not recognize the full advanced-practice nurse model because of limited documentation choices in record systems. Nurse practitioners need to be very clear in their own minds and in their communication about the nature of their practice. This might require adapting record keeping to allow documentation of interventions such as health counseling.

Busy clinicians often say there is no time or place for nursing diagnoses in their practice. Encounter forms are designed and printed to maximize billing and streamline documentation. However, when nurse practitioners reflect on how they spend their time, they often discover that they spend many hours listening to patients, supporting them, and teaching them about problems that are not strictly medical diagnoses. How prevalent are nursing diagnoses in primary care? A database developed by one university to track the clinical experiences of their adult nurse practitioner students revealed that nursing diagnoses were identified during 57 percent of patient visits. The most common nursing diagnosis was pain (16.8%), followed by health-seeking behaviors (13.9%), altered health maintenance (9.3%), unspecified knowledge deficit (6.4%), altered tissue perfusion (4.7%), and others. The most frequently cited medical diagnosis was hypertension (12.7%). The system was set up to allow students to record both medical and nursing diagnoses (O'Connor, Hameister, & Kershaw, 2000). Billing for health counseling is appropriate for many of the nursing diagnoses.

Intervention and Outcome Classifications

The study by O'Connor and others (2000) also revealed that adult nurse practitioner students used nursing interventions as codified by the Nursing

Intervention Classification. The most frequently cited nursing interventions were patient education, drug management, information management, and risk management. The use of nationally and internationally recognized data sets is important for nurse practitioners who need to continually describe and differentiate their practice. Documenting only those skills that are printed on an encounter form prevents research on the aspects of nurse practitioner practice that are most effective. Nurse practitioners are more than substitutes for physicians. As nurses, they have their own body of knowledge and skills that are used to help improve patients' health. The use of accepted language to describe those skills is essential. Outcomes of nurse practitioner practice may be different from outcomes of physician practice. Identifying patient outcomes such as "Knowledge: Medication... Pain Control Behavior...Health Promoting Behavior...Urinary continence" (Johnson & Maas, 1997, p. xxi) and tracking which intervention accomplishes these outcomes, and for whom, are necessary to justify the argument for nurse practitioners' emerging role in health care.

Advanced-Practice Roles and Judgment

Traditionally, the advanced-practice role that predominated in hospitals was that of the clinical nurse specialist. This role differed from the nurse practitioner role in that it was based in the hospital system, usually in the department of nursing. The clinical nurse specialist used advanced knowledge and skill to improve the care delivered by an institution. The traditional roles of the clinical nurse specialist include educator, researcher, change agent, direct-care provider, and consultant. Usually the direct-care aspect of the role was only part of the clinical nurse specialist's responsibility, whereas the nurse practitioner focused on direct care and carried out the other roles of advanced practice to a lesser degree. Clinical nurse specialists focused on a specialty area of practice, such as oncology, cardiology, or orthopedics. They developed management plans for complex patients and consulted with medical and nursing staff on patient care. They also helped to establish patient education and discharge planning systems for groups of patients. In many settings, the case management role has assumed responsibility for the disease management focus.

A recent study comparing practice patterns between nurse practitioners and clinical nurse specialists shows continued differences in role activities (Lincoln, 2000). This study showed the differences in practice patterns that persist. In this sample of advanced-practice nurses in Minnesota, there seems not to be a merging of the roles, as has been suggested by some. Another study conducted in the United Kingdom using the Delphi technique showed that most of the competencies of both clinical nurse specialists and nurse practitioners were built on registered nurse competencies, but that nurse practitioners were required to assess and diagnose in both the nursing and medical domains and to manage and evaluate care for medical and nursing problems. This distinguished the practice of nurse practitioners, although some clinical nurse specialists used many of these skills as well (Roberts-Davis & Read, 2001).

Clinical nurse specialists and nurse practitioners, as well as nurse midwives and nurse anesthetists, are all considered advanced-practice nurses. The scope of judgment for each of these roles is considered more specialized than that of the basic registered nurse. Educational programs for each of these roles prepare the nurse to exert judgments and act independently with a unique scope of practice. The range of issues covered by each role varies somewhat, but each can be seen as working from a core of interpersonal relationship, in a practice that requires clinical judgment. Many of the skills described in this book apply to roles other than that of the nurse practitioner and can be adapted for use. For example, history taking and documentation are required of all roles. Clinical specialists have advanced education and experience in working with a special group of clients and frequently are involved in complex system support roles. They may have clinical management responsibilities for their patient population that transcend settings and may include clinics, in-hospital units, and departments. They are frequently involved in quality improvement in the system and develop specialized training programs for staff nurses to ensure quality of care. Their judgments are for both individual patients and populations of patients. Certified Nurse Midwives manage pregnancy and labor-related issues. They specialize in supporting healthy pregnancies and offer teaching, support, and holistic care. Nurse anesthetists are authorized to provide anesthesia care, including preanesthesia assessment, administration of various anesthetic agents, management of recovery, and consultation with pain services. All of these skills require judgment. The basic elements of clinical judgment, if not the particular content, are common to each of these advanced nursing practice roles. The processes of establishing a relationship, determining patient problems and potential for health improvement, selecting from a variety of interventions (some of which are unique to the advanced-practice role), and evaluating the quality of care are basic to all.

Certification

Graduates of nurse practitioner programs must meet certification and regulatory requirements before they can practice in the expanded nursing role. These regulations affect the scope of clinical judgments that nurse practitioners in a particular jurisdiction can perform and for which they are held accountable. Each state sets its own requirements for authorization for advanced practice, and these requirements may vary by type of preparation. For example, nurse practitioners may be regulated differently from clinical nurse specialists. Psychiatric clinical nurse specialists, because they have always had direct patient care as their primary orientation, may be handled differently from other types of clinical nurse specialists. It is the nurse practitioner's responsibility to determine the requirements of the state in which he or she wishes to practice. Each state Board of Nursing has a website that can be accessed to determine specific requirements.

Most states require certification by a nationally recognized certifying board in order for a nurse to practice in the expanded nursing role. Students need to determine which certifying board they wish to use. Several of the organizations listed in Table 9–1 provide certification examinations. Requirements for sitting for the examination may vary. Most now require the master's degree or a post-master's degree program as preparation. Although some specialties have only one exam to choose from (neonatal, gerontological, acute care, school nurse practitioner), others offer more than one option. The American Academy of Nurse Practitioners (AANP) certifies adult and family nurse practitioners, using a paper-and-pencil test offered three times a year in locations around the country. The American Nurses Credentialing Center (ANCC) now offers computer-based testing only. It is affiliated with the American Nurses Association, which offers discounts to members. ANCC examinations include separate tests for acute care, adult, family, gerontology, pediatric, adult psychiatric and mental health, and family psychiatric and mental health. Pediatric examinations are also offered by the National Certification Board for Pediatric Nurse Practitioners and Nurses (NCBPNP/N). To sit for this examination, the nurse must be a graduate of a program that this group approves (Miller, 1999a).

Legal Considerations

Nurse practitioner practice is controlled by individual state laws and by the rules and regulations that each state's board promulgates. A wide variety of practice restrictions currently exists. Each January the journal *The Nurse Practitioner: The American Journal of Primary Health Care* publishes its annual legislative update, which lists each state's legal practice authority and allowable reimbursement and prescriptive authority. For example, some states allow nurse practitioners to prescribe any class of

TABLE 9—1

Selected Organizations for Nurse Practitioners

American Academy of Nurse Practitioners (AANP)

P. O. Box 12846

Austin, Texas 78711

512-442-4262

www.aanp.org

American Association of Occupational Health Nurses, Inc.

2920 Brandywine Road, Suite 100

Atlanta, Georgia 31341-5539

770-455-7757

www.aaohn.org

American College of Nurse Midwives (ACNM)

818 Connecticut Avenue NW, Suite 900

Washington, DC 20006

202-728-9860

www.midwife.org.

American College of Nurse Practitioners (ACNP)

1111 19th Street SW, Suite 404

Washington, DC 20036

202-659-2190

www.acnpweb.org

American Nurses Association (ANA)

600 Maryland Avenue SW, Suite 100W

Washington, DC 20024-2571

1-800-274-4262

www.nursingworld.org

American Nurses Credentialing Center (ANCC)

600 Maryland Avenue SW, Suite 1001W

Washington, DC 20024-2571

1-800-274-4262

http://nursingworld.org/ancc/

Association of Advanced Practice Psychiatric Nurses (AAPPN)

555 33rd Avenue NE

Seattle, Washington 98105

1-888-308-7336

www.aappn.org

TABLE 9–1

Selected Organizations for Nurse Practitioners

Association of Nurses in AIDS Care (ANAC)
3538 Ridgewood Road
Akron, Ohio 44333
1-800-260-6780
www.anacnet.org

Association of Women's Health Obstetric and Neonatal Nurses (AWHONN)
2000 L Street NW, Suite 740
Washington, DC 20036
1-800-673-8499
www.awhonn.org

National Alliance of Nurse Practitioners
P. O. Box 40326
Washington, DC 20016
202-675-6350

National Association of Neonatal Nurses (NANN)
4700 W. Lake Avenue
Glenview, Illinois 60025-1485
1-800-451-3795
www.nann.org

National Association of Nurse Practitioners in Women's Health (NPWH)
503 Capitol Court NE, Suite 300
Washington, DC 20002
202-543-9693
www.npwh.org

National Association of Pediatric Nurse Practitioners (NAPNAP)
100 King's Highway N, Suite 206
Cherry Hill, New Jersey 08034-1912
1-877-6NAPNAP
www.napnap.org

National Certification Board of Pediatric Nurse Practitioners and Nurses
(NCBPNP/N)
800 S. Frederick Avenue, Suite 104
Gaithersburg, Maryland 20877-4151
1-888-641-2767
www.pnpcert.org

(Continued on following page)

TABLE 9—1 *(Continued)*
Selected Organizations for Nurse Practitioners
National Conference of Gerontological Nurse Practitioners (NCGNP) P. O. Box 232230 Centreville, Virginia 20120 710-802-0088 *www.ncgnp.org*
National Organization of Nurse Practitioner Faculties 1522 K Street NW, # 702 Washington, DC 20005 202-289-8044 *www.nonpf.com*
Nurse Practitioners Associates for Continuing Education (NPACE) 5 Militia Drive Lexington, Massachusetts 02421 781-861-0270 *www.npace.org*

drug and to practice without a physician's supervision, but others restrict prescriptive authority and require a supervisory arrangement with a physician. Another important issue is whether nurse practitioners are regulated by nurses alone or partly by a physician board (Pearson, 2002). It is vital for nurse practitioners to safeguard their authority to practice and to promote further development in states where full authority is not yet allowed.

Influencing Policy

A recent paper (Pruitt, Wetsel, Smith, & Spitler, 2002) described a survey of nursing organization leaders who had achieved legislative success in their respective states. The survey showed that legislative work is a long process that requires careful planning, a coherent message, and the establishment of personal relationships with legislators. Successful initiatives involved not only nurse practitioners but also clinical nurse specialists, certified nurse midwives, and certified registered nurse anesthetists. Many of the nursing leaders worked with professional lobbyists, many of whom had nursing backgrounds. To have the greatest impact, the nursing groups sometimes delayed action because of elections, budget concerns, and other hot legislative topics. A research study (Martin & Hutchinson, 1999) that used the qualitative research methodology grounded theory to uncover a problem that nurse practitioners faced when dealing with legislative and regulatory issues describes the process of "discounting." This process results in marginalization of nurse practitioners. Marginalization means that the staff preparing legislation and regulations disregarded the communication and concerns of nurse practitioners. Nurse practitioner practice was described from a negative perspective. The authors intend that, by recognizing the process of discounting, nurse practitioners can minimize its effect as they work on legislative issues. Some means that nurse practitioners can use are repeating concerns, supplying facts, and building support by constituents.

The nurse practitioners surveyed by Pruitt and others (2002) reported a sense of satisfaction in participating in the legislative process. Some started their policy initiatives as a commitment they felt as they completed graduate school. The skills involved in this complex process required many types of individual efforts, from research and writing to meeting the public and the legislators. There is room for everyone's contribution to support this important work. Another national survey (Oden, Price, Alteneder, Boardley, & Ubokudom, 2000) of nurse practitioners' involvement in the policy process found that because of the complexity of the task of influencing legislation, teamwork was necessary. Most nurse practitioners were involved in three or fewer activities. The most common activities were voting (most prevalent) and contributing to political campaigns. Lack of time was cited as a barrier to more policy involvement.

Nurses need to develop a strong voice so that their perspective is heard at the national level where health system delivery is designed and regulated. Nurses are eligible for policy fellowships through such programs as the Robert Wood Johnson Health Policy Fellowship. These year-long programs provide a perspective on the health policy process and experience in researching and taking a position on policy issues such as legislation, funding, and regulation. Information on the Robert Wood Johnson program is available at *http://www4.nas.edu/iom/hppf/hppfhome.nsf* (Sharp, 1999).

Active involvement in the state's legislation and regulation, as well as participation in professional organizations, can support these efforts. The message to legislators should not be about what is good for the nurse practitioner, but what is good for the health of the legislator's constituents. Communication needs to be based in research, such as the effectiveness and safety of advanced-practice nurses, but also on the policies and regulation of neighboring states. Pruitt and others (2002) suggest that all legislative work needs adequate funding for paying lobbyists, developing written materials, and conducting research. Professional organizations and fund raising are important supports. Finally, after successful legislation is passed and signed by the governor, another event that may need support, the administrative or regulation phase of the process, begins and needs monitoring.

Organizational Involvement

All the issues discussed in this chapter require an organized effort and voice in order to be addressed in the policy arena. Individual effort makes a difference, but real influence comes from activities with other professionals. (See Table 9–1 for professional organizations that nurse practitioners can join in order to have a larger influence on the policy debate.) Nurse practitioners may also identify health needs for their patient populations that they can better address by organizing and speaking in a united front with other nurses and health professionals. This type of action may require political action. Membership in advanced-practice organizations such as the American Academy of Nurse Practitioner or the American College of Nurse Practitioners can support work at the policy level.

International Licensure Issues

A conference held in Dublin, Ireland in August 2002 brought together nurses and policy makers from 12 countries to discuss development of the nurse practitioner role. The meeting was sponsored by the Royal College of Nursing and the Irish Nurses Organization. Attendees from Africa, Asia, North America, Australia, and New Zealand participated. Thirty different countries are considering implementing the nurse practitioner role as a cost-effective means of providing for health care. Differences in the roles are noted by country. For example, the role of nurse practitioner in the United States was first developed to provide primary care, whereas nurse practitioners in the Netherlands are developing hospital-based roles that support continuity of care. Representatives from the International Council of Nursing presented information on worldwide health concerns that nurses are needed to address (Zimmer, 2002). Individual nurse practitioners can become involved through activities of the International Nurse Practitioner/Advanced Practice Nurse Network. Their website address is *http://icn-apnetwork.org/*. Annual conferences are planned.

⊚) GETTING PAID FOR NURSE PRACTITIONER WORK

One of the different aspects of nurse practitioner practice is the independence that it affords. Rather than the nurse practitioner being a shift employee, the practice arrangements for nurse practitioners involve a professional practice model. There are a variety of models for nurse practitioner practice, and factors such as payment systems, whether the nurse practitioner will maintain a caseload of patients, and how patients are scheduled are important. A recent paper described the importance of having local data on prevailing payment practices, which can assist in negotiations. Several factors were found to affect salary, including experience, the practice setting, geographical location, and certification. The most influential factor in determining salary was experience (Hayes, Allen, Gruen, Wilson, & Kalmakis, 2001).

Obtaining the First Nurse Practitioner Position

Obtaining the first position as a nurse practitioner is a major concern of graduating nurse practitioner students. Some areas with well-established educational programs may experience an oversupply of nurse practitioners, whereas in other areas, the nurse practitioner role may not be well established. Either situation can present problems in obtaining the first position. Presenting oneself in a competent way can help any nurse practitioner find the right position. There are a variety of strategies for finding the ideal position, including taking a position with a practice that you used as a preceptor site as a student, taking a part-time position in a practice while maintaining a staff nurse position for the transition, or using connections from former employers and faculty members.

Interviewing for positions can begin before graduation. Many student nurse practitioners obtain employment at their student practice site. The members of the practice come to know them, and the orientation experience is simplified. Open positions are frequently filled through networking and are not publicized for long, if at all. Networking opportunities can be found in professional organizations and continuing education conferences for nurse practitioners, and through school alumni. The website *http://www.npcentral.net* lists available positions and is a general resource for nurse practitioners (Miller, 1999b). Professionals tend to use a curriculum vitae (CV) rather than a resume, which is shorter. See Box 9–1 for pointers on preparing the CV. After developing the CV, the nurse practitioner should invite a friend or colleague to critique it. CVs should always be kept current, including the latest presentations, publications, leadership experiences, and professional organization work. A CV reflects an individual's career development. Nurse practitioners can use the CV as a barometer to judge their trajectory.

Once an individual is hired, the transition from student to practitioner

---

Box 9–1   *Preparing a Curriculum Vitae (CV)*

A CV differs from a resume in that it is more detailed.
It should include:
• Types of skills and experiences of the NP program
• Various clinical sites in the NP program
• Patient populations served
• Clinical sites where staff nurse or other clinical skills were developed
• All higher educational accomplishments
• Leadership and program development experience
• Community service connections
• Professional memberships and honor societies
• Certifications
• Publications
• Presentations
• Foreign language skills
• Offer a separate sheet that lists reference contact information
  Consider developing different forms of CVs to emphasize experiences
that are most relevant for a particular position:
• Community-based position: Emphasize community or volunteer contacts.
• Hospital-related position: Emphasize contacts in acute care.

---

involves several major adjustments. Transitions from one status to another
are often the cause of disequilibrium and stress. Emotional responses
should be anticipated and interpreted as such. Brown and Olshansky
(1997) conducted a longitudinal interview study to better understand this
transitional process. They described four broad stages in the transition
from student to practitioner (Table 9–2). The metaphor of building a
house was used by one of the study participants. It connotes a long process
of many stages and smaller tasks that need to be planned and followed.
When one stage is accomplished, the skills available to tackle the tasks of
the next stage can be developed. As the stages advance, the nurse practitioner's attention moves from his or her own performance and status to
larger system issues that have an impact on effectiveness. Stage 1, "laying
the foundation," has variable length because certification, credentialing,
and finding a first position may take months. Stage 2, "launching," takes
about 3 months while the nurse practitioner gets oriented to the first position. Stage 3, "meeting the challenge," involves gaining confidence and
building support systems. This competence builds over the next 6 to 9
months. By the end of the first year, the broadened perspective of stage 4
emerges, and nurse practitioners know how to make the system work for

---

TABLE 9–2

Transitional Stages from Student to Nurse Practitioner

Stage 1	Recuperating from school
Laying the foundation	Negotiating the bureaucracy
	Looking for a job
	Worrying
Stage 2	Feeling real
Launching	Getting through the day
	Battling time
	Confronting anxiety
Stage 3	Increasing competence
Meeting the challenge	Gaining confidence
	Acknowledging system problems
Stage 4	Developing system savvy
Broadening the perspective	Affirming oneself
	Upping the ante

Source: Brown, M., & Olshansky, E. (1998). Becoming a primary care nurse practitioner: Challenges of the initial year of practice. *The Nurse Practitioner: The American Journal of Primary Health Care*, 23 (7), p. 52, with permission.

them and their patients. Maintaining a relationship with a mentor, possibly a faculty member or experienced nurse practitioner on site, can assist the student throughout this process (Brown & Olshansky, 1998).

Another study (Kinner, Cohen, & Henderson, 2001) of the transition from student to nurse practitioner that used focus groups determined that nurse practitioner graduates generally felt prepared for their role, but felt guilt and uncertainty about not knowing everything they felt they should know. Difficult responses, such as feeling a loss of personal control of time, changes, or losses in relationships and feelings of isolation were balanced by feelings of special bonding with their clients (Kelly & Mathews, 2001). A study designed to uncover the barriers to nurse practitioner practice in the first 3 years in California showed that lack of public understanding of the role, unavailability of positions, and low salary were barriers to initial practice.

Practice Arrangements

Carolyn Buppert, a nurse attorney, suggests that nurse practitioners get involved in deciding important economic questions regarding their practice and its compensation (Buppert, 1999). Such questions as whether nurse practitioners are reimbursed directly for their work or whether employing or collaborative physicians are compensated for their work, the correct pricing of nurse practitioner services, and who should profit from the difference in what is currently paid between physician and nurse practitioner rates all must be addressed. For example, if it is cheaper to employ a nurse practitioner than a physician, and if services are reimbursed close to physician rates, the employer makes a profit. If the third-party payor pays much less for nurse practitioner care, employing a nurse practitioner is not a good business decision for a practice group and the nurse practitioner is not paid well for his or her work (Buppert, 2001). Health-care policy decisions regarding what the provider is paid and at what level will be shaped in the years to come through regulators and the people who have influence on them. An individual nurse practitioner has little clout, but an organized group of nurse practitioners may. Individual nurse practitioners can support professional organizations in addressing these issues.

Nurse practitioner students who have always worked as staff nurses in hospitals or clinics may never have thought about how they are paid. They are employees of either a large or small organization. Nurse practitioners, however, frequently work for independent practice groups. As a result, their compensation can vary widely from one practice to another. Nurse practitioners have several options for payment, which they determine through negotiation. The options include straight salary, productivity-based salary, or a partnership arrangement that involves sharing in the group's profits and losses. Each option has benefits and drawbacks. Straight pay or salary offers income security, but work hours can be long with no additional recognition or remuneration for contributions to the overall practice. This arrangement also considers the nurse practitioner as part of overhead, as a cost rather than as a revenue generator, which could place the nurse practitioner in a vulnerable position during an economic downturn.

A productivity-based salary takes into account how much income the nurse practitioner brings into the practice. On the surface, the concept is that the harder one works, the more income one brings to the practice, and the more one is compensated. The arrangement is not, however, as simple as it might seem. Nurse practitioners must be careful that they are not charged directly for tests or interventions selected, which can create an ethical dilemma for them in providing quality care. For example, a patient with a recurring headache that has been unresponsive to standard therapy might need magnetic resonance imaging (MRI) for full evaluation. How does the cost of that MRI reflect on the practice or on the nurse practitioner's salary or bonus? At an even more subtle level, does an incentive plan reward the nurse practitioner for seeing more patients and thereby spending less time with the patients who are seen? If the nurse practitioner specializes in caring for complex patients, such as newly diagnosed diabetics, will the lengthy care delivered decrease the salary or bonus at the end of the year? Of course, traditional fee-for-service models rewarded providers for ordering or performing services whether they were truly needed or not. This practice had economic and quality costs, as do the limits of managed care (Buppert, 2000).

Naturally, new nurse practitioners are not as productive as experienced nurse practitioners. They require more consultation and are not as efficient in seeing patients or completing documentation. Consequently, productivity-based salaries are more appropriate for experienced nurse practitioners. When considering this type of compensation, the nurse practitioner and prospective employer should discuss the following questions: Who decides which provider is assigned new patients? Are services available so that the nurse practitioner is not filing, drawing blood, and performing immunizations, using time away from productive hours? Does pressure to see more patients in a shorter time affect the quality of the relationships that are established with patients and the quality of clinical judgments that are made? (Buppert, 2002).

Buppert (2002) notes that there is a difference between being paid for a percentage of billed services and being paid for a percentage of receipts. The latter depends on the effectiveness of the practice in collecting its fees from third-party payors or direct-pay patients. Of course, using good documentation and coding practice ensures that the nurse practitioner is more likely to be paid for all the services truly provided. Does the practice have a good record of collecting on its billing? Has it negotiated a good contract with the many payors who cover their patients' services? These things may be beyond the control of the individual nurse practitioner, but they will affect overall income to the practice as well as the earnings of the nurse practitioner who receives productivity-based compensation.

A partnership is a legal entity that provides for shared decision making and shared risk and profit from the activities of the partnership. Some states allow a limited liability company to reflect shared decision-making, profit, and liability responsibility, but limit the liability of individual members for losses of the company. For example, if the practice had to pay a malpractice claim, the individual members' responsibility would be limited. A professional corporation is a business entity with a board of directors. A lawsuit against the corporation would be limited to corporate assets, not personal assets. Some states do not allow members of different disciplines to form a professional corporation (Buppert, 1999).

Payment Systems

All practice arrangements must deal with the issue of receiving payment from insurance, government health programs such as Medicare or Medicaid, or private sources. Just as Medicare reimbursement of home care is moving to Prospective Payment Systems, where an agency is reimbursed a specific rate for an episode of care at a rate determined by the illness event and comorbidities, regardless of the actual cost of that care, more and more institutions are establishing a capitation system. This pays the practice for the total care of the patient. In this system, prevention of complications, building good self-management skills, and delivering quality outcomes can result in reduced costs of care and therefore more profit for the practice. Most practices have a combination of patients who are under capitated systems and who are billed on a fee-for-service basis.

Billing Medicare

The Department of Health and Human Services reported that, since 1997, the number of services paid by Medicare to nonphysician providers has increased fourfold according to 1999 figures. These providers include nurse practitioners, clinical nurse specialists, and physician assistants (Wall Street Journal, August 7, 2001, cited in NPWN July Aug 2001, p. 24). Services are delivered in primary-care offices and in homes. Often individual physician-nurse practitioner relations are cordial, based on mutual respect and trust. National organizations, however, often act out of group self-interest, and nurse practitioners must maintain vigilance, individually and collectively, to maintain practice privileges and to maintain funding sources that support nurse practitioner practice.

Currently, nurse practitioner care to Medicare patients is paid at 100 percent of the physician rate as long as the nurse practitioner's care is "incident to" the care of the physician. This means that the physician who initiates care for the patient supervises the care. If the nurse practitioner initiates care, services are reimbursed at 80 percent of the rate that would have been paid to a physician. The resource-based relative value scale is used by Medicare to assign a value for services to Medicare patients. Several reported studies used a method of assigning value to nurse practitioner work similar to the method that had been used for physicians. It showed that nurse practitioners provided similar services to those of physicians and additionally provided patient evaluation and education with a consideration of social factors. Their care was consistent with the Medical Fee schedule. Ways of identifying and reimbursing nurse practitioners for the full range of their services need to be developed (Sullivan-Marx, Happ, Bradley, & Maislin, 2000; Sullivan-Marx & Maislin, 2000).

Marketing

Many people, including potential patients and other health-care providers, do not fully understand what the nurse practitioner can offer to the health-care system in general, or to them in particular. An information-sharing plan that includes marketing principles can improve understanding of nurse practitioner contributions. Marketing strategies include representation of product, price, place, and promotion (Gallagher, 1996).

In the case of care delivery, product means the service provided. What is the practice's particular niche? What services are needed in the community? Is there competition for this market segment? Price determination is not as clear in health care as it is in retail. The cost to the patient for care is affected by insurance coverage, co-payments, and network service limits. The price of a nurse practitioner's salary to a practice is offset by the new business that he or she can generate. Additionally, in capitated payment systems, decreased hospitalization as a result of improved preventive care results in decreased costs of care. Place is related to the location of delivered services. This might include satellite clinics or home-based care that would add benefit to both patients and a busy practice.

Promotion includes the activities that are planned after clarifying the issues relating to the first three principles. Marketing a practice, whether it is an independent practice or a niche in an established practice, can be a new activity for the nurse practitioner. Not all marketing campaigns require expensive television or radio time. One can volunteer to do free public lectures in local hospitals, senior centers, or other community agencies. Specialty consultations can also be donated to develop a niche. Such consultations might address weight management, incontinence, perimenopause, or chronic pain problems. One must have expertise in these areas, but in order to begin a niche practice, donating free time and then demonstrating effectiveness to referral sources can help to establish a practice. For example, community groups need speakers for programs. Volunteering to speak on health issues and describing service availability can help to develop a practice.

Written materials, such as brochures or business cards, can help nurse practitioners market their practice. Patients can take brochures home to share with family and friends. Brochures can also be left in prominent public locations to further spread the practice's message. As with any patient-targeted material, reading level and type size should be checked to ensure that the information is accessible and accurate. Business cards can be given out at professional and lay gatherings. Nurse practitioners should also keep a set of cards in their offices and in waiting and examination rooms so that patients can take them easily. Visibility is the key to keeping nurse practitioner services accessible to potential patients (Miller, 2000a).

Nurse practitioners need to develop national marketing campaigns. Recent prescription drug advertising frequently includes such language as "only your doctor can prescribe..." Regardless of whether one approves of such advertising, this is an error that excludes providers other than physicians from consideration. One of the reasons why drug companies exclude nurse practitioners from their campaigns is that, according to their market surveys that track who is prescribing their drugs, nurse practitioner prescriptions are frequently reported under the name of a supervising physician. This makes nurse practitioner work invisible. Nurse practitioners need to argue for recognition of all aspects of their practice. They can do so by having prescription pads with their own name listed and, if the state allows, using their own name only (Edmunds, 2002). A Nurse Practitioner National Marketing Campaign is supported by five nurse practitioner organizations. It uses public relations strategies to inform federal and state legislators, third-party payors, and major employers of the advantages of supporting nurse practitioner practice. The campaign website is *http://www.npcentral.net/mc/*.

Managed Care

Managed care is part of America's health-care scene. In an active practice, patients may come from a variety of health plans, all of which have a unique pattern of costs and benefits. Some plans use guidelines that promote and/or restrict the use of screening and other laboratory tests. Many have drug formularies that reflect the health-care system's review of the effectiveness and cost of specific drugs. All these issues affect the decisions that nurse practitioners make about assessing and managing the health of their patients. In many cases, managed care actually promotes quality care by setting out prevention and screening programs based on evidence of cost effectiveness. For the vast majority of patients, general guidelines work well. For some individual patients, however, general guidelines might not apply. For example, a patient with a history of Crohn's disease will need screening colonoscopies earlier and at more frequent intervals than a specific plan's guidelines allow. As a result, the nurse practitioner may need to argue for coverage for particular patients. If there seem to be systematic problems with benefit programs, the nurse practitioner needs to advocate individually or as part of a group for more adequate coverage.

The major issues of health care are cost, access, and quality. Achieving any two is relatively easy. If costs are reduced and access increased by a national program, one can expect that quality of care will be difficult to maintain. If quality and access are priorities, keeping costs down will be difficult (personal communication, J. Vessey, May 16, 2001). As costs for health care continue to increase, employers will shift the costs of insurance to their employees, restricting benefits or requiring higher individual contributions. Patients may need advice on evaluating their options. Nurse practitioners can be part of the public dialogue on controlling health-care costs and ensuring benefits for patients (Partnerships for Quality Education, 2001). Managed-care organizations are rated based on Health Plan Employer Data Set (HEDIS), which allows employers to compare the quality of the managed-care plans that they are considering contracting. The National Committee for Quality Assurance (NCQA), a nonprofit organization with a mission to improve heath care quality, administers the program. HEDIS performance measures are consistent with quality screening and prevention activities, and nurse practitioners contribute to overall quality ratings for their patients by providing immunizations; smoke cessation interventions; breast and cervical cancer screening; and appropriate care for asthma, cardiac, and diabetic patients. Information on keeping up with the ever-changing performance measures is found at *http://www.ncqa.org* (Miller, 2000b).

Managed care is changing as health-care systems merge and gain bargaining clout. More costs are being shifted to patients in employee contributions and three-tier drug-charge systems, in which different prices are charged for generic drugs, cheaper brand-name drugs, and premium brand-name medications. Health plans are loosening their preapproval restrictions in order to avoid managed care "backlash." As employer and employee costs continue to rise, more employees will be closed out of the health insurance system (Strunk, Ginsburg, & Gabel, 2001).

)) MEDICAL ERRORS

Medical errors are an important concern for nurse practitioners. Although medical errors have many causes, they commonly result from transcription errors (caused by poorly written prescriptions), mistakes in medication administration, or predictable risks of therapy, such as bleeding in patients on anticoagulation therapy. System errors, which include mistakes in transcription or medication delivery, can be prevented through careful review and management of underlying problems. In this book, the most relevant type of medical error involves judgment. In two recent studies of 3000 residents in 18 nursing homes (Gurwitz, Field, Avorn, et al., 2000), and 30,000 patients in a practice group (Gurwitz, Field, Harrold et al., 2003), researchers found that preventable medication-related errors occurred in 18.9 per 1000 resident-months in the nursing home setting and 50 per 1000 person-years in the ambulatory setting. Errors were caused by ordering mistakes, including ordering incorrect doses; failing to consider foreseeable drug interactions; and choosing the wrong medication. Other errors involved problems with monitoring, such as missing medication overloads. As usual, considering the total patient situation, including all of their medications would help to prevent errors related to drug interactions. Nurse practitioners need to use great care to prevent medical errors and to seek out systemic problems that can contribute to error. For example, they should make sure that prescriptions are written clearly and in a way that prevents tampering. They should also ensure that pharmacists can easily reach them or the physician to clarify confusing or interacting prescriptions.

Following the classic article (Knaus, Draper, Wagner, & Zimmerman, 1986) that showed that intensive-care patients matched for disease severity survived better when cared for in a unit with good nurse-physician communication, research on collaboration has shown benefits in many other areas. A joint meeting of the Council on Graduate Medical Education and the National Advisory Council on Nurse Education and Practice found that "patient safety cannot be accomplished without interdisciplinary practice approaches" (2000, p. 1). Meeting participants further found that revolutionary changes would be required to make substantial impact on current rates of medical error. One of the problems with the current system is that it perpetuates discontinuity. For example, every time a message must be communicated from one person or system to another, the potential for error is increased. The very culture of care needs change, which includes how members of the system communicate, how reporting and accountability structures are established, and customs such as how error is reviewed. Furthermore, beyond nurse-physician collaboration, the patient must become an active participant in making health-related decisions and carrying out the health plan. Patients must be supported as they learn to orchestrate their own care which may include challenging the system, as well as being assertive in getting the help they need from individual nurses and physicians.

The practice needs to develop an attitude toward error that treats such events as learning opportunities. Blame and retribution only force practitioners to hide mistakes and prevent the development of new systems. Any errors, which can include both procedural and judgment errors, should be treated as a systems problem, and everyone involved should have an opportunity to offer suggestions to improve the system to prevent the error from occurring again.

Practices need to invest in high-quality management systems, and that can sometimes be expensive. However, is a computerized system that prevents errors in transcribing orders worth the cost if it prevents negative patient outcomes? Systems can be used to structure documentation and to offer guidelines-based care. Nurse practitioners and physicians, together with therapists and others, can contribute to optimal patient-care guidelines. To support quality care, each team member's contribution to care should be documented so that individual practice can be studied and improved. Outcomes management provides an opportunity to measure collaborative efforts. Shared responsibility for outcomes and recognition of individual contribution to care can enhance collaboration (Grady & Wojner, 1996). Systems must be developed with all users' perspectives in mind (Simpson, 1998).

The Committee on the Quality of Health Care in America was appointed by the Institute of Medicine in 1998 to develop new approaches to improving quality of health-care delivery. Its second work, *Crossing the Quality Chasm* (2001), suggests several approaches to systemic problems in delivering the quality of health care that is theoretically possible. Many of these recommendations will reduce medical error. They suggest new approaches for educating professionals for new models of care. These are summarized in Table 9–3. The National Coordinating Council for Medical Error Reporting and Prevention (a group of independent organizations) has developed a taxonomy of medical error and has standardized how reporting occurs. (Helpful information and reporting forms can be found at the website: *www.nccmerp.org*). The philosophy behind reducing medical error holds that any error, even a potential one, becomes a source of system correction in that it points out a flaw in the system and should be studied. By clustering reports from many sources, patterns of error can be determined. For example, if two medications have similar names and/or appearances, the chance for error is increased. Product design might need to be altered.

TABLE 9–3
Approaches to Health-Care Provider Education
Different focus of patient encounters including the use of technology
Preparation for the ability to summarize scientific evidence for decision making in understandable terms
Use of evidence, population and patient preference in choosing treatments
Open communication between patient and provider/Open patient records
Use/development of decision support systems
Identification of error and hazards of care
Understanding patient experience of illness and health
Continuous quality monitoring and improvement
Team collaboration
Design of care processes and measurement of outcomes
Development of new knowledge related to care provision
Research on the determinant of health and appropriate role of health-care provider

Source: Adapted from Preparing the Workforce, *Crossing the Quality Chasm*, Committee on the Quality Health Care in America, 2001.

⟨⟩ HEALTH-CARE WORKFORCE

The nursing shortage that is currently present and that threatens to intensify in the years ahead challenges the ability of all health professionals to deliver care (American Association of Colleges of Nursing, 2000). It has been said that the nurse is the "glue that holds the health-care system together." For advanced-practice nurses, the shortage of registered nurses has several implications. In primary care, many offices do not have access to the services of registered nurses. This means that triage, health teaching, and such aspects of practice as immunizations will either fall to less qualified persons or become the responsibility of advanced-practice nurses. Although it is true that advanced-practice nurses can step in and administer immunizations, the practice as a whole must ask whether this is the best use of the advanced-practice nurse's time.

In acute-care settings, the nursing shortage is already affecting the quality of care that can be delivered, stretching the nurses who are present to cover more patients. Hospitals with high patient occupancy rates end up holding patients in emergency or recovery departments longer than desirable because beds cannot be opened because of short staffing. Advanced-practice nurses can offer creative solutions by providing urgent-care support, freeing up emergency department space, or getting involved with predischarge preparation using the transition care model tested by Naylor and others (2000), thus offering tertiary institutions a solution to full units with fewer staff members.

Naylor and others (2000) report that the holistic nature of advanced-practice nurse support focuses on physiologic and health behavior problems as well as emotional responses to illness. Advanced-practice nurses focused on surveillance as a major intervention and differed from home-care nurses in that they performed more advocacy and referral and fewer direct-care treatments. The value placed on initial assessment and ongoing monitoring functions by the advanced-practice nurses in the study shows the importance of clinical judgment. There are more than 149,000 nurses registered at the advanced-practice level in the United States, and more than 94,000 are nurse practitioners (Pearson, 2002). The impact of this large group of advanced-practice nurses needs to be measured and publicized.

))) GRANT WRITING FOR PROGRAM DEVELOPMENT

Experienced nurse practitioners frequently identify service needs that are not being met and develop new programs of care. Box 9-2 lists important elements of developing a program plan. These can range from community-based practices that are free standing to specialized practices within an internal medicine or hospital setting. Nurse practitioners know their patients and are in an excellent position to identify unmet service needs. Political and economic skills can be obtained through consultation in order to develop a strong plan. Grant-funding agencies exist to promote good work that is consistent with the foundation's stated purpose. The Internet and local public libraries have listings of grant-making organizations. Librarians can assist in developing searches to find funding sources for projects. Searches by key words can support locating available funding sources. For example, children's health can be entered as a key word to streamline the process of finding a funding source. Grants must be written to conform to each agency's specific guidelines, but answering the questions listed in Box 9-2 is a first step in the process. Consulting with a local school of nursing or other agency that has engaged in grant writing can also help the nurse practitioner to focus the search. In addition, nurse practitioners should communicate with the contact person at the grant-funding organization. Although there are no funding guarantees, the agency's staff members can help the nurse practitioner develop a quality proposal. Nurse practitioners should not be discouraged if they are not successful after the first try. Most foundations do not provide detailed feedback on proposals, but the agency contact person should be able to say which projects were funded. Once

---

Box 9–2   *Program Development*

Needs Assessment:
- How many potential patients would benefit from the proposed service?
- Where else do these patients receive care?
- What is the history of service provision in this area?
- Who are the necessary supports in the community?
- Who would be a valuable member of an Advisory Board?

Business Plan:
- How will the care be funded?
- Are start-up costs going to need support before an income stream begins to cover costs?
- How will services be valuated?
- Where are the key referral linkages?
- Is an umbrella organization available that can help with start-up?
- What would be the first year's budget?

---

nurse practitioners receive funding, they should provide all necessary reports to the funding agency and be sure to use the grant money in the way that was proposed.

))) EDUCATION

Precepting Students

The relationship between the student nurse practitioner and the preceptor is vital to student learning. The student needs to remember that the preceptor has responsibilities to the practice setting for managing a reasonable number of patients and overseeing the student's own use of time so that the workflow is not interrupted. If a student spends an hour obtaining a patient's health history, patients who are scheduled after that patient will be delayed. The student needs to remember that a good history is a focused history and that structuring the interview is appropriate. Sometimes students who cannot come to a clear diagnosis engage in "fishing expeditions," hoping that the answer will come if they continue to ask more questions. This approach rarely helps to either make a diagnosis or establish trust with the patient. It is acceptable for the student *not* to know the diagnosis for the patient. The preceptor will not think badly of the student if he or she reports the approaches used and the diagnoses that were considered but not chosen. Of course, with experience, the student will become more adept at diagnosis.

From the preceptor's point of view, having a student can be a rewarding experience. Being able to share the wisdom of one's practice with a
new person entering the profession is an honor and a privilege. Good
practice cannot be learned from books or simulations. There is no substitute for guided clinical experience. Sometimes, however, a practice setting
puts pressure on potential preceptors not to take students because of the
time and the use of examination rooms by students, which are then un-
available to other providers. In actuality, the time invested in students
early in an experience can be recovered after they become more proficient
and can offer skills to the practice in areas such as teaching and quality improvement.

In a typical arrangement, the student takes a history and performs a
physical examination while the preceptor does a visit with his or her own
patient. The student then presents major findings to the preceptor, who
then sees the patient to clarify history issues and verify physical findings.
The preceptor is, of course, not limited to the direction that the student
took. Early in the experience, the student may not be able to propose a
treatment approach, but later, the student will engage in dialogue with the
preceptor on a therapeutic regimen. The student can then write prescriptions and orders for cosignature, make telephone referrals, and finalize
teaching.

Patient Selection

Ideally, students should conduct follow-up visits with patients whom
they have previously seen in order to develop relationships and to see the
outcomes of their decisions. These visits support students' development of
judgment by providing direct feedback on actions taken. Another consideration in patient selection involves "special patients" whom preceptors do
not wish to share, perhaps because of the fragile nature of the relationship
or the particular follow-up that the patient needs. Students need to understand that they are temporary members on the scene and trust the preceptor's judgment. If students feel that they are not given access to patients
with whom they would like to work, they should discuss this with the preceptor and with their faculty member.

Preceptor Recognition

Practice settings and educational institutions have much in common.
They have shared goals of recruiting and preparing the best possible practitioners who will provide quality, cost-effective care. Faculty members can
assist the transition for students and preceptors by maintaining a meaning-

ful practice of their own. This is a rewarding experience for faculty members, but the pressures on them to generate research funding in addition to teaching and committee work can result in overloading. Many schools have clinical faculty lines that recognize the importance of clinical expertise in the practice discipline and that allow faculty members to support the school through their practice rather than through research grant writing. Many practice settings are under increasing pressure to manage more patients in order to remain economically viable. To maintain a good list of preceptors for their students, schools offer a range of recognition programs, including titles, continuing education or credit course tuition waivers, or access to university resources such as libraries. Preceptors can negotiate with schools on receiving appropriate support so that they can justify their time spent with students. Open dialogue about the pressures and priorities on all players, faculty, preceptors, and students can help each party find a balance that meets the needs of all.

Doctoral Education

Nurses with master's degrees are equipped to function in the advanced-practice role, providing direct care to individuals, families, and communities. For many, this is the culmination of their education, and they are happy to stay at this level. In the last decades of the 20th century, however, more doctoral programs in nursing became available, many with a focus on clinical nursing research. Nurse practitioners may want advanced research skills to answer questions that arise from clinical practice, or they may feel motivated to perform large-scale research that shows the cost effectiveness of nurse practitioner practice. They may also engage in interdisciplinary research as a member of a team or find that teaching is rewarding. All these skills are supported by doctoral education in nursing. Only 2 percent of American nurses hold a doctorate in nursing or any other area. For nurse practitioners to participate fully in research and evaluation of nurse practitioner practice, doctoral preparation is required. There is a need for skilled clinicians to be educated with a research degree. True interdisciplinary collaboration is supported by equality of education. Box 9–3 shows questions to consider when considering doctoral study.

))) RESEARCH FOR NURSE PRACTITIONERS

Research skills are best developed in doctoral and postdoctoral education programs, but the source of research questions is an active clinical practice

---

Box 9–3   *Considering Doctoral Education*

Investigate the doctoral programs of interest carefully:
- Are the costs of education borne by the institution?
- Will you be free to pursue the type of research that you want? Some schools steer students away from qualitative research; others are open to it. Some schools focus on policy research, whereas others focus on research with individual patients.

Faculty:
- Are they engaged in the types of research that interest you?
- Are they available to meet with you as an applicant?
- Are they available to students?
- Do you want a program that allows interdisciplinary education or would you rather focus on the disciplinary question in nursing?
- Do you want to study with a strong theorist, or is that not of interest to you?

Program Format:
- Do you need the convenience of weekend or evening classes?
- Is part-time study allowed or supported?

---

where real-world problems present themselves. Research skills that are learned in master's degree programs can assist nurse practitioners in determining the major health risks of their particular populations, the interventions most frequently offered to subpopulations of the practice, and the outcomes of health that can be delivered. Partnerships with faculty for local schools of nursing can provide a mix of research skills that can provide answers to these and other questions. See Box 9–4 for sample quality improvement questions.

Research on Nurse Practitioner Effectiveness

The effectiveness of nurse practitioners in providing quality health care has been tested, but much research needs to be done. Many studies on the effectiveness of nurse practitioner practice (Mundinger et al., 2000) report success as equivalence with physician care. Do nurse practitioners provide additional benefits for patients, and if so, for whom? From the patient's perspective, what is most valued in the primary-care relationship? What might be missing from care as it is practiced now? Nurse practitioners need to ask the questions that will improve their practice. Partnering with

---

Box 9–4   *Quality Improvement Questions*

Quality improvement questions can be analyzed with a variety of research tools:

- How long does it take for a new patient to get an appointment?
- What is the waiting time once a patient arrives at the office?
- How many insurance or Medicare claims are denied and for what reason?
- What is the patient's satisfaction with care at the setting?
- Which patients cost the practice or the system the most money?
- Can care be more cost effective with the same or improved level of quality outcomes?
- What proportion of patients is up to date on immunizations?
- What proportion of patients uses available health resources such as classes or help lines?

---

doctorally prepared nurse researchers in this endeavor will promote the development and recognition of nurse practitioner practice.

》 SUMMARY

The development of the nurse practitioner movement continues. Issues that affect the larger system of care have implications for the clinical judgment activities of nurse practitioners. Payment and documentation systems shape certain aspects of practice. Legislation and regulations directly affect the practice of nurse practitioners and vary from state to state. Active participation in shaping such legislation is the responsibility of the advanced-practice nurse. Assisting the next generation of nurse practitioners through education is the responsibility of the experienced nurse practitioner. Research into local practice patterns and patient outcomes that can be achieved through nurse practitioner intervention needs to be conducted and the information disseminated. Collaboration with other nurses locally, nationally, and globally can enhance one's own practice. Interdisciplinary collaboration grows when the nurse practitioner functions in the full range of professional activities.

The issues raised in this chapter may not be the primary concerns of the new nurse practitioner student, but they should be considered before graduation from school. The first years of practice will provide opportunities for nurse practitioners to increase their influence on the structures and system that affect their clinical judgment.

REFERENCES

American Association of Colleges of Nursing (1995). *Position statement: Interdisciplinary education and practice.* Washington, DC: Author.

American Association of Colleges of Nursing (2000). *Report of the Community Advisory Commission Meeting.* Washington, DC: Author.

Brown, M., & Olshansky, E. (1997). From limbo to legitimacy. *Nursing Research, 46*(1), 46–51.

Brown, M., & Olshansky, E. (1998). Becoming a primary care nurse practitioner: Challenges of the initial year of practice. *The Nurse Practitioner: The American Journal of Primary Health Care, 2*(7), 46, 52, 54–56, 58, 61–62, 64, 66.

Buppert, C. (1999). *Nurse practitioner's business practice and legal guide.* Gaithersburg, MD: Aspen Publishers, Inc.

Buppert, C. (2000). *The primary care provider's guide to compensation and quality.* Gaithersburg, MD: Aspen Publishers.

Buppert, C. (2001). Who should profit from nurse practitioners? *Nurse Practitioner World News, 6*(5), 1, 19.

Buppert, C. (2002). Let's talk money: Productivity-based compensation. *Nurse Practitioner World News, 7*(2), 1, 16.

Committee on the Quality Health Care in America, Institute of Medicine (2001). *Crossing the quality chasm: A new health system for the 21st century.* Washington, DC: National Academy Press.

Council in Graduate Medical Education and National Advisory Council on Nurse Education and Practice (2000). *Collaborative education to ensure patient safety.* Obtained from *http://www.cogme.gov/jointmtg.pdf.*

Draye, M. A., & Brown, M. A. (2000). Surviving the proving ground: Lessons in change from NP pioneers. *The Nurse Practitioner: The American Journal of Primary Health Care, 25*(10), 65–71.

Edmunds, M. (2002). Are your prescriptions part of a disappearing act? *The Nurse Practitioner: The American Journal of Primary Health Care, 27*(6), 54.

Gallagher, S. (1996). Promoting the nurse practitioner by using a marketing approach. *The Nurse Practitioner, 21*(3), 30, 36–37, 40.

Grady, G. F., & Wojner, A. W. (1996). Collaborative practice teams: The infrastructure of outcomes management. *AACN Clinical Issues, 7,* 153–158.

Gurwitz, J. H., Field, T. S., Avorn, J., McCormick, D., Jain, S., Eckler, M., Benser, M., Edmondson, A. C., & Bates (2000). Incidence and preventability of adverse drug events in nursing homes. *American Journal of Medicine, 109,* 87–94.

Gurwitz, J. H., Field, T. S., Harrold, L. R., Rothschild, J., DeBellis, K., Seger, A. C., Cadoret, C., Fish, L. S., Garber, L., Kelleher, M., & Bates, D. W. (2003). Incidence and preventability of adverse drug events among older persons in the ambulatory setting. *Journal of the American Medical Association, 289,* 1107–1116.

Hayes, E., Allen, J., Gruen, S., Wilson, J., & Kalmakis, K. (2001). Forces of change: Nurse practitioner practice patterns, compensation, and professional organization participation: Western Massachusetts. *Clinical Excellence for Nurse Practitioners, 5*(1), 52–60.

Hooker, R. S., & McCaig, L. F. (2001). Use of physician assistants and nurse practitioners in primary care, 1995–1999: Non-physician providers often spend more time with patients and order fewer tests. *Health Affairs, 20,* 231–238.

Hurtado, M. P., Swift, E. K., & Corrigan, J. M. (Eds). (2001). Envisioning the national health care quality report. Washington, DC: National Academies Press.

Johnson, M., & Maas, M. (Eds.). (1997). *Iowa Outcomes Project: Nursing outcomes classification.* St. Louis: Mosby.

Kelly, N. R., & Mathews, M. (2001). The transition to first position as nurse practitioner. *Journal of Nursing Education, 40,* 156–162.

Kinner, K., Cohen, J., & Henderson, M. J. (2001). Comparison of past and current behaviors to novice nurse practitioner practice: The California perspective. *Clinical Excellence for Nurse Practitioners, 5,* 96–101.

Knaus, W. A., Draper, E. A., Wagner, D. P., & Zimmerman, J. E. (1986). An evaluation of outcome from intensive care in major medical centers. *Annals of Internal Medicine, 104,* 410–418.

Lee, M., & Pulcini, J. (1998). Barriers to independent practice: Mandatory collaboration between nurses and physicians. *Clinical Excellence for Nurse Practitioners, 2,* 172–173.

Lincoln, P. E. (2000). Comparing CNS and NP role activities: A replication. *Clinical Nurse Specialist, 14,* 269–277.

Martin, P. D., & Hutchinson, S. A. (1999). Nurse practitioners and the problem of discounting. *Journal of Advanced Nursing, 29*(1), 9–17.

Miller, S. (1999a). Choosing a certifying board. *Patient Care for the Nurse Practitioners, 2*(5), 53.

Miller, S. (1999b). Finding that first position. *Patient Care for the Nurse Practitioner, 2*(8), 53.

Miller, S. K. (2000a). Marketing your practice. *Patient Care for the Nurse Practitioner, 3*(11), 52–53.

Miller, S. K. (2000b). Reporting on managed care: What do the NCQA performance measures mean? Marketing your practice. *Patient Care for the Nurse Practitioner, 3*(12), 69.

Mills, A. C., & McSweeney, M. (2002). Nurse practitioners and physician assistants revisited: Do their practice patterns differ in ambulatory care? *Journal of Professional Nursing, 18*(1), 36–46.

Moody, N. B., Smith, P. L., & Glenn, L. L. (1999). Client characteristics and practice patterns of nurse practitioners and physicians. *The Nurse Practitioner: The American Journal of Primary Health Care, 24*(3), 94–96, 99–100, 102–103.

Mundinger, M. O., Kane, R. L., Lenz, E. R., Totten, A. M., Tsai, W., Cleary, P. D., Friedewald, W. T., Siu, A. L., & Shelanski, M. L. (2000). Primary care outcomes in patients treated by nurse practitioners or physicians: A randomized trial. *Journal of the American Medical Association, 283*(1), 59–68.

Naylor, M. D., Bowles, K. H., & Brooten, D. (2000). Patient problems and advanced practice nurse interventions during transitional care. *Public Health Nursing, 17,* 94–102.

O'Connor, N. A., Hameister, A. D., & Kershaw, T. (2000). Developing a database to describe the practice patterns of adult nurse practitioner students. *Journal of Nursing Scholarship, 32,* 57–63.

Oden, L. S., Price, J. H., Alteneder, R., Boardley, D., & Ubokudom, S. E. (2000). Public policy involvement by nurse practitioners. *Journal of Community Health, 25,* 139–155.

Partnerships for Quality Education (2001). Storm clouds gathering for health care, downloaded 12/3/01, *http://www.mceconnection.org/mce/*.

Patel, V. L., Cytryn, K. N., Shortliffe, E. H., & Safran, C. (2000). The collaborative health care team: The role of individual and group expertise. *Teaching & Learning in Medicine, 12,* 117–132.

Pearson, L. (2002). Fourteenth annual legislative update. *The Nurse Practitioner, 27,* 10–12, 15, 19–20, 22.

Pruitt, R. H., Wetsel, M. A., Smith, K. J., & Spitler, H. (2002). How do we pass NP autonomy legislation? *The Nurse Practitioner, 27,* 56, 61–65.

Roberts-Davis, M., & Read, S. (2001). Clinical role clarification: Using the Delphi method to establish similarities and differences between nurse practitioners and clinical nurse specialists. *Journal of Clinical Nursing, 10*(1), 33–34.

Ryan, J. W. (1999). Collaboration of the nurse practitioner and physician in long-term care. *Lippincott's Primary Care Practitioner, 3,* 127–134.

Sharp, N. (1999). Wanted: Nurse leaders to craft health policy. *The Nurse Practitioner, 24*(10), 85–86, 89.

Simpson, R. L. (1998). The role of technology in interdisciplinary practice. *Nurse Manager, 29,* 20–22.

Strunk, B. C., Ginsburg, P. B., & Gabel, J. R. (2001). Tracking health care costs. *Health Affairs Web Exclusive*, International Standard Serial Number 0278–2715.

Sullivan-Marx, E. M., Happ, M. B., Bradley, K. J., & Maislin, G. (2000). Nurse practitioner services: Content and relative work value. *Nursing Outlook, 48,* 269–275.

Sullivan-Marx, E. M., & Maislin, G. (2000). Comparison of nurse practitioner and family physician relative work values. *Journal of Nursing Scholarship*, 32(1), 71–76.

Zimmer, P. A. (2002). New shores, new horizons: Inaugural conference of the International Network of Nurse Practitioners and Advanced Practice Nurses. *Nurse Practitioner World News*, 6(7), 1, 3, 26.

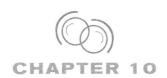

CHAPTER 10

Philosophical Considerations in Nurse Practitioner Practice

Pamela J. Grace, APRN, BC, PhD

For more than a century, nursing as a discipline has struggled to define the special nature of its purposes and the knowledge necessary to fulfill those purposes. Schlodtfeldt (1989) asserted that a priority for nursing "is that of identifying, structuring, and continually advancing the knowledge that underlies the practices of professionals in the field" (p. 35). This is important to nurses because, in general, we do believe that we provide a unique service not duplicated by other disciplines. The problem is that we also use knowledge from a variety of sources, such as medicine, psychology, sociology and anthropology, among others, to inform our practice.

What, then, makes nursing in general, and advanced-practice nursing in particular, both unique and important to individuals in society? To answer that, nursing must consider the following philosophical questions: What makes nursing special? How is advanced-practice nursing related to nursing as a discipline? How can nursing maintain its own identity and resist becoming assimilated into either medicine or another human science field? For whom is it important that nursing maintain its own identity? Will advanced-practice nursing contribute to nursing's demise by virtue of its inclusion of skills previously considered to be the exclusive domain of medicine? Or will it, by virtue of its superior ability to provide holistic care, help strengthen nursing's position as a profession?

This chapter discusses these questions and explores the historical and philosophical development of nursing as a discipline and profession. Because expanded practice roles are nonetheless *nursing practice* roles, nurse practitioners must both grasp and ascribe to the philosophical foundations of the discipline in order to resist becoming a subgroup of medicine. Advanced-practice nurses are morally obligated to maintain a nursing focus on the health or well-being of each unique individual, but doing so may be difficult when pressures such as limiting the language that nurses use to describe their practice to medical terms or reducing the length of visits allowed from a medical or economic model impinge on practice. However, by firmly understanding nursing's professional commitments and philosophical foundations, advanced-practice nurses can resist pressure from others with different goals.

)) PHILOSOPHICAL INQUIRY

Philosophical inquiry involves questioning the underlying nature of the world and humankind's place in the world. It is a search for wisdom about the universe and its workings. Philosophical questions, as Sarvimaki (1999) notes, "are questions that cannot be answered by empirical observations—or rather by empirical observations alone" (p. 10). According to Beck (1969), there are four main activities of philosophy: "the speculative, the descriptive, the normative, and the analytic" (p. 2).

Speculative philosophy tries to make sense of the world as an integrated entity. It promotes ideas about the world and its working that transcend (are outside of) our experiences but that are based partly on our observations. *Descriptive* philosophy characterizes the world as objectively as possible while recognizing that we are sensory creatures who experience the world subjectively. *Normative* philosophy attempts to answer questions about how humans should live. It has been used to formulate guidelines and standards for behavior. *Analytic* philosophy allows us to question underlying assumptions made either as a result of, or preceding the other three facets of philosophy. For example, moral philosophy is concerned with questioning how people do or should relate to each other and to other aspects of the environment. It includes both *descriptions* of actions and *normative* (prescriptive) appraisals of actions. Analytic philosophy helps us to dissect such actions in order to discover hidden assumptions. It permits a "critical assessment of ... assumptions or presuppositions and of the methods upon which common sense, the sciences, and even philosophy rely" (Beck, 1969, p. 2). Table 10–1 lists examples of activities of philosophy.

In addition to knowing the four facets of philosophy, nurse practitioners must also understand the philosophical concepts of *ontology, epistemology,* and *ethics.* The work implied by these terms has proved important for nursing's scholars, theorists, and researchers to undertake in attempting to delineate the meaning and nature of nursing as a practice discipline. Sarvimaki (1999) asserts that questions such as what is the essence of our being when we assume the role of nurse practitioner, how we know what

TABLE 10–1

Activities of Philosophy

Activity	Definition	Example
Speculative Philosophy	Integrates concepts related to the world	Developing an understanding of how culture affects health belief for patients and practitioners
Descriptive Philosophy	Clarifies essential concepts and processes	Learning the phases of adjustment to the diagnosis of a chronic health problem in a patient
Normative Philosophy	Develops standards for how persons should live	Developing a code for nurse practitioner practice as part of a professional organization
Analytic Philosophy	Questions underlying assumptions	Questioning the basis for policies that determine how to classify nurse practitioner activities

we know as practitioners, and how we decide for the good when we make any clinical judgment must be investigated in order to "construct comprehensive views of nursing" (p. 11).

Ontology

Ontology is concerned with understanding the nature and essential characteristics of things. It answers the question "What is this"? A broad ontological question asked by many ancient philosophers was "What is being"? More discrete ontological questions about humans might be formulated as "What does it mean to be human?" "What is the essential nature of humans?" "What is it that demarcates humans from other beings?" Aristotle's answer to this last question was that man is distinguished from other animals by his reasoning abilities. Ontological questions about nursing, then, might be formulated as "What is nursing?" or, as Fry (1999) phrases it, "What is the nature of nursing practice? Is it an art, a science, or a type of presence?" (p. 6). Ontological questions are important to address because they permit nursing to identify its proper focus for inquiry and to defend its significance to society.

Epistemology

Epistemology is philosophical inquiry about what constitutes knowledge. "Among its questions are, What is the nature of knowledge? What is the source of knowledge?" (Beck, 1969, p. 3). An additional question of contemporary importance asks whether there is such a thing as absolute truth. Many philosophers, especially those of the American Pragmatist School (Charles Saunders Peirce, 1839–1914; William James, 1842–1910; John Dewey, 1859–1952), have concluded that truth is an evolutionary concept; that is, what is considered to be truth changes as circumstances or the environment changes. They believe that we, as humans, can never know whether there is absolute truth. The reason for this assertion is that humans are subjective beings whose view of the world is necessarily distorted by sensory perception. Thus, to the pragmatist, the search for absolute truth is a misbegotten quest.

An additional epistemological question concerns what criteria we can use to make judgments about what does or does not constitute knowledge. Feminist philosophers have also challenged the warrants for knowledge because they believe that traditional views devalue intuitive and experiential knowledge in favor of principled knowledge. Alcoff and Potter (1993) have written about the epistemological concerns of contemporary feminist philosophers that "women's ways of knowing" and "women's experiences" (p. 1) have been left out of philosophical theories of knowledge and what is knowable.

Ethics

Ethical inquiry is also known as moral philosophy or value theory. It concerns the study of human actions and their causes. Chapter 11 discusses in detail the nature of ethical inquiry and the nature of nursing actions as these are directed towards furthering a good.

⊙⟫ PHILOSOPHICAL ROOTS OF HELPING PROFESSIONS

The philosophical roots of helping professions are imbedded in the idea that humans are not solely self-interested individuals but also have the capacity for altruism. That is, besides being interested in our own welfare, we understand that others' projects, beliefs, values, and desires are as important as our own (Nagel, 1970, 1991). Hume (1974/1748) commented on this fact that we can have "sympathy" with others. This sympathy can move us to actions on behalf of those others. Historically, religious ideals have also provided a strong impetus for a life of service to others. Many of the so-called "professions" emerged from roots in religious service to the needy in a given society. Gradually, though, **professions** separated from their ecclesiastical ties. Carr-Saunders & Wilson (1933) note that "surgeons, apothecaries, ... notaries, and common lawyers" (p. 291) were the first groups to distance themselves from their religious ties.

Ambiguity and controversy remain about the purposes of professions. Some (Carr-Saunders & Wilson, 1933) have noted that professions (such as medicine and law) are subject to the criticism that, although they ostensibly exist to serve a need, they are primarily self-serving. They cite observations including the fact that professions such as medicine and law are elitist, exclusionary, and self protectionist. In comparison to medicine, nursing is a new, young, and immature profession whose development was influenced by religious and virtuous ideals in its premodern and early modern eras and did not achieve the professional status it has until fairly recently. However, it, too, has been criticized as having self-interested motives (Bernal, 1992). Bernal, a hospital ethicist, suggested that nursing's claim of patient advocacy was linked to a desire for autonomy of practice, which she took as a self-interested maneuver by the profession. Others

(Gaylord & Grace, 1995) have challenged Bernal's argument, citing a misunderstanding of nursing's purposes in this regard. Generally, nursing has not been perceived by the general public as a self-serving profession.

Flexner (1915) noted that, in order for a group to be recognized as a profession, the following would be evident from its activities:

◎ Assumption of responsibility for using intellectual processes
◎ Ongoing engagement in scientific knowledge development (this seems to exclude lawyers as professionals)
◎ A practice (or practical skill) orientation
◎ Specialized education of members
◎ Self-organization and self-consciousness of the group as a profession with a given purpose
◎ Interest in furthering the "good" of the society

More recently, Kepler (1981), a medical historian, asserted:

Professions are organized; the physicians have their medical organizations and the lawyers have their bar associations. A high level of education is necessary to provide knowledge not readily available or capable of being understood by all. Professions normally interact with clients for whom they provide services rather than goods (pp. 17–18).

One might ask why it would be important to categorize a group as a profession. The importance lies in the idea that professions are sanctioned by society. In return for specialized services, society awards **professions** and professionals a certain standing. It places a high value on the information and skills that professionals contribute. Society supports the education of professionals through subsidizing their training costs. They are trusted to provide what they promise in exchange for financial or other types of compensation. In return, professionals are held to standards of practice that support the betterment of society as a whole.

One important facet of human services professions is that they have "codes of ethics" outlining what, in essence, are their promises of service to society. A significant consequence of these ethical codes, which serve as guides to practice, is that professions and their members can be held accountable by the public through such agencies as professional licensure boards for these "promises." Newton (1988) asserted that a profession's members are accountable for practices that are

... inadequate at any stage of the rendering of the service: if the client the ultimate consumer is unhappy; if he is happy but unknowing, badly served by shabby products or services; or if he is happy and well served by the best available product but the state of the art is not adequate to his real needs. (Newton, 1988, p. 49)

Thus, if members of a profession promise, via their code of ethics, to be able to care for any societal member, regardless of that person's circumstances, they can be criticized by society or by other professions to the extent that they fail to fulfill this self-asserted obligation. For nurse practitioners, professional membership means that nursing—not an associated discipline—remains the foundation for practice.

HISTORICAL ROOTS OF NURSING PRACTICE AND NURSE PRACTITIONER PRACTICE

Nursing Practice

The development of nursing as a profession has had a more troublesome course than that, say, of medicine. There are several well-documented reasons for this. First, nursing remains a predominantly female discipline; therefore its progress has echoed that of the status of women in society. Second, there are different levels of educational preparation for nurses. This has led to one of the most vital problems for nursing leaders, that is, how to unify the profession. Unity is crucial because without it there is little power to effect change or gain practice autonomy, which is necessary for nursing to fulfill its goals in regard to its commitment to improve the health of people. Third, although historically nursing has enjoyed a positive image, at times it has been held in low regard. For example, a negative image of nursing involves the nurse as "servant" (Flaherty, 1982, p. 68). This ignominious period in nursing's history, according to Flaherty, ran from the "sixteenth to the nineteenth" century. The unflattering image of the nurse was personified in fiction by Charles Dickens' slovenly, alcoholic Sarah Gamp, who nursed as a last resort to earn money, but had no pretensions to any expertise. Because of its reputation as the occupation of "low" women, nursing was not considered suitable employment for most women.

It was during the Victorian era, an era of great scientific progress, that nursing, under the influence of Florence Nightingale, began its reformation and developed into an occupation suitable for gentlewomen. In 1836, the first modern hospital was established in Kaiserwerth, Germany. It provided a 3-year training course for women of good "moral standing" in principles of hygiene, current scientific knowledge, pharmacology, and religion (Deloughery, 1977). This institution had a powerful influence on Nightingale, who was a frequent visitor.

As is commonly known, Nightingale went on to establish training schools for nurses in England. The influence of her model of nurse training was present also in the United States. As documented by Fitzpatrick (1983), "while the medical profession was busily placing the nursing role in a passive and subservient position, Florence Nightingale was carving a unique independent role for nursing" (p. 63). Her model (Nightingale, 1859) was based on the idea that one had to manipulate the environment to promote the body's natural healing. Additionally, in training nurses for this work, she believed that schools of nursing had to influence both the minds and character of those being trained.

In the years since Nightingale, nursing in the United States has seen an evolution from hospital-based training to instruction in places of higher education. There have been many changes in nursing as it has struggled to develop its professional autonomy. Nurses have evolved (and are still struggling to evolve) from obedient physicians' helpers to professionals with their own purposes and goals distinct from those of medicine, yet in some ways also complementary to these. More recently, the problems of an economically focused health-care environment have been impinging on nurses' development of more autonomous practice. Indeed, as Nagel (1999) points out, "in view of fiscal constraints and the increasingly technical environments of health care, the essential and unique contributions of all health-care providers, including nurses are being challenged" (p. 71).

Nurse Practitioner Practice

The development of advanced-practice nursing, especially the nurse practitioner role, has posed both new problems and new possibilities for the nursing profession. Although some nursing scholars have criticized the expansion of nursing practice to include extended practice roles, Cockerham (1989) and others think that the nurse practitioner role might be the key to achieving status as a profession. The recently agreed-on criterion of a master's degree as a minimum preparation for this role and the formulation of curriculum guidelines supports this hope (American Association of Colleges of Nurses [AACN], 1996; National Organization of Nurse Practitioner Faculty [NONPF], 2002). Despite the support for graduate education for nurse practitioners, it should be noted that there are many nurse practitioners who are not yet educated to the master's level because early programs were not developed in graduate programs. The nurse practitioner role is the most recent of the four advanced-practice roles: certified nurse midwife (CNM), certified registered nurse anesthetist (CRNA), clinical nurse specialist (CNS), and nurse practitioner (NP).

Komnenich (1998) notes that the nurse practitioner movement "arose against the backdrop of the 1960s and in response to needed changes in the health care environment" (p. 30). During this time, there was a proliferation of nursing master's level education programs. In addition, there was also increased public concern about the distribution of resources, including health-care resources that often left out the poor and marginalized, and the lack of available physicians. "President Lyndon Johnson declared the war on poverty" (Komnenich, 1998, p. 31), and there was an emerging emphasis on preventing disease as well as on promoting health. Thus a window of opportunity opened.

Loretta Ford (1995) is credited with being one of the founders of the nurse practitioner movement. She noted that the nurse practitioner role emerged successfully, in part, because dedicated groups of faculty members collaborated on a model for master's education in nursing, identifying and emphasizing appropriate clinical content. According to Komnenich (1998), Ford dates the inception of nurse practitioner education to 1965, when the first nurse practitioner student was admitted to the University of Colorado. Ford has repeatedly tried to dispel some of the pervasive myths, such as the idea that nurse practitioners were physician substitutes, surrounding the emergence of the nurse practitioner role. She affirms that the nurse practitioner role was firmly founded in nursing ideals because the American Nurses Association (ANA) criteria for clinical practice served as the model for the role. As Komnenich (1998) confirms, "the emphasis was on professional, direct client care, health and wellness, collegiality with physicians, and prevention-oriented care, including consumer education" (p. 32).

In spite of this focus and clarity of purpose, the nurse practitioner movement struggled to gain acceptance from professional nursing associations. However, as Komnenich reports, private foundations and specialty organizations provided support through conferences and position statements and through the development of credentialing mechanisms that affirmed the importance of nursing educational preparation, which permitted the slow but steady progress of faculty support for the nurse practitioner movement. Initially, as Komnenich notes, faculty had feared medical control of the education of these students. The following section explores what this means philosophically for nurse practitioner students as they work toward assuming a more independent practice role.

⟩⟩ PHILOSOPHICAL ROOTS OF NURSING PRACTICE

What Is Nursing's Purpose?

Contemporary developments in nursing and the movement of nursing toward professional maturity have occurred partly because nursing's scholars, theorists, and even researchers have been willing to ask the hard questions about nursing. They have been willing to ask, "What is it that we are doing when we are doing nursing? How is what we do different from what other professions do? What is our unique purpose? Although scholars differ about the goals of nursing and what sorts of things do or do not constitute nursing, they agree (both implicitly and explicitly) that nursing is concerned with the four metaparadigm concepts: person, environment, health, and nursing. What this means, roughly, is that nursing has to do with assisting humans, who are viewed as complex individuals who interact with their environment and have health needs that nursing can address. However, nursing philosophers and theorists disagree about the definitions of the metaparadigm concepts. It is doubtful that unity in answering this question can be achieved, given different philosophical views regarding the nature of humans. However, many (Newman, 1996) have argued that, although unity at this level would be difficult, this is not necessarily problematic for the nursing profession. Indeed, it may foster creativity by opening the dialogue to multiple views of nursing and inclusivity in providing care in a variety of settings and contexts. Definitions of the metaparadigm concepts emerge from both the scholars' personal philosophy regarding these concepts and the context of these scholars' original practice arenas. Therefore, although the health needs of nursing's population will be addressed by all of the proposed nursing models and theories, the manner in which this occurs may differ according to the lens through which the scholar views the phenomena of concern. For example, the scholar who views the person as a unitary being will view patterns of the whole as important in working with a patient, whereas the scholar with a systems view of the person will focus on functioning of systems and subsystems in the person's life. Both views offer a useful perspective. Advanced-practice nurses who develop their thinking regarding the nursing metaparadigms concepts will be able to offer flexible responses to the range of situations that patients present.

The implication of these discussions for the nurse practitioner students is that they must take time to explore their personal beliefs about the nature of humans and examine their philosophy of nursing and its purposes. Attention should also be paid to the particular context of the specialty practice, with an emphasis on how practice in this area can be nursing focused. Reviewing the works of the various nursing theorists and philosophers may prove helpful in this regard. Theory-based practice generally leads to consistency in purpose and action (Grace, 2002). However, it is incumbent on the nurse practitioner student to choose a model or theory that not only fits both personal philosophical views on persons and nursing, but is also appropriate for the practice setting as an environmental consideration. Because most master's programs in nursing now include a course on the conceptual basis for nursing practice, faculty members should be able to help students determine appropriate theories of nursing for the desired setting. A nurse practitioner student who understands his or her personal beliefs regarding nursing, and who bases practice on nursing concepts, is better able to resist pressures from other disciplines or from economic constraint to take shortcuts. He or she will be able to maintain focus on the patient as a complex being and to justify the need to address system or institutional inadequacies or obstacles.

Indeed, it can be reiterated here that the nurse-patient relationship is as pivotal to advanced-practice nursing as it is to nursing practice in general. How the nurse practitioner approaches this relationship will depend on the nurse practitioner's perspective on the metaparadigm concepts described previously. The experienced nurse practitioner will develop a perspective that provides the basis for action for both individuals and society as a whole.

What Knowledge Is Needed for Nurse Practitioner Practice?

Nursing's epistemological task involves discovering how the basic phenomena of the discipline can be known. Among the nursing epistemological questions that might be asked, as Fry (1999) notes, are the following, "Is there knowledge used by nursing that is unique to nursing? If so what is its nature and structure, and how is its truth evaluated?" (p. 7). Another question concerns the controversy about whether nursing knowledge is primarily practical or theoretical. It is crucial that nursing continues to ask such questions because the environment in which nursing practice occurs is evolving and subject to rapid change. For example, changes in health-care delivery systems, societal needs, and the political climate all affect nursing and, in turn, the knowledge needed for practice. As may be observed from a variety of nursing curricula, much knowledge used in nursing practice is derived from other disciplines: scientific, sociologic, and human sciences. What is it, then, that permits us to take this knowledge and make it peculiarly nursing knowledge? How does knowledge for advanced nursing practice differ from nursing knowledge, or does it? What is it that makes advanced-practice nursing advanced?

It should be emphasized that the issue of synthesizing knowledge from other disciplines for a particular use is not solely a problem for nursing. Other disciplines also use knowledge developed in disparate arenas. For example, medicine uses knowledge developed by chemists, physicists, engineers, and others. Medicine is clear, though, about the distinct goal of this borrowed knowledge, which is to cure disease. For nursing and for advanced-practice nursing, the issue is to be clear about the focus of the knowledge, which is to provide holistic care of a patient, who is viewed as interactive with his or her environment. Care of the patient—which involves facilitating health, addressing health needs, or assisting the patient to find meaning in illness—will be influenced by both the nurse's and the patient's beliefs, values, or philosophies and by the setting. Finding meaning in illness is a sense of claiming a purpose or acceptance of accommodations that illness requires and that can change the values and perspective of a person's life. Thus, the epistemological question for an individual nurse practitioner is, "What knowledge do I need to provide **nursing** care for these patients in this setting?" The particular knowledge needed for a given advanced-practice setting will be assimilated into the broader knowledge needed for general nursing practice.

Carper (1978), in a seminal work on nursing knowledge, identified four interrelated patterns of knowing in nursing: empirical, esthetic, personal, and ethical. Nurses, she believes, use all four in the work of nursing. Empirical knowing is derived from nursing science—from research on "health and illness in relation to human life processes" (p. 14). Esthetic knowing is related to the art of nursing; it involves creativity in approaching patient care for a particular patient. This, in turn, requires an "engaged" knowing of the patient (Benner, Tanner, & Chesla, 1996). Engaged knowing results from attention to **this** patient in all of his or her particularities. Personal knowing in nursing, Carper notes, is probably both the hardest to master and to teach, but is necessary for authentic relationships with others. Although she does not say this exactly, genuine self-reflection—a willingness to question one's motives and beliefs—is an important part of this personal knowing. Personal knowing is seen as essential to the therapeutic use of self, which has been viewed as an essential component of nursing practice. Ethical knowing involves discernment of the good in a particular situation and will be addressed more fully in Chapter 11. Table 10–2 lists examples of patterns of knowing.

It is essential to note that these patterns of knowing overlap. For example, Carper notes that "… personal knowledge is essential for ethical

TABLE 10–2

Carper's Patterns of Knowing

Pattern	Definition	Example
Empirical	Abstract and systematic explanations of phenomena	Describing the natural history of addictions; describing how relationships between nurse practitioner and patient are formed
Esthetic	Creative responses to particular patient issues	Developing a management plan that assists an older person to live independently through the use of nontraditional community resources
Personal	Interpersonal processes, using the authentic self, investment	Developing a trusting relationship that enables a woman to leave an abusive relationship
Ethical	Discernment of what ought to be done	Balancing patient autonomy with preventing harm when considering support for independent living

Source: Adapted from: Carper, B.A. (1999). Fundamental patterns of knowing in nursing. In J. W. Kenney (Ed.). *Philosophical and theoretical perspectives for advanced nursing practice* (2nd ed., pp. 5–13). Sudbury, MA: Jones and Bartlett.

choices in that moral action presupposes personal maturity and freedom" (p. 22). In other words, the four patterns of knowing are interrelated and dependent upon each other. Consequently, personal and professional growth is dependent on the development of all four "patterns" of knowing.

FURTHER PHILOSOPHICAL QUESTIONS FOR NURSE PRACTITIONER PRACTICE

Because nurse practitioner practice is a relatively new role for nursing, some of the philosophical questions such as what is appropriately considered nursing and what knowledge is essential to its practice have not been fully explored. However, master's education prepares nurses to ask their own questions about the implications of their role. Both nursing theory and practice are dependent on each other. For example, nursing theory focuses on the scope and limits of nursing practice, which in turn depends upon theory for guidance. Yet knowledge gained in practice is essential for refining and even revising nursing theory. Thus nurse practitioner input is essential to further develop the role through shaping regulations that govern practice. Demonstrating nursing's unique contribution to the health of people is an important task ahead. Nurse practitioner research that is focused on particular patient groups in primary and specialty settings will be an important part of theory refinement. Additionally, further development of the nurse practitioner role as the provision of holistic nursing care (rather than merely treatment of disease) to those who otherwise may not receive care is essential to nursing's goals and purposes.

⟩⟩ SUMMARY

Assuming the role of nurse practitioner requires thoughtful consideration of how this new role includes, but is unique from, previous roles held in nursing. Beyond learning new assessment techniques, specifics about diagnosing human conditions and designing treatments, philosophical questions about the elements of advanced nursing practice, the nature of humans and their health, and the nurse's position as a person who assists patients in improving their health must be addressed. This chapter has provided definitions for ontology, the essence of being a nurse practitioner; epistemology, the knowledge that nurse practitioners use to support their practice; and the philosophical roots of the profession. It illustrates enduring questions about the nature of nursing. Addressing these issues will offer the nurse practitioner a broader array of perspectives for understanding and for making clinical judgments surrounding health.

REFERENCES

Alcoff, L., & Potter, E. (1993). *Feminist epistemologies.* New York: Routledge.

American Association of Colleges of Nursing (1996). *Essentials of master's education for advanced practice nursing.* Washington, DC: Author.

Beck, R. N. (1969). *Perspectives in philosophy* (2nd ed.). New York: Holt Rinehart, & Winston.

Benner, P., Tanner, C. A., & Chesla, C. A. (1996*). Expertise in nursing practice: Caring, clinical judgment and ethics.* New York: Springer.

Bernal, E. W. (1992). The nurse as patient advocate. *Hastings Center Report, 22*(4), 18–23.

Carper, B. A. (1978). Fundamental patterns of knowing in nursing. *Annals of Nursing Science, 1*(1), 13–24.

Carper, B. A. (1999). Fundamental patterns of knowing in nursing. In J. W. Kenney (Ed.). *Philosophical and theoretical perspectives for advanced nursing practice* (2nd ed., pp. 5–13). Sudbury, MA: Jones and Bartlett.

Carr-Saunders, A. M., & Wilson, P. A. (1933). *The professions.* Oxford, UK: Clarendon.

Cockerham, W. C. (1989). *Medical sociology* (4th ed.). Englewood Cliffs, NJ: Prentice-Hall.

Delougherty, G. L. (1977). *History and trends of professional nursing.* St. Louis: C. V. Mosby.

Fawcett, J., & Malinski, V. M. (1999). On the requirements for a metaparadigm: An invitation to dialogue. In J. W. Kenney (Ed.). *Philosophical and theoretical perspectives for advanced practice nursing* (2nd ed., pp. 111–116). Sudbury, MA: Jones & Bartlett.

Fitzpatrick, M. L. (1983). *Prologue to professionalism.* Bowie, MD: Prentice-Hall.

Flaherty, M. J. (1982). Nursing's contract with society. In L. Curtin & M. J. Flaherty (Eds.). *Nursing ethics: Theory and pragmatics* (pp. 67–78). Bowie, MD: Brady Communications.

Flexner, A. (1915). Is social work a profession? In *Proceedings of the National Conference of Charities and Corrections* at the Forty-Second Annual Session (pp. 578–581), Baltimore, May 12–19. Chicago: Hildmann.

Ford, L. C. (1995). Nurse practitioners: Myths and misconceptions. *Journal of New York State Nurses Association, 26*(1), 12–13.

Fry, S. T. (1999). The philosophy of nursing. *Scholarly Inquiry for Nursing Practice: An International Journal, 13*(1), 5–15.

Gaylord, N., & Grace, P. (1995). Nursing Advocacy: An ethic of practice. *Nursing Ethics, 2*(1), 10–18.

Grace, P. J. (2002). Philosophies, models, and theories: Moral obligations. In M. R. Alligood & A. M. Tomey (Eds.). *Nursing theory: Utilization & Application* (2nd ed., pp. 63–79) St. Louis: Mosby.

Hume, D. (1974). An enquiry concerning human understanding (original publication 1748). In *The Empiricists: Locke, Berkeley & Hume.* New York: Doubleday, Anchor Press.

Kenney, J. W. (1999). *Philosophical and theoretical perspectives for advanced nursing practice* (2nd ed.). Sudbury, MA: Jones & Bartlett.

Kepler, M. O. (1981). *Medical stewardship: Fulfilling the Hippocratic legacy.* Westport, CT: Greenwood Press.

Komnenich, P. (1998). The evolution of advanced practice in nursing. In C. M. Sheehy & M. C. McCarthy (Eds). *Advanced practice nursing: Emphasizing common roles* (pp. 8–46). Philadelphia: F. A. Davis.

Maclean, U. (1974). *Nursing in contemporary society.* Boston: Routledge and Kegan Paul.

Nagel, N. M. (1999). A matter of extinction or distinction. *Western Journal of Nursing Research, 21*(1), 71–82.

Nagel, T. (1970). *The possibility of altruism.* Oxford: Clarendon.

Nagel, T. (1991). *Equality and partiality.* New York: Oxford University.

National Organization of Nurse Practitioner Faculty (2002). *Advanced nursing practice: Building curriculum for quality nurse practitioner education.* Washington, DC: Author.

Newman, M. (1996). Prevailing paradigms in nursing. In J. Kenney (Ed.). *Philosophical and theoretical perspectives for advanced practice nursing* (pp. 302–308). Sudbury, MA: Jones and Bartlett.

Newton, L. H. (1988). Lawgiving for professional life: Reflections on the place of the professional code. In A. Flores (Ed.). *Professional ideals* (pp. 47–56). Belmont, CA: Wadsworth.

Nightingale, F. (1859). *Notes on nursing: What it is and what it is not.* London, UK: Harrison Reprint.

Sarvimaki, A. (1999). Answering philosophical questions facing contemporary nursing practice. *Western Journal of Nursing Research, 21*(1), 9–15.

Schlodtfeldt, R. (1989). Structuring nursing knowledge: A priority for creating nursing's future. *Nursing Science Quarterly, 1*(1), 35–38.

CHAPTER 11

Ethics in the Clinical Encounter

Pamela J. Grace, APRN, BC, PhD

CHAPTER OUTLINE

This chapter investigates and supports the idea that ethical practice is in many ways synonymous with "good" clinical practice, as has been discussed throughout preceding chapters. Additionally, it offers strategies for uncovering and analyzing ethical issues prevalent in advanced-practice nursing.

⟩⟩ CLINICAL AND ETHICAL JUDGMENT AS INSEPARABLE CONCEPTS

Good or "ethical" nursing practice results from the use of theoretical, conceptual, and practical knowledge in formulating clinical judgments, acting on these judgments, and evaluating ensuing actions for their ability to meet patient needs. Although conceptual or theoretical knowledge may be derived from other disciplines as well as nursing, it should always be synthesized through a nursing perspective. Included in the knowledge base necessary for "good" nursing practice is an understanding of the general language, principles, and methods of ethical reasoning.

Although a distinction is often made in general philosophy and ethics literature between the terms "ethical" and "moral," this distinction is dependent on the context of discussion. For the purposes of this chapter, with its emphasis on nursing practice, these terms will be used interchangeably. That is, "ethically" sound clinical judgments and their ensuing actions are aimed at benefiting a patient or patients (providing for a patient's good), and for this reason they may equally be referred to as "morally" sound clinical judgments.

In health care, "ethics" is concerned with evaluating actions or possible actions, including lack of action. Actions may be judged "good" or "bad," "right" or "wrong," "mandatory" or "prohibited" (or, more weakly, "permissible") when measured against particular standards, or when analyzed using the methods of moral decision making. Guidelines for appraising nursing actions include the American Nurses Association's (ANA's) ethical code (2001) and appropriate (for specialty) advanced nursing practice standards. Additionally, nursing actions can be appraised to the extent that their intent is to optimally address the health-care needs of the person to whom they are directed.

The accepted standards, both of nursing practice and ethical conduct of that practice, have been formulated over time as a result of formal and informal discussions among nursing's scholars and its membership. These discussions are based on the idea that nursing's purpose is to promote the health or well-being of people or, in the case of terminal illness, a comfortable death. These are moral goals, and therefore it may be claimed both that nursing practice is a moral endeavor and that clinical judgments have inseparable moral content.

Beside the intrinsically moral nature of clinical nursing, advanced-practice nurses also encounter morally troubling situations in their daily work. There are two categories of moral issues that nurses (and other health-care providers) face: dilemmas and problems. Ethical dilemmas involve a situation for which there is no good solution but in which a choice must be made between unsatisfactory alternatives. For example, an 8-year-old child with a terminal illness keeps asking what is wrong with him, but his parents are adamant that he not be given this information. Alternatively, a psychiatric patient in a counseling session with her nurse practitioner divulges her intent to harm her ex-boyfriend. In this second case, the choice is between conflicting ethical principles (nonmaleficence) or the duty to prevent harm (to the ex-boyfriend) and confidentiality (warning the boyfriend). Weston (1997) argues, though, that true dilemmas are rare, and that viewing a seemingly impossible situation from a different angle or perspective often allows one to see other possible avenues of action.

In the first example, understanding the source and nature of the parents' misgivings may facilitate resolution of the issue. In the second example, there may also be an alternative solution, but if not, the clinician is faced with a true dilemma in which neither action is good and the nurse must decide on the least harmful alternative. Dilemmas often require consultation with peers, allied professionals, or an ethics resource person because of their difficult nature. Of course, if this is the case, it remains important to maintain patient confidentiality unless there is a strong reason (e.g., potential harm to self or others) not to do so.

In advanced-nursing practice, the issues encountered more frequently are not dilemmas. An ethical problem exists any time a practitioner is obstructed in formulating or carrying out sound nursing judgment. Obstructions may be internal (lack of knowledge, experience, reflective ability, or emotional capacity) or external (institutional, economic, regulatory, or supervisory). It is important that nurse practitioners recognize that these issues of everyday practice are also moral in nature because they interfere with the ability to provide a "good" for the patient and should be addressed.

⟩⟩ NURSING'S CODE OF ETHICS: APPLICABILITY TO ADVANCED-PRACTICE NURSING

Codes of ethics are generally conceived over time and in response not only to the development of the profession but also to environmental and societal changes (Grace, 1998; Grace & Gaylord, 1999). "Nursing, like other professions, is an essential part of the society from which it has grown and within which it continues to evolve" (ANA, Nursing's Social Policy Statement, 1995, p. 2). It is important to note, however, that the philosophy and goals of any practice discipline provide the basis for that group's ethical code. Thus, nursing's ethical code is not an externally imposed guideline, even though it is influenced, at least indirectly, by society. Nursing may be said to "own" its code in the sense that it reflects what nurses have proposed that they **can** accomplish with regard to individual and societal health or well-being.

Since the beginning of the 20th century in the United States, nursing scholars such as Isabel Robb (1990) and Isabel McIsaac (1900) have struggled to formulate guidelines about what constitutes good nursing conduct. However, it was not until 1950 that the ANA's first *Code of Ethics for Nurses* was published. Since then, the code has been revised several times. In 2001, the most recent revision was completed. It currently serves as the standard of moral conduct for nurses practicing in the United States (ANA, 2001). It is also non-negotiable (ANA, 1994). This means that it applies to all professional nurses and cannot be subverted by institutional demands or employer mandates. In other words, institutions or employers cannot legitimately make demands on a nurse that conflict with codal guidelines. For example, in a correctional setting, nurses cannot be required to shift their focus from furthering the health of inmates to controlling behavior and maintaining discipline.

Although nurse practitioners appear to have wider-ranging ethical responsibilities to provide optimal patient care than nurses practicing in more traditional roles, the same guidelines for moral conduct apply to them. Simply put, the ANA's Code of Ethics for Nurses is relevant for nurse practitioners because advanced practice is, nevertheless, **nursing** practice. However, this does not deny the special nature of nurse-patient relationships in advanced-practice roles, in which nurses often serve as the primary and coordinating health-care provider.

In addition to utilizing theoretical knowledge, clinical experience, an understanding of specialty practice standards, and the ANA Code for Nurses in the interests of quality patient care, it is also important that the nurse practitioner have a grasp of ethical theory and its language. This is necessary for several reasons. It permits recognition of the moral content of ambiguous situations, facilitates analysis of complex problems, and enhances communication between involved professionals. This next section provides a brief description of the nature of ethics as a branch of philosophical inquiry (often referred to as moral philosophy) and shows how this relates to ethics in professional activity.

⟩⟩ ETHICS AS PHILOSOPHICAL INQUIRY

Ethics is a branch of philosophical inquiry that is also often referred to as "value theory." This is because it investigates what humans value in their relationship with the world and the reasons for these values. When ethics is discussed in relation to nursing, the scope of inquiry is narrowed from discovering what is good in human relations with others and the environment in general to what constitutes good practice given the knowledge and goals of the profession. Many of the principles of value theory are useful in helping us to determine what is good practice. However, ethical theories, perhaps unlike nursing theories, cannot be used exclusively to determine what constitutes good care in a particular practice setting. This is because the several ethical theories have radically differing ideas about a variety of concepts. For example, one type of ethical theory known as "deontology" gives individual well-being preference in decision making, whereas another ethical theory called "utilitarianism" places a higher value on societal well-being. In addition, ethical theories disagree about what constitutes the ultimate "good" for, or main purpose of, persons. The ultimate "good" for persons (or that which persons should or do strive for as an end in itself) has been conceptualized variously as happiness (Bentham, 1967/1789; Mill, 1967/1863), duty (Kant, 1967/1785; Ross, 1930), the cultivation of virtue (Aristotle, 1967; MacIntyre, 1984), or something else. More will be said about this later. This difference is a result of fundamentally contrasting beliefs about the nature of human beings and their place and purpose in the world as discussed in Chapter 10.

Nevertheless, in health-care ethics, principles inherent in a variety of ethical theories serve as useful tools with which to examine the implications of different proposed courses of action. They permit clarification of hidden issues or facets. An understanding of ethical principles commonly used in health-care ethics decision making also permits better communication between the advanced-practice nurse and others involved in decision making, thus enhancing the decision-making process. These tools cannot be used effectively in the absence of contextual considerations because it is often just these contextual considerations that determine the relevant principle. For example, a woman is being pressured by her family to have a surgical procedure that she does not want. The nurse who is familiar with ethical reasoning realizes that what is at issue here is the person's "autonomous" choice. Clinical judgment (including ethical considerations) would permit an assessment to determine what interventions might be most helpful in facilitating her autonomy.

Traditional Ethical Theory and Ethical Principles

The earlier discussion regarding nursing ethics portrayed ethics as a set of guidelines or standards formulated by a group. In this case the group was the nursing profession, but other groups may also have implicit or explicit rules about conduct, which would be termed the ethics of the group. Most professional groups have their own codes of ethics that reflect the values of the society as well as discipline-specific values.

However, another meaning of "ethics" is "field of inquiry." Ethics as a field of inquiry studies the foundations for distinguishing good from bad and right from wrong in human action. It is also known as moral philosophy. "Applied" ethics is the practice of using ethical theory that has been developed or derived from moral philosophy to evaluate or resolve actual problems. Nursing ethics, medical ethics, and health-care ethics are types of applied ethics that seek to promote the good for the population concerned.

What constitutes the main "good" for humans varies according to the particular theory and its philosophical foundations. For example, utilitarian theories like those of Jeremy Bentham (1748–1832) and John Stuart Mill (1806–1873) are focused on maximizing overall happiness for a society and minimizing pain or unhappiness. Because of their focus on overall good, there are implications to these theories that many would find troubling. Such theories, it has been argued, might permit withholding an expensive but life-saving drug from a critically ill patient in order to provide health screening for 100 persons. These theories are subject to the criticism that the mistreatment of individuals may occasionally be permissible if the interests of the larger society (which is, after all, made up of individual persons) are at stake.

Alternatively, duty-based or deontological theories like that of Immanuel Kant (1724–1804) and, to a certain extent, W. David Ross (1930) focus on the idea that something other than consequences provides the moral driving force for action. This "something" is duty. The philosophical underpinning of this theory is that man is a rational entity. The hallmark of humans is innate reasoning ability. Therefore humans have the capacity (and for this reason should make efforts) to determine what duty requires in any given situation that has a moral component. Duty requires that the "Categorical Imperative"(CI) be used to frame questions (Box 11–1).

Interestingly, it is this capacity of humans to determine right and wrong actions that makes them worthy of respect as individuals and underlies the principle of autonomy, which will be discussed subsequently. Duty-based theories are also subject to criticism for a variety of reasons. Sometimes duties seem to conflict. If I have a duty to do no harm but telling the truth would cause pain to someone, I have two conflicting categorical imperatives. There is no valid way to decide between these competing duties in a duty-based theory such as Kant's. These are just a few examples of how moral theories can pose more problems than they solve.

In health-care practice, what is "good" is assumed by the services provided and professional goals. We do not have to decide what constitutes the ultimate good for humans as much as decide what is good for this pa-

---

Box 11–1

The Categorical Imperative
(Kant, 1967/1785)

- Requires the human capacity to reason and to self-govern.
- Relies on the idea that there are absolute truths (e.g., lying is wrong).
- Humans can determine right action by posing a question.
- The answer to the question is the morally correct answer (the action that must or must not be taken). The question is a universally valid formal rule (to be applied when reasoning about action).
- "I ought never to act except in such a way that I can also will that my maxim should become a universal law" (Kant, 1967/1785, p. 318) or, more simply put,
- "Could any other person in the same or similar circumstances also take this action or refrain from this action?"
- If the answer is "no," **duty** demands that I not do it (regardless of consequences).
- If the answer is "yes," **duty** demands that I do it (regardless of consequences).
- The CI has no content of its own but serves as a format by which rational individuals can determine morally correct actions by using their reasoning abilities (e.g., it is a CI that one never tell lies because if people could lie occasionally, no one could be trusted to be truthful and communication would break down—an irrational consequence [note that it is not so much the consequence of the single action that is the problem as the irrationality of willing it]).

---

tient in these circumstances. This requires knowledge about the patient and the use of our professional knowledge and expertise. Similarly, we cannot rely on a particular moral theory taken as a whole because it may direct us to actions that do not benefit the patient. (Utilitarian theory might direct us to consider social costs at the expense of an individual patient's good, and duty theories might give conflicting directions.) However, general principles derived from such theories have proved helpful both in facilitating the inclusion of relevant considerations during the decision-making process and in deciding which considerations might carry the most weight and under what circumstances. A selection of principles that have proved particularly helpful in health-care decision making are discussed in more detail subsequently, with examples from the advanced-practice environment.

Feminist Ethics and the Ethic of "Care"

Currently, feminist philosophers suggest that moral decision making often requires more than the use of moral theory and reasoning; it requires also the unearthing of buried assumptions about the influences of power in relationships and situations (Donchin & Purdy, 1999; Tong, 1997; Warren, 2001). Feminist concerns about uneven power relationships within many social and institutional settings are especially appropriate in problems arising in settings where nursing is practiced. Feminist ethics is also concerned with understanding the context of a situation and the interrelationships of those involved. This is different from the focus of many traditional ethical theories in which the emphasis is on the isolated individual viewed as an autonomous entity. Davis et al. (1997) note that Gilligan's research on moral development revealed women's moral concerns to be focused more "on care and responsibility in relationships rather than on the application of abstract principles such as respect for individual autonomy and justice" (p. 58).

"Care" is a concept that has appealed to feminists and nursing scholars over the last couple of decades. This is partly because care represents the more relational aspects of human interactions. Feminist philosophers have explored the traditional ethical treatment of persons as isolated and atomic entities and find that perspective inadequate for describing daily life. Although viewing persons this way was thought to allow just treatment and to permit generalization, feminist philosophers such as Baier (1985), Noddings (1984), and Sherwin (1992) think that this does not "capture" women's reality (or men's, for that matter). They do not think that viewing individuals as totally autonomous beings helps in analyzing ethical aspects of problematic situations in part because humans are social beings who depend on others and, in turn, have others who depend on them. Thus decisions never involve only one individual, but rather have a ripple-type effect on others within the individual's circle of relationships.

From a literature review on care, Fry (1990) has identified three models of caring: cultural, feminist, and humanistic. She defends the humanistic model as most appropriate in describing care as an aspect of nursing practice. Generally, care might be described as the idea that human relationships are complex webs of interdependencies and interrelationships. A person cannot successfully be extricated from this complex web and treated as an isolated entity. For example, a focus on pathophysiology is liable to miss nonphysiologically based contributing aspects of illness or ill health. Thus a physiologic cure is effected, but the patient is left vulnerable to other sequelae. Care as a facet of nursing practice requires an engagement on the part of the nurse with the patient in a relationship that permits the meaning and context of the patient's needs to be exposed. It also requires that the nurse be willing to address those needs from the patient's perspective wherever possible. Moreover, it requires nursing knowledge as a foundation to addressing these needs. Thus, in nursing care is a concept requiring an engaged knowing of the patient. Benner, Tanner, & Chesla (1996) note that care is "the dominant ethic found in [nurses] stories of everyday practice" (p. 233).

Unlike traditional moral theories that treat humans as isolated individuals whose ethical concerns should be addressed impartially and objectively to ensure just actions, "an ethic of care grounds moral reasoning and responses in the particularity of the situation" (Liaschenko, 1999, p. 36). Women's approaches are "rooted in receptivity, relatedness and responsiveness" to particular others (Noddings, 1984, p. 2). That is to say, care requires attention to **this** particular patient and his or her unique characteristics and situation. Care in nursing is seen as the nurse's knowledgeable and skilled responses to a given patient's needs based on an interpersonal relationship with that patient that reveals the complexity of the situation. Fry (1989) has noted that the nurse's caring actions are focused on the involved individual and are guided more by personal and professional goals and attitudes than by formal "rights" and "principles" (ethical theory), which some consider a limitation of care. Criticisms of care viewed as an ethic of practice include the problem of moral predictability or certainty (Nelson, 1992). That is, if there are no criteria for right and wrong, how can one be assured of the morally correct action in a given situation? It may be argued that a morally correct action is one that emerges as a result of nursing judgment based both on previous knowledge or experience and an engaged relationship with the patient. However, another criticism is that the "care" ethic does not permit a moral critique of such things as poor institutional practices or poor interprofessional relationships (Nelson, 1992). Additionally, an ethic of care might preclude moral consideration for other involved persons such as family members. An ethic of care and principles derived from traditional moral theory may **both** be needed for decision making in situations posing a moral problem for the nurse practitioner and his or her patients. It should be affirmed here, then, that the purpose of ethical inquiry in practice settings is to gain clarity about moral issues arising in the practice context. Ethical inquiry cannot solve all problems, but it can facilitate appropriate and in-depth data gathering, permit the uncovering of hidden agendas and interests, and focus us on the most salient aspects of a particular problem, thus enhancing clinical judgment.

)) ETHICAL PRINCIPLES IN ADVANCED NURSING PRACTICE

Although the tenets of nursing's "codes of ethics" and "standards of practice" provide some guidance about the nature of practice and the manner in which services will be provided, they tend to be vague and nonspecific, often leaving some ambiguity about the best course of action in morally troubling situations.

Using principles derived from a variety of ethical theories along with an ethic of care in exploring morally troubling situations may provide a richer picture of a given problem by including salient aspects of the given patient's (or patients') life (or lives). As Beauchamp and Walters (1999) note, "principles provide a starting point for moral judgment and policy evaluation, but more content is needed than that supplied by principles alone" (p. 19). In other words, principles such as "autonomy," "beneficence," and "justice" often serve as helpful starting points in teasing out the tangled elements of complex issues, but taken alone, they are usually insufficient to permit moral problem solving in health-care environments. What has to be decided is which principles are important to consider in a given case, and this requires an exploration of the case. Additionally, tenets of the Code for Nurses (ANA, 2001) and other ANA position statements provide guidance regarding what a nurse's moral responsibilities are in a particular type of situation.

Autonomy

Perhaps the most powerful moral principle underlying social and political systems in many Western societies is that of respect for autonomy. This principle asserts that persons have the capacity to make choices for themselves (as in Kant's idea of the human as a rational entity). Thus they should not be subject to external coercion in making these choices, with the possible exception of cases in which free action on the part of an autonomous agent harms, or is likely to harm, others. To make autonomous choices, individuals must have appropriate information to permit decision making, along with intact mental capacities and no coercive influences (Beauchamp & Childress, 2001). The autonomy principle is also known as "respect for persons" because, in honoring it, we are acknowledging the moral importance of a person's right to self-determination. Autonomy, viewed as informed, uncoerced, and reasoned action, is therefore an ideal. Many of us, and probably most of the time, fall short of the ideal because we are products of our various previous environments, subject to misconceptions and psychological blind spots, and often hold inconsistent values and beliefs (a deficit of reasoning or self-reflection). Nevertheless, autonomy remains an important moral consideration because, all other things being equal, an individual may be presumed to know better than anyone else what course of action will best serve his or her interests.

Respect for autonomy is what underlies the idea of "informed consent" to various treatments, research, and procedures. Informed consent should be thought of ideally as an ongoing process, especially when the risks of consenting may be high, as in drug research. It has been documented that people do not grasp information well when they are in stressful situations or when the information is complex (Broadbent, 1971; Degner & Sloan, 1992; Edwards, 1954; Janis & Mann, 1977; Redelmeier, Rozin, & Kahneman, 1993; Schaeffer, 1989).

To ensure patient autonomy, the advanced-practice nurse must consider the patient's unique characteristics when deciding what constitutes adequate information to facilitate the patient's decision making. This is no easy task. Time constraints prevail in many settings. Creativity may be required. Some activity on the part of the nurse (perhaps in concert with others) may also be required to ensure that the environment is made more conducive to autonomous decision making when obvious barriers to this exist. That is, if the nurse sees the same problems (e.g., stringent time constraints, inadequate staffing, lack of patient privacy) recurring, he or she may need to consider addressing the problem at a more institutional or political level. This may seem like a tall order, but if nurse practitioners are genuinely interested in furthering the goals of their profession with regard to their patient population, there is no escape from this obligation. No other professionals are better equipped to recognize and address such problems. Such problems may be best addressed with the help of the specialty nursing organization, the state nursing association, or other appropriate venues.

Exceptions to Autonomous Decision Making

Certain populations are considered less than fully autonomous for a variety of reasons. For example, patients with Alzheimer's disease and other dementias have cognitive deficits that can prevent adequate comprehension. Incarcerated persons are restricted in their choices and may be subject to subtle or not-so-subtle coercion. Children are considered less than fully autonomous because they are not developmentally mature. Additionally, patients with certain mental illnesses such as psychoses or bipolar disorders may be incapable of decision making in alignment with previous life goals. The importance of such considerations in advanced-practice settings cannot be overstated. Any conclusions about patient capacity for decision making have to consider the criteria for autonomy. The President's

Commission (1982) formed to look at health-care decision making has noted that the minimum capacities needed for competent decision making are: "1. Possession of a set of values and goals, 2. the ability to communicate and to understand information, and 3. the ability to reason and deliberate about one's choice" (p. 57). These criteria are still generally accepted as a basic minimum (Beauchamp & Childress, 2001). Thus it may be that some children do understand the implications that a given course of treatment holds for them and other persons with cognitive impairments may nevertheless be deemed competent to make certain decisions. Buchanan and Brock (1989) have argued persuasively that the capacity to make autonomous choices is not an all-or-nothing condition. They remind health-care professionals that competency determinations are usually made for a given decision or task and thus should be relative to that task. Moreover, they affirm that competency for decision making occurs along a continuum. Thus, a person may vacillate between competency and noncompetency, depending on either the task at hand or the person's physical or psychological status during the period when a decision must be made.

Generally, when advocating decision making for a cognitively impaired person, the nurse practitioner considers the risk of permitting the decision versus the benefits to the patient of overriding his or her choice. That is, if the risk of injury is high and it is obvious that the patient does not grasp this fact, he or she may be overruled in decision making. The idea behind this is that either we are preserving the patient's autonomy so that he or she may engage in decision making at a future time (and presumably death truncates autonomy), or that severe suffering is likely to occur and the patient has not taken this into consideration. This is an example of paternalism that will be discussed in more detail subsequently in relation to the principle of beneficence. In high-risk situations, paternalistically overriding the patient's decision is permissible only if it serves the patient's best interest.

Proxy Decision Making

When children are involved, it is often the parent or guardian to whom we turn for permission to treat. Nevertheless, in pediatric settings it is incumbent on the nurse practitioner to gain assent from the child also after providing information in language that the child can grasp. Pediatric advanced-practice nurses may have to weigh the risks and benefits of proceeding with interventions in the absence of a child's assent to treatment. Together with a risk/benefit assessment, the nurse practitioner should try to ascertain the extent to which the child understands the purpose, risks, and benefits of refusing treatment. For those who are cognitively impaired, the nurse practitioner must make a similar assessment. When adult patients are deemed incompetent to make their own decisions (a legal determination), a proxy decision for or against treatment must be made.

There are three types of surrogate or proxy decision making. The legal processes for surrogate or proxy decision vary from state to state. It is necessary that nurse practitioners be familiar with state laws before offering guidance to patients in a given state. For example, in Massachusetts the legally accepted form of surrogate decision making is a "Health Care Proxy." This means that an individual, while competent, can designate the person he or she considers most appropriate to make proxy health-care decisions in the event of temporary or permanent incapacity. Patients should be counseled that the best proxy may be, but is not necessarily, the person with whom he or she is most intimately acquainted. The best decision maker may be a trusted friend who can set aside personal feelings in the interest of determining what one's most likely preferences would be. Patients need to know that their wishes in regard to designated proxies and/or written directives may be changed at any time when the patient has the capacity and is competent to communicate new instructions.

More generally, of the three types of proxy decision making (Table 11–1), the one most reflective of the patient's desires (most likely to resemble a patient's "autonomous" choice) is the one in which previous information exists about what the patient would want in either a written document or verbal expression **and** there is a previously designated health-care proxy (in some states the designated person is recognized as holding "durable power of attorney" for the health care of the patient) who can use these written or verbal expressions to determine which course of action is appropriate. Second, in the absence of verbal or written directives and of a designated proxy, a surrogate decision maker may be appointed (usually by family and/or friends' consensus) to give a "substituted judgment" of what the patient would want. This surrogate helps the health-care provider to institute a course of action directed toward furthering the patient's best interests as the patient would most likely see them. It is expected that the substituted judgment would be predicated on knowledge of the patient's life goals, beliefs, and values, and thus is supposed to most closely approximate what the patient would want if competent. When there is doubt whether the surrogate decision maker actually has the patient's best interests in mind, it may be necessary for the health-care provider or team to seek legal advice. In this case, and when there is little knowledge about a person's background history and life, a "best interest" standard is used. "Best interests" are predicated on the idea that "quality of life" considerations are important and that the benefits and burdens of treatments or actions must be factored into the decision-making process (Beauchamp & Childress, 2001). The "reasonable person" standard basically directs us to provide the treatment that most rational people would choose after due consideration of the details.

TABLE 11–1 Proxy Decision Making	
Type	**Explanation**
A. Autonomy based–Person's previously expressed wishes	• *Written* Living will, advance directives • *Substituted Judgment*: 1. Durable Power of Attorney for health care (person appointed to provide information about a patient's previous wishes expressed while having decision-making capacity) 2. Informal (family member, friend, significant other)
B. Best interests	• Surrogate determines the "highest net benefit among available options" (Beauchamp & Childress, 2001, p. 192). This is a quality-of-life (QOL) evaluation—it may or may not be based on a person's previously expressed desires. Previous values, beliefs, and wishes are considered to the extent that they give information about what would constitute QOL for the person. • This may permit overriding a Durable Power of Attorney's decision that does not seem to further patient best interests and when there are no written instructions (from the incapacitated patient) to support the proposed course of action.
C. Reasonable person	• A standard used when neither A nor B is applicable. It asks, "What would a reasonable person want?" The typical patient was never competent (e.g., baby or cognitively impaired) and/or previous wishes cannot be determined. For example: 1. Some permanently unconscious patients who might be said to have no interests and who cannot be "benefited" or "burdened." 2. Incapacitated, dying patients left on life support to preserve organs for transplantation (Medical College of Georgia, 2000)

These are the ideals of proxy decision making. The nurse practitioner should be aware, however, that circumstances of proxy decision making are often less than ideal. The proxy may not be able to separate his or her own desires, beliefs, and values from those of the patient. There may be family strife that interferes with rational decision making. Written documents may not have instructions for the situation at hand (Box 11–2).

It is important that advanced-practice nurses help their patients to determine *in advance* what therapeutic measures they would wish for should they become unable to decide for themselves. This may be called preventive ethics. Advanced-practice nurses have an important role to play in empowering their patients to plan for such things as the type of end-of-life care they would like. Advanced planning should be part of holistic primary

---

Box 11–2

The Case of Mr. B.: A Failure of Proxy Decision Making

Mr. B. is a nursing home patient with early Alzheimer's disease who has lucid periods and is generally capable of making decisions about his health care. He has developed pneumonia, become more forgetful and confused, and is deemed currently not capable of making his own health-care decisions. As a result of ongoing discussions with his nurse practitioner, he has appointed a health-care proxy and left written instructions concerning his wishes not to have his life prolonged through "heroic measures" should he suffer a respiratory or cardiac arrest. His proxy (a grandson) decides that "no heroic measures" means "no antibiotics." The nurse practitioner, who has an ongoing relationship with Mr. B., does not think that in this case Mr. B. would consider antibiotics "heroic measures." He was still generally enjoying life and liked to participate in unit activities. What should the nurse practitioner do?

Possible strategies:

1. Ensure that assessment of the situation is accurate (clinical judgment).
2. Assess the likelihood of treatment success (benefits and burdens).
3. Discuss with colleagues and ethics resource (local hospital, committee, or person associated with the nursing home). JCAHO requires that long term care facilities have resources for the resolution of ethical issues.
4. Discuss with the proxy your reasoning why, in this particular instance, it is in Mr. B.'s best interest (given his own previously stated beliefs and values) to be treated with antibiotics.

---

care and is best discussed before patients become seriously ill. However, the limitations of advanced planning also need to be understood because not all eventualities can be foreseen or planned for. Knowledge of the patient can help the nurse practitioner understand what sorts of things are congruent with previous beliefs and lifestyle preferences.

Since 1991, the Patient Self Determination Act (PSDA) has been in effect. This act essentially makes legal the moral rights of persons to determine whether they will accept or refuse treatment, thus adding force to the concept of such rights (Box 11–3). Wolf (1991) notes that "the goal of the statute is to encourage but not require adults to fill out advance directives" (p. 411). The implications of the PSDA are important for nurse practitioners working in institutions or with institutionalized patients because they may be responsible for ensuring that the "spirit" of the PSDA is supported by the institutions with which they are associated. This is a moral responsibility of patient care; it facilitates patients' control over decisions even when they become incapacitated.

Box 11–3

The Patient Self Determination Act (PSDA)

The PSDA of 1991 was designed to encourage communication about end-of-life issues. It required changes in public policy, public and professional education, and institutional policy, and was expected to facilitate social awareness about end-of-life care problems.

It relies on state law and merely mandates that individuals are provided with details of the state laws regarding end-of-life care on admission to an institution that caters to Medicare or Medicaid patients, regardless of whether the individual himself or herself is a recipient of Medicare or Medicaid.

The PSDA requires that:

- Written information be given to admitted patients about their rights under the law to make their own treatment decisions.
- Patients be informed and given written policies about their rights to complete state-allowed advance directives.
- There is documentation of a patient's advance directive.
- The patients know that care is not conditional on the existence or absence of an advance directive.
- There be staff education about advance directives and patient rights.

Further information may be accessed at *nursingworld.org/ethics*

Confidentiality

Autonomy is also the principle underlying confidentiality. The idea is that persons have the right to determine who shall be privy to information about them. In certain situations, the status of confidentiality between a person and others such as clergy is considered a privilege and is shielded from exposure by (or to) the legal system. In health care, confidentiality does not carry as strong a status as clergy/supplicant or lawyer/client privilege. Nevertheless, because it is a necessary ingredient of trust, in health-care settings there are strong sanctions against breaching confidentiality. In theory, the principle of confidentiality may be overridden only in situations in which extreme harm to self or others is imminent. In practice, confidentiality is breached frequently. In hospital settings, many persons have access to the patient's information. Insurance companies demand access to patient information before payment for services is made. Additionally, there has recently been a push to institute a nationwide medical information bank. The ethical implications of this are many, and such implications are the subject of current debates in the ethics literature (Etzioni, 1999; Gostin, 1997; Hodge, 2000; Goldberg, 2000).

Additionally, in outpatient settings, barriers to privacy may include the fact that office personnel are personally acquainted with the patient. In rural practice it is not unusual for practitioners to be approached by a member of the office staff who is curious about an acquaintance or family member's health problems. They may ask for information about a patient with whom they have a personal acquaintance or, alternatively, want access to the chart of a neighbor or family member. In such settings, advanced-practice nurses have the responsibility to address confidentiality issues with the staff members they supervise. As members of the community in which they practice, nurse practitioners may be approached outside the practice facility, for example in the grocery store, for information about a person who has been secretive about an illness. It is often very difficult to respond diplomatically while maintaining the patient's privacy.

The new "privacy rule" governing patient information provides legal guidelines about disclosure, but the nurse practitioner is responsible for using clinical judgment in deciding what level of detail to share. A rule of thumb for this would be: "disclose only as much information as is necessary to permit optimal care **and** only information that is pertinent to the situation." Disclosure of patient information may require a balancing of the risks of information sharing with the benefits in terms of treatment.

Adolescents often provide nurse practitioners with very difficult confidentiality issues. As Bandman and Bandman (2002) note, most adolescents are torn between wanting to challenge authority and assert independence and needing the "help and support of effective parents" (p. 195). The results of risk-taking behavior, such as drug and alcohol experimentation and risky sexual activity, as well as normal health-care needs, often lead the teenager to seek the assistance of a nurse practitioner. Thus nurse practitioners frequently find themselves in the position of trying to maintain the adolescent's autonomy and confidentiality needs while mediating between the teenager and parental figures who feel that they have a right to information about the child for a variety of reasons. The nurse practitioner can find himself or herself caught in the tension "between the anger and perceived duties of the parent and the defensiveness and vulnerability of the adolescent" (Bandman & Bandman, 2002, p. 200).

Although federal and state laws, in addition to (and as a result of) ethical considerations, generally serve to protect the privacy and autonomy of adolescents, the nurse practitioner's professional obligations have a broader goal than mere protection. The nurse practitioner is concerned with facilitating the adolescent's health; therefore his or her responsibilities include helping the adolescent to grasp his or her authentic options and rights, facilitating interaction between the adolescent and parents or guardians, maintaining trust, and conserving confidentiality.

However, nursing judgment (which includes ethical judgment) is important in determining risk. For example, if the nurse practitioner determines that the risk of preserving the adolescent's privacy is high, based on all pertinent and available evidence such as the presence of sexual or physical abuse, he or she may decide to disclose this information to *appropriate authorities*. It is understood that mandatory reporting laws exist. Such laws are important for the general protection of a society's citizens. However, there may be rare occasions when a nurse practitioner's clinical judgment is that the legal obligation will cause more harm than good. In such circumstances, the nurse practitioner has two separate considerations: risking his or her professional standing and license versus providing for the patient's good. There is no easy resolution of such problems; however, if the situation is not an emergency, the nurse practitioner should try to solicit appropriate advice from a peer, a counselor, or an ethics expert/resource. In any case, it remains the nurse practitioner's responsibility to handle the situation in a manner that preserves trust and provides ongoing support. This ongoing support may be provided by the nurse practitioner and/or by appropriate allied services.

There are also occasions when family members ask a nurse practitioner to be deceptive. They request information on an adolescent patient's health status but do not want the adolescent to know that they have made this request (Box 11–4).

The responsibility to maintain patient confidentiality related to the sharing of medical records and other health information has recently been

---

Box 11–4

The Case of the Deceptive Father

A nurse practitioner student presented a case for "ethics discussion" during his clinical practicum. His preceptor had asked him to begin the physical examination for an adolescent male patient (16 years old) who wished to resume football practice after an injury. After the assessment, the nurse practitioner student planned to draw some blood for a variety of routine tests. When the student left the room, the boy's father followed him and asked if he could "get a drug screen" on the blood work but not tell his son what he was doing. He was very worried that his son was under the influence of a "bad group of friends" whom he suspected both took drugs and used alcohol. If he knew for sure, he would make efforts to get help for his son, but he did not want to seem "untrusting" if there were no problem–they had had some trust problems before. The student was taken aback. He had never previously encountered such a request. He knew that "confidentiality" was not the only issue but wasn't sure how best to respond. What should the nurse practitioner student do?

Discussion

The nurse practitioner student is right to take time to think this through. With the help of his preceptor, he was able to identify that the situation involved both confidentiality and a breach of the fiduciary (patient/provider) relationship. The fiduciary relationship is one of trust. A patient is in the position having to trust that the health-care provider is going to maintain a focus on his or her best interest. Moreover, the father-son relationship is not facilitated by deception. Finally, even if the drug screen were carried out, the father would not necessarily have the right to the information in the absence of his son's permission. The student watched as the preceptor explored with the father ways to approach his son that would both further the father-son relationship and facilitate an ongoing patient-nurse relationship.

There are occasions when even seasoned professionals are presented with problems that they are not sure how to resolve. Because nurse practitioners often work in isolation from peers, it is important to build a network of colleagues with whom to discuss difficult problems. It is helpful if these colleagues are from a variety of specialty areas.

---

reinforced legislatively. A "Privacy Rule" (45 Code of Federal Regulations [CFR] Part 160, 164 subparts A & E) was developed as a result of the Health Insurance Portability and Accountability Act (HIPAA) of 1996. The "Privacy Rule" became law in April 2003. This rule has implications for nurse practitioner practice as well as for all health-care providers and researchers (Table 11–2). Aspects of the privacy rule require interpretation (clinical and ethical judgment) on the part of the nurse practitioner so that the intent of the rule is upheld. That is, the best interests of the patient are served.

TABLE 11–2
HIPAA Final Privacy Rule (45 CFR 160, 164—Subparts A & B)

Intent	• Ensure that individuals' health information is properly protected while allowing the flow of health information needed to provide and promote high-quality health care and protect the public's health and well-being (Privacy Summary).
	• Protect the privacy of individually identifiable health information related to advances in electronic technology (HHS Fact Sheet).
	• Limit the ways in which "health plans, pharmacies, hospitals, clinics, nursing homes, and other covered entities (e.g., physicians, nurse practitioners)" can use patients' medical information (HHS Fact Sheet).
	• The limitations extend to any identifiable information: written, oral, or computerized (HHS Fact sheet).
Patient Protections	• Patients have the right to access their medical records.
	• "Covered entities" (see glossary) should inform patients in what ways their information may be used and their rights under the privacy regulations. Information generally would be shared only on a "need-to-know" basis. Patient must authorize other uses.
	• Providers must make efforts to ensure that communications with patients also remain confidential (e.g., in what manner important communications between provider and patient should be handled—can the nurse practitioner call the patient's home? Should the nurse practitioner leave a message?).

TABLE 11–2

HIPAA Final Privacy Rule (45 CFR 160, 164—Subparts A & B)

Special Considerations	• Privacy Rule does not supersede state laws about privacy when these are more stringent.
	• "Covered Entities" must develop written privacy policies and train their employees (*implications for NPs in supervisory roles*).
	• Civil and criminal penalties apply to "covered entities" who misuse information.
Glossary: Covered Entity	• Any institution or individual responsible for providing patient care (anyone "covered" by the rule).
HIPAA	• The Health Insurance Portability and Accountability Act of 1996. This act included "Administrative Simplification" provisions which mandated that the HHS "adopt national standards for electronic health care transactions." Meanwhile, there was a recognition of potential associated problems. The privacy rule was formulated in response.

HHS=Health and Human Services
Sources: HHS Fact Sheet: *Protecting the privacy of patients' health information.* Accessed 8/3/03 from *www.hhs.gov/news/facts.privacy.html*
The Privacy Rule Summary. Accessed 8/3/03 from *www.hhs.gov/privacysummary.pdf*

Veracity

Veracity or truth telling is another principle that has *prima facie* (on first reflection) strength in the nurse-patient relationship. In general, veracity is a very important consideration because it involves trust, which is the basis of nurse-patient relationships. Veracity or truthfulness in giving patients information about their health-care needs facilitates autonomous choice and enhances patient decision making. There are times, however, when health-care professionals are tempted to withhold certain details from the patient, especially when it is seen as in the patient's best interests or when family members demand it. It is sometimes difficult for health-care providers to determine both how much information and which types of information will best serve patient needs. For example, explaining too many of the possible side effects of antihypertensive drugs can confuse patients or unduly alarm them.

The nurse practitioner must use good clinical judgment based on knowledge of the patient in supplying adequate information to support a given patient's autonomous decision making. One way to do this is to give the appropriate information for this patient while acknowledging that certain undesirable effects may occur. For example, when prescribing a medication, the nurse practitioner would inform the patient that, because individuals respond differently to drugs, there is a chance that rare side effects may occur, and these should be reported immediately. Making decisions about the amount and type of information to be given to a patient in a variety of circumstances is more one of good clinical judgment based on knowledge of the patient than purely a problem of veracity. However, deliberately withholding information so that a patient agrees to a treatment that the nurse practitioner considers important is a problem of veracity. It is tempting to avoid the longer route around such problems (patient education, understanding patients' motives, and so forth), but this eventually undermines trust and constitutes a moral problem. Veracity is compromised when the clinician withholds information that a patient has a right to know. Veracity has some cross-cultural implications in that various cultures have not traditionally valued truth telling in the case of terminal illnesses or cancer diagnoses. Decision making about whether to honor veracity in such cases must take into consideration what is known about the culture, the particular patient, the strength of his or her personal and cultural beliefs, and whether there is evidence about what sorts of things the patient would like to know.

The absence of veracity on the part of the nurse practitioner may interfere with a patient's autonomous action. In the case of terminal illness, it may deprive the patient of the ability to plan the remainder of his or her life. It is rare, but may be possible, that a patient does not want to know a certain diagnosis or a given trajectory. If this is known in advance (and validated in writing), it may prove an exception to the rule of veracity (e.g., patient waiver of the right to know gained before testing).

Nonmaleficence

Allied with the principle of autonomy is the principle of nonmaleficence. In general society, this principle constrains people from harming others. In health-care settings, it prohibits clinicians from harming patients. This may seem odd on two accounts. First, we expect that clinicians do not usually intend harm to patients. Second, some harms seem unavoidable. For example, it may be necessary to cause discomfort to an individual by placing an intravenous catheter to give fluids when the person is dehydrated and unable to ingest nutrients. Also, a nurse practitioner may feel that he or she is doing harm when performing a procedure on a protesting child. In this case, the nurse practitioner relies on self-reflection, critical thinking, and nursing knowledge to be sure that the overall intent of the discomfort caused is to provide a good result that can be achieved only through these interventions. In other words, nurse practitioners are accountable for their nursing judgment that the intervention will bring the desired result. Therefore, more than just the intention **not** to do harm is required.

The nurse practitioner can inadvertently do harm through ignorance or incompetence, through referral to another provider who is incompetent or inappropriate, by inadequate supervision or training of those under one's supervision, and so on. A health-care professional who genuinely attempts to minimize "harms" that are necessary to provide a greater good (beneficence) cannot truly be said to be causing harm if what results is more benefit than harm. Alternatively, even if greater harm than good did actually ensue, or if it could not have been anticipated based on available information and the clinician's competent judgment, the action was not maleficent. For example, a patient develops anaphylaxis after an antibiotic was prescribed for an infected spider bite. The patient reported that she had not taken the particular drug before and had never had a drug reaction, and moreover, the nurse practitioner kept her under observation as a precaution. Nevertheless, she had to be hospitalized and was mechanically ventilated for a few hours (until treatment reversed the shock). Her life was endangered by the treatment.

The idea is that the main objective of the agent is therapeutic. However, the duty of nonmaleficence does mean that clinicians are accountable for foreseeing the consequences of their actions wherever possible. This places obligations on the practitioner to thoroughly evaluate the problem in its rich contextual facets. A thorough and informed evaluation, in turn, requires professional competence. Harm caused through careless, indifferent, or expedient decision making and ensuing actions violates the principle. Therefore both deliberate harm and harm caused by indifferent or incompetent decision making should be considered maleficent and are morally problematic.

Beneficence

The principle of "beneficence" concerns the duty a person has to benefit another under certain conditions. Beneficence, unlike nonmaleficence, is not **necessarily** a moral requirement of action on the part of societal members toward each other. Whether beneficence is viewed as a moral requirement of societal members very much depends upon philosophical beliefs and the ethical theory (perspective) ascribed to (if any). That is, as an ordinary citizen, I am not necessarily morally required to go out of my way to help or benefit someone who is not in danger. If someone is in danger and I do not try to prevent harm when the risk to me is minimal, I violate the principle of nonmaleficence. However, exceptions include the actions of parents on behalf of their children and guardians on behalf of their wards.

The principle of "beneficence" in health-care settings does require that actions taken serve the patient's best interests as well as preferences (where possible). In contrast to ordinary members of society, health-care professionals have augmented duties of beneficence because their professional goals involve meeting health-care needs and thus are aimed at providing a "good." For such reasons, beneficence is a moral expectation of health-care professionals.

Conflicts with Autonomy

Occasionally the principles of beneficence and autonomy seem to conflict in a given situation. Take, for example, a patient who refuses antibiotics for pneumonia. In this case it seems that harm is caused if he or she is permitted to refuse—indeed, the patient may be risking his or her life. What is the clinician's responsibility? Duties of beneficence seem to mandate treating the patient against his or her will, ensuring that the "good" of health is facilitated but violating the principle of autonomy. Preserving the patient's life so that he or she can make autonomous decisions in the future may be required by beneficence. Therefore, in this case, beneficence demands a temporary overruling of autonomous choice.

However, it can be argued that beneficence takes precedence over autonomy only in cases in which the choice is not truly autonomous. Therefore we have to explore how autonomous the choice is. First, there has to be evidence that a choice has been made. In this case, a choice between accepting antibiotic treatment and not accepting antibiotic treatment was made. Second, the reasonableness (or rationality) of the decision has to be discerned. That is, it must be ascertained whether the patient has really grasped the implications of refusing treatment. The reasons given for the treatment refusal, then, should illuminate gaps in information delivery or processing. Finally, it must be determined whether there are any external or internal coercion factors impinging on the decision. Perhaps the patient feels that he or she cannot afford the medicine (external) or perhaps he or she has a mistrust of antibiotics because of a previous experience (internal).

Agich (1998) has noted that competent decision making requires, among other things, that the person be in possession of adequate information, an understanding of benefits and costs of alternative treatments or plans, and knowledge of personal values and beliefs and the effects of these on the decision. He is expressly discussing decision making in nursing-home settings, but these ideas are applicable to patient decision making in all types of settings and perhaps especially in correctional facilities. These criteria can be used to permit clinicians to distinguish informed decisions from those that cannot be considered autonomous or when special measures must be taken to control coercive factors. When a decision cannot be said to be "informed," the principle of beneficence directs us to decide treatment based on the patient's best interests. Generally, beneficence does not trump autonomy unless there is a question regarding the autonomous nature of the decision. On such occasions beneficence may permit (or preserve) future autonomous decision making. For example, if we see an unknown person about to jump off a tall building, we do not stop to ask if this is an autonomous decision on the individual's part because jumping efficiently ends all future decision making. We beneficently stop them from committing suicide until it can be determined whether or not the person has a psychiatric (or other) illness that is interfering with rational thought processes. If it turns out to be an autonomous decision, many would say we have no right to interfere.

Paternalism

The attempt (or intent) to interfere with an autonomous decision is commonly termed "paternalism." Beauchamp and Childress (2001) define paternalism as "the intentional overriding of one person's known preferences ... where the person who overrides justifies the action by the goal of benefiting or avoiding harm to the person (in question)" (p. 178). "Paternalism" has negative connotations in health care because historically it was assumed (by physicians and others) that superior medical knowledge and skills permitted physician decision making on behalf of patients without patient involvement. In contemporary health-care settings, the principle of autonomy has to a great extent revealed paternalistic attitudes on the part of physicians as problematic. Beauchamp and Childress (2001), however, although agreeing that paternalistic actions must be justified, note that "beneficence" does sometimes provide grounds for justifiably restricting autonomous actions as well as nonautonomous ones" (p. 181). The difficulty for the nurse practitioner lies in this process of justification. It is most important to resist relying on one's own beliefs or values as justification for paternalism. Equally, one needs to guard against expediency as a motivation. Paternalism is warranted only if it will serve the patient's best interests as grasped through an understanding of that patient's beliefs and values **and** if the risks of not intervening are high, as in life-threatening situations. What is warranted is the provision of adequate and appropriate information for the patient to make his or her own decision. When autonomy or competence for decision making is not ensured, an attempt to discover what the person would have wanted must be made (see previous discussion under autonomy).

Justice

Another major principle used to provide guidance for health-care decision making is justice. The term "justice" is used in many different ways. For the purposes of this chapter, the discussion is about social justice. Social justice has to do with any formal or informal systems existing within a given society to determine what will be the distribution of "goods" such as health, education, food, and shelter. The social justice arrangements in a society are indicative of what the society values. In democratic societies, the requirements of social justice generally include equitable distribution of the benefits and burdens of societal life. This is also known as "justice as fairness" reflecting the ideas behind Rawls' (1971) *A Theory of Justice*, in which he discusses a hypothetical method for deciding how a society's institutions should be arranged to provide for fairness. A main concept in the theory is that any unequal burdens viewed as necessary to improve overall conditions will be slanted to benefit the most disadvantaged.

Justice issues in health care have to do with such things as ensuring access to care and addressing the needs of the vulnerable, or deciding where resources are to be directed. An emphasis on justice in health-care settings is sometimes called the "impartialist" perspective in that it considers the needs of all who fall under its umbrella. For example, within the prison system, this view of justice would mandate access to care for prisoners in need. Thus, it would not permit arbitrary obstacles to access (such as requiring good behavior or favors) that might be presented by prison officers or other prisoners in order to exert physical or psychological control. Justice would also require improved access to care for the poor and underprivileged, both in terms of receiving care and transportation and local availability of services.

Although justice might require consideration of the special needs of a disadvantaged group, it does so impartially. That is, it does not distinguish among the particulars of individuals; each member within the group has an equal right to whatever is proposed. The requirements of "justice as fairness" sometimes pose problems for the nurse practitioner. For example, he or she may feel a need to advocate that a particular patient receive an expensive treatment not normally covered by insurance. However, this could divert resources away from the needs of others in the society. It is part of the health-care professional's responsibility to advocate for justice. But in an economically, and often for-profit, driven health-care system, injustices occur at both the local and societal levels.

Many have argued that the United States health-care delivery system has become inherently unjust because of the business model approach to the provision of services (Brock, 1990; Brock & Buchanan, 1987; Daniels, 1991; Drevdahl; 2002; Gray, 1991; Kassirer, 1995; Pellegrino, 1995; Relman, 1992; Wong, 1998). The business model treats patients as commodities. The incentives of a business model are to reduce costs and increase profits. Gostin (1999) and others have noted the many problems associated with applying market theory to the provision of health care. He notes that "no health care system outside of the United States has demonstrated the worth of managed competition in promoting quality and constraining medical inflation" (p. 397). The implication is that we have no reason to suppose that the United States health-care system will fare any better than other health-care systems in this regard.

However, the constraints that managed-care companies place on the autonomous practice of clinicians sometimes pressure the nurse practitioner to be less than truthful about a patient's symptoms to insurance companies. This is seen as necessary by the clinician in whose judgment the tests or treatments are necessary for the care of this patient even though the patient does not meet criteria for receiving the treatment as set by the managed-care or insurance company. Unfortunately, the practice of misrepresenting the patient's condition to obtain needed services, which Morreim (1991) has termed "gaming the system," further complicates the problems caused by health care that is primarily economically driven versus being patient or health centered. Additionally, it compromises the health-care provider's integrity. The ANA Code of Ethics for Nurses tenet No. 5 asserts that the nurse has a "responsibility to preserve integrity" (p. 18). If managed-care practices do not serve patients well, they should be challenged by those who recognize and can describe the problem using experience, research, or other scholarly literature to back up their claims. This is a moral requirement of "justice as fairness."'

⟩⟩ EXPANSIONARY NATURE OF MORAL RESPONSIBILITY IN ADVANCED PRACTICE

Because advanced-practice nurses oversee the patient's total care, it might be claimed that they have greater moral responsibilities than nurses who share oversight with other health-care professionals. For example, when nursing care is delivered in concert with what might reasonably be termed "medical" care, as is often the case in traditional nursing, the ethical responsibilities are generally shared by two or more persons. However, when a nurse is the primary health-care provider responsible for ordering and/or carrying out necessary "medical" interventions (e.g., prescribing drugs, delivering anesthesia, inserting invasive tubes) as part of holistic nursing care of the patient, his or her clinical, and thus ethical, responsibilities may be augmented.

Although nurse practitioners, along with all nurses, are accountable for understanding the limits of their own knowledge base, in advanced practice there are additional obstacles and obligations related more specifically to the role of primary health-care provider or specialist health-care provider. These responsibilities include, but are not limited to:

- ◎ Choosing wisely one's consulting physicians (or the allied health-care specialists with whom one collaborates)
- ◎ Making appropriate referrals to competent and qualified specialists
- ◎ Identifying and addressing conflicts of interests and the sources of these
- ◎ Participating in advocacy or political activity (alone or in concert with others) when obstacles to providing good care prove recalcitrant or intractable to remedy
- ◎ Ensuring congruence between professional philosophy of practice and the philosophy of a given workplace

The idea that "good" nursing practice is ethical practice, then, presents the advanced-practice nurse with a variety of challenges. The practitioner must be diligent not only in exploring what is best practice in difficult situations, but also in uncovering and challenging more subtle barriers to good care such as restrictions placed on practice by their employers, certain managed-care companies, or economic conditions. Furthermore, all nurses as professionals have responsibilities to forecast future needs when possible and to anticipate the preventive measures required for furthering the health of the society. Because many nurse practitioners provide care in relative isolation from peers, these responsibilities can appear onerous. However, such responsibilities fall to us because, in many cases, we are the ones in the best position to recognize problems that perhaps are not obvious to patients or to the public in general.

For example, there are times when managed-care companies, in the absence of intense lobbying on the part of the health-care provider, pay only for care that is suboptimal or not state of the art. For example, it was reported to me by a variety of different nurse practitioners in the state where I taught Family Nurse Practitioner (FNP) students that a certain managed-care company, contracted to provide services to Medicaid patients in that state, would pay only for an allergy drug that had drowsiness as a side effect even though other more expensive drugs were available that did not have this side effect. Drowsiness is undesirable for working adults; it is even more problematic for children. It puts the children at risk for poor learning or inability to concentrate on lessons. A nurse practitioner and physician coalition was eventually successful in persuading the company to change its policies. However, there are numerous other instances in which future health needs have been identified, but preventive or screening practices are not instituted because of economic incentives that weigh against long-term savings in the interest of the economic "quick fix" (Baer, Fagin, & Gordon, 1996; Daniels, Light, & Caplan, 1996; Howe, 1995; Jecker & Jonsen, 1997; McCullough, 1997; Mechanic, 1996; Nordgren, 1995; Richman & Fein, 1995; Rodwin, 1993; Wong, 1998; Zoloth-Dorfman & Rubin, 1995).

It may seem an impossible task for already harried advanced-practice nurses to address the social and political issues surrounding health-care delivery. However, if we as a group do not find ways to do this, we do a disservice to both our patients and to ourselves. There is a disservice to our patients because they have put their trust in us and expect us to provide good care. We serve ourselves ill because, if we are powerless to change poor practices, there is nothing to stop the domination of our practice by those who give higher priority to economic interests than to health interests. This is not to say that management of costs is not also necessary, but it should be second to health concerns and should focus on permitting improved care for the society. One strategy to assist nurse practitioners in political and advocacy activities on behalf of patients and patient groups concerns collaboration with peers and allied professionals to address political and social concerns and the formation of ethics discussion groups in which peers can reflect with others on difficult cases, problematic situations, or obstacles to good practice. Additionally, formal professional organizations such as the ANA and state nurses' organizations (SNOs), as well as practice specialty organizations, are all important sources for collective political action on behalf of nursing's population of concern.

⊚⟩⟩ SELF-REFLECTION, VALUES CLARIFICATION, AND REFLECTION

Gaining confidence in one's moral decision making is a slow process. However, nurse practitioners can enhance their confidence by ensuring that the following five elements are present in their daily practice.

1. A genuine willingness to (a) examine personal values and beliefs for origin and consistency and (b) identify and revise inconsistencies. Nurse practitioners must guard against being unduly influenced by their own biases and values in cases in which decision making primarily concerns furthering the interests of others. This is not to say that the nurse practitioner's personal integrity is not important—it is. Maintaining both personal and professional integrity is essential to good practice. Integrity has to do with a sense of wholeness of the self and consistency of actions with truly examined beliefs and values. "Nurses have both personal and professional identities that are neither entirely separate nor entirely merged, but are integrated" (ANA, 2001, p. 19). Tenet 5 of the ANA *Code of Ethics for Nurses with Interpretive Statements* (2001) validates the nurse's preservation of integrity in those situations where he or she feels that personal integrity is compromised. It notes that "where a particular treatment, intervention, activity or practice is morally objectionable to the nurse ... the nurse is justified in refusing to participate on moral grounds" (p. 20). When this involves risk to the patient, though, other arrangements must be made to safeguard patient care.

A true examination of beliefs and values requires a willingness to admit that these may not always be justifiable—they may be remnants from childhood indoctrinations of various sorts. For example, the ideas that certain other ethnic groups are inferior in some way, or that one should not question authority, cannot logically be defended and are not supported by nursing's knowledge base or its Code of Ethics. An honest and ongoing examination of one's values and biases permits one to control these in situations in which personal values and biases are irrelevant to, or worse, interfere with, the care of patients.

2. An understanding of how personal beliefs and values are either congruent or liable to interfere with the task at hand. In any given situation, the nurse practitioner must ask himself or herself, "What are my beliefs and biases in this situation?" For example, a nurse practitioner may believe that a patient with an alcohol problem should have been able to control his or her drinking; perhaps the nurse had an alcoholic relative whose lifestyle caused family grief. Such biases are not uncommon. What is important, though, is that the nurse practitioner recognize this attitude as a bias and not allow it to interfere with decision making in this situation and for this patient. As another example, perhaps the nurse practitioner believes that his or her below-poverty-level, depressed, obese, diabetic patient who smokes is responsible for the poor healing of his or her own leg ulcer and thus is less inclined to provide assistance to this patient than to a so-called "compliant" patient. It is incumbent on the nurse practitioner to examine the consistency of this belief with nursing knowledge about the effects of poverty and disease on the patient's motivations.

3. An understanding of the nature of ethical theory, its strengths, limitations, and language (this facilitates interdisciplinary communication). This chapter has provided a foundation for understanding ethical language as it applies in health care. It has also discussed some of the main principles that have been derived from a variety of ethical theories and are applicable to patient situations as well as to the broader ethical concerns of health-care provision for society. Additionally, the importance of including a broader contextual understanding of morally problematic situations in health care was emphasized. This broader view of the crucial importance of context, as well as ethical principles, in examining morally troubling situations is especially relevant to the environments in which advanced-practice nursing occurs.

4. Experience in examining situations for their moral implications using a framework for data gathering and analysis. When trying to gain clarity on morally troubling situations, nurse practitioners must consider a framework of questions as part of the ethical decision-making process (Box 11–5). A variety of frameworks are available in both nursing and medical ethics texts. The framework offered here is synthesized from the nursing process and from other sources, including my own experiences, but it also includes cultural and contextual considerations in accordance with insights from feminist ethics. No framework will give definitive answers to all moral problems or dilemmas. What a framework can do is promote clarity by highlighting essential or important factors, ensuring thorough fact finding, determining what data are missing, and revealing important contextual aspects such as institutional or societal obstacles to good care.

5. Opportunities to discuss problematic situations after the fact with colleagues and experts on ethical decision making (i.e., clinical ethicists) Confidence in moral decision making is gained when nurse practitioners have the opportunity to reflect on the situation and discuss its handling and outcome with colleagues and/or clinical ethicists. Additionally, reflection and discussion with others help isolate those intractable or recurrent problems that require addressing at a local, institutional, or societal level.

))) SUMMARY

Discussion in this chapter has been focused on the particular ethical responsibilities and concerns of nurse practitioners, but is applicable to other advanced-practice nurses. Although the emphasis has been on **moral** decision making in advanced practice, moral and clinical decision making may

---

Box 11–5

Ethical Decision-Making Process

For nurse practitioners, decision making has an inseparable moral component. Thus, the careful exercise of experience, skill, and knowledge is warranted when trying to formulate the best course of action for a given
individual or to resolve a particular situation. In usual health-care situations,
thoughtfulness, pertinent data gathering, and careful consideration of the
options are required. In situations that are more complex, in which no good
options seem to exist or obstacles to providing care arise, a more in-depth
analysis of contributing factors is needed. The following framework can help
nurse practitioners make sound ethical decisions in daily practice situations.
It is also important to recognize when a problem is beyond one's personal
expertise so that assistance may be sought.

Steps	Questions
1. Identify the major problem(s).	• What ethical principles are involved? (Is the patient being prevented from making an autonomous decision? Might coercion [psychological or cognitive] be involved? Is beneficence being trumped by economic concerns, e.g., is treatment being denied?)
	• What are the power influences? Obstacles?
	• Who has an interest in maintaining power imbalances?
2. Determine who is involved.	• Who has, or who thinks he or she has, a stake in the outcome?
	• Who else beside the patient is important (e.g., other patients, family members, significant other)?
3. Determine the prevalent values.	• What are the values held by the patient, the institution, and you?
	• What are the value conflicts? Are these conflicts interpersonal, inter- or intraprofessional, or personal versus professional?
	• Are cultural influences present?
	• Who can help sort out cultural beliefs?
	• Who is the most appropriate interpreter (knowledgeable and neutral)?

Box 11—5 (Continued)

Steps	Questions
4. Identify information gaps.	• Do you need more information? • From whom or where might you obtain this information?
5. Identify possible courses of action and probable consequences.	• Which course of action is likely to be most beneficial and least harmful to those involved (including you)?
6. Implement the selected course of action and evaluate the outcome.	• Does the actual outcome correlate with the anticipated outcome? If not, what was unexpected? Was this foreseeable given more data? • Do similar problems keep reoccurring? If so, why? Does the problem need to be addressed at a higher institutional or public policy level? How can you alert appropriate officials about the problem?
7. Engage in self-reflection and peer discussions.	• Could you have done things differently? • Would consulting with other professionals have altered your conception of the problem or the course of action taken? • What insights can you and your peers glean from this problem that may be applicable to similar situations in the future?

---

realistically be viewed as different aspects of the same process. Both are based on the ideal of furthering a "good" for individuals and society. This "good" is the goal of nursing and is generally agreed by the profession to be focused on improving health and relieving suffering for individuals and society using a holistic approach. This approach views persons as complex relational beings. The chapter is intended to give the nurse practitioner a basis on which to improve his or her confidence in moral decision making. Further reading on ethical issues associated with a given specialty area is recommended.

REFERENCES

Agich, G. J. (1998). Respecting the autonomy of elders in nursing homes. In J. F. Monagle & D. C. Thomasma (Eds.). *Health care ethics: Critical issues for the 21st century.* Gaithersburg, MD: Aspen.

American Nurses Association (1994). *Position Statements: The nonnegotiable nature of the ANA code for nurses with interpretive statements.* Washington, DC: Author.

American Nurses Association (1994). *Position statements: Risk versus responsibility in providing patient care.* Washington, DC: Author.

American Nurses Association (1995). *Nursing's Social Policy Statement.* Washington, DC: Author.

American Nurses Association (2001). *Code of ethics for nurses with interpretive statements.* Washington, DC: Author.

Aristotle (1967). The Nichomachean Ethics, books I, II, III (chapters 1-5), VI & X (Trans. W. D. Ross). In A. I. Melden (Ed.). *Ethical theories: A book of readings* (2nd ed., pp. 88–142). Englewood Cliffs, NJ: Prentice-Hall. (Date of original work uncertain.)

Baer, E. D., Fagin, C. M., & Gordon, S. (1996*). Abandonment of the patient: The impact of profit-driven care on the public.* New York: Springer.

Baier, A. C. (1985). What do women want in a moral theory? *Nous, 19*(1), 53–63.

Bandman, E., & Bandman, B. (2002). *Nursing ethics through the lifespan* (4th Ed.). Upper Saddle River, NJ: Prentice-Hall.

Beauchamp, T. L., & Childress, J. F. (2001). *Principles of Biomedical Ethics* (5th ed.). New York: Oxford University.

Beauchamp, T. L., & Walters, L. (1999). *Contemporary Issues in Bioethics* (5th ed.). Belmont, CA: Wadsworth.

Benner, P., Tanner, C. A., & Chesla, C. A. (1996). *Expertise in nursing practice: Caring, clinical judgment and ethics.* New York, NY: Springer.

Bentham, J. (1967). An introduction to the principles of morals and legislation. In A. I. Melden (Ed.). *Ethical theories: A book of readings* (2nd ed., pp. 367–390). Englewood Cliffs, NJ: Prentice-Hall. (Original work published 1789.)

Bowden, P. (2000). An 'ethic of care' in clinical settings: encompassing 'feminine' and 'feminist' perspectives. *Nursing philosophy, 1*(1), 36–49.

Broadbent, D. E. (1971). *Decision and stress.* New York: Academic Press.

Brock, D. (1990). Medicine and business: An unhealthy mix? *Business and Professional Ethics Journal, 9*(3&4), 21–37.

Brock, D. W., & Buchanan, A. E. (1987). The profit motive in medicine. *Journal of Medicine and Philosophy, 12,* 1–35.

Buchanan, A. E., & Brock, D. W. (1989). *Deciding for others: The ethics of surrogate decision making.* New York: Cambridge University.

Caplan, A. L. (1994). Can money and morality mix in medicine? *Academic Emergency Medicine, 1*(1), 73–81.

Daniels, N. (1991). The profit motive and the moral assessment of health care institutions. *Business and Professional Ethics Journal, 10*(2), 3–30.

Daniels, N., Light, D. W., & Caplan, R. L. (1996*). Benchmarks of fairness for health care reform.* NY: Oxford University.

Davis, A. J., Aroskar, M. A., Liaschenko, J., & Drought, T. S. (1997). *Ethical dilemmas & nursing practice* (4th ed.). Upper Saddle River, NJ: Appleton & Lange.

Degner, L. F., & Sloan, J. A. (1992). Decision making during serious illness: What role do patients really want to play? *Journal of Clinical Epidemiology, 45*, 941–950.

Donchin, A., & Purdy, L. (Eds.) (1999). *Embodying bioethics: Recent feminist advances.* Lanham, MD: Rowman and Littlefield.

Drevdahl, D. (2002). Social justice or market justice? The paradoxes of public health partnerships with managed care. *Public Health Nursing, 19*(3), 1611–1619.

Dubler, N. N. (1988). Patient rights in an emerging AIDS crisis. *Journal of Prison & Jail Health, 7*(1), Spring/Summer.

Edwards, W. (1954). The theory of decision making. *Psychological Bulletin, 51*, 380–417.

Etzioni, A. (1999). Medical records: Enhancing privacy, preserving the common good. *Hastings Center Report, 29*(2), 14–23.

Fowler, M. (1997). Nursing ethics. In A. J. Davis, M. A. Aroskar, J. Liaschenko, & T. S. Drought (Eds.). *Ethical dilemmas and nursing practice* (4th ed., pp. 17–34). Stamford CT: Appleton and Lange.

Fry, S. T. (1989). Toward a theory of nursing ethics. *Advances in Nursing Science, 11*(4), 9–22.

Fry, S. T. (1990). The philosophical foundations of caring. In M. M. Leininger (Ed.). *Ethical and moral dimensions of care* (pp. 13–24). Detroit: Wayne State University Press.

Gilligan, C. (1982). *In a different voice: Psychological theory and women's development.* Cambridge, MA: Harvard University.

Gilligan, C. (1993). Reply to critics. In M. J. Larrabee (Ed.). *An ethic of care: Feminist and interdisciplinary perspectives* (pp. 207–214). New York, NY: Routledge. (Reprinted from *Signs: Journal of Women in Culture and Society, 11*, 1986, pp. 324–333.)

Goldberg, I. V. (2000). Electronic medical records and patient privacy. *Health Care Manager, 18*(3), 63–69.

Gostin, L. O. (1997). Personal privacy in the health care system: Employer-sponsored insurance, managed care and integrated delivery systems. *Kennedy Institute of Ethics Journal, 7*(4), 361–376.

Gostin, L. O. (1999). Securing health or just health care? The effect of the health care system on the health of America. In T. L. Beauchamp & L. Walters (Eds.). *Contemporary issues in bioethics* (5th ed., pp. 393–400). Belmont, CA: Wadsworth.

Grace, P., & Gaylord, N. (1999). Transcendental health care ethics: Beyond the medical model. *Ethical Human Sciences and Services, 1*(3), 243–253.

Grace, P. J. (1998). A philosophical analysis of the concept 'advocacy': Implications for professional-patient relationships. *UMI Dissertation Abstracts*, 9923287.

Gray, B. H. (1991). *The profit motive and patient care: The changing accountability of doctors and hospitals.* Cambridge, MA: Harvard.

Heidegger, M. (1962). *Being and time* (Trans. J. Macquarrie and E. Robinson,). San Francisco, CA: Harper & Row. (Original work published 1927.)

Henderson, V. (1966). *The nature of nursing: A definition and its implications for practice, research and education.* New York: Macmillan.

Hodge, J. G., Jr. (2000). National health information: Privacy and new federalism. *Notre Dame Journal of Law, Ethics, & Public Policy, 14*(2), 791–820.

Howe, E. G. (1995). Managed care: "New moves," moral uncertainty, and a radical attitude. *The Journal of Clinical Ethics, 6*(4), 290-305.

Janis, I. L., & Mann, L. (1977). *Decision making: A psychological analysis of conflict, choice and commitment.* New York: Free Press.

Jecker, N. S., & Jonsen, A. R. (1997). Managed care : A house of mirrors. *The Journal of Clinical Ethics, 8*(3), 230–241.

Kant, I. (1967). *Foundations of the metaphysics of morals* (Trans. L. W. Beck). In A. I. Melden (Ed.). *Ethical theories: A book of readings* (2nd ed., pp. 317–366). Englewood Cliffs, NJ: Prentice-Hall. (Original work published 1785.)

Kassirer, J. P. (1995). Managed care and the morality of the marketplace. *New England Journal of Medicine, 333*(1), 50–52.

Liaschenko, J. (1999). Can justice coexist with the supremacy of personal values in nursing practice? *Western Journal of Nursing Research, 2*(1), 35–50.

MacIntyre, A. C. (1984). *After virtue: A study in moral theory* (2nd ed.). Notre Dame, IN: University of Notre Dame Press.

McCullough, L. (1997, March). Medicine and money: Past, present, future. In *The ethics of managed care.* Kennedy Institute of Ethics Course, Georgetown University, Washington, DC.

McIsaac, I. (1900). Ethics in nursing. *American Journal of Nursing, 1*(7), 488–490.

Mechanic, D. (1996). Reconciling the demand and provision of health services. In P. Day, D. M. Fox, R. Maxwell, & E. Scrivens (Eds.). *The state, politics and health: Essays for Rudolph Klein.* Cambridge, MA: Blackwell.

Medical College of Georgia (2000). *Ethics syllabus glossary.* Accessed August 4, 2003 at *www.mcg.edu/gpi/Ethics/ph1sylbus/bioethic.htm*

Mill, J. S. (1967). Utilitarianism. In A. I. Melden (Ed.). *Ethical theories: A book of readings* (2nd ed., pp. 391–434). Englewood Cliffs, NJ: Prentice-Hall. (Original work published 1863.)

Morreim, E. H. (1991). *Balancing act: The new medical ethics of medicine's new economics*. Dordrecht, Netherlands: Kluwer Academic.

Nelson, H. (1992). Against caring. *The Journal of Clinical Ethics, 3*(1), 8–15.

Nicholson, L. J. (1993). Women, morality and history. In M. J. Larrabee (Ed.). *An ethic of care: Feminist and interdisciplinary perspectives* (pp. 87–101). New York, NY: Routledge. (Reprinted from *Social Research, 50*, 1983, pp. 514–36.)

Noddings, N. (1984). *Caring: A feminine approach to ethics and moral education*. Berkeley: University of California Press.

Nordgren, R. A. (1995). The case against managed care and for a single-payer system. *Journal of the American Medical Association, 273*(1), 79–82.

Pellegrino, E. D. (1995). Interests, obligations and justice: Some notes towards an ethic of managed care. *Journal of Clinical Ethics, 6*(4), 313–317.

President's Commission for the Study of Ethical Problems in Medicine and biomedical and Behavioral research (1982). *Making Health Care Decisions*. Washington, DC: US Government Printing Office. 33. PB83236703.

Rawls, J. (1971). *A theory of justice*. Cambridge, MA: Harvard University Press.

Redelmeier, D. A., Rozin, E., & Kahneman, D. (1993). Understanding patients' decisions: Cognitive and emotional perspectives. *Journal of the American Medical Association, 270*, 72–76.

Relman, A. S. (1992, March). What market values are doing to medicine. *Atlantic Monthly*, pp. 99–106.

Richman, J. B., & Fein, R. (1995). The health care mess: A bit of history. *Journal of the American Medical Association, 273*(1), 69–71.

Robb, I. A. H. (1990). *Nursing ethics: For hospital and private use*. New York: E. C. Koeckert.

Rodwin, M. A. (1993). *Medicine, money and morals: Physician's conflict of interest*. New York: Oxford.

Ross, D. (1930). *The right and the good*. Oxford: Oxford University Press.

Schaeffer, M. H. (1989). Environmental stress and individual decision-making: Implications for the patient. *Patient Education and Counseling, 13*, 221–235.

Sherwin, S. (1992). *No longer patient: Feminist ethics and health care*. Philadelphia, PA: Temple University.

Tong, R. (1997). *Feminist Approaches to Bioethics: Theoretical Reflections and Practical Applications*. Boulder, CO: Westview Press.

Warren, V. L. (2001). From autonomy to empowerment: Health care ethics from a feminist Perspective. In W. Teays & L. Purdy (Eds.). *Bioethics, Justice, & Health Care* (pp. 49–53). Belmont, CA: Wadsworth.

Weston, A., (1997). *A practical companion to ethics*. New York: Oxford.

Wolf, S. M. (2001/1991). Sources of concern about the Patient Self Determination Act. In W. Teays & L. Purdy (Eds.). *Bioethics, justice, & health care* (pp. 411–419). Belmont, CA: Wadsworth. (Reprinted from *New England Journal of Medicine* [1991], *325*, 23, 1666–1671.)

Wong, K. L. (1998). *Medicine and the market place.* Notre Dame, IN: Notre Dame.

Zoloth-Dorfman, L., & Rubin, S. (1995). The patient as commodity: Managed care and the question of ethics. *The Journal of Clinical Ethics, 6*(2), 339–357.

Index

An "f" following a page number indicates a figure; a "t" following a page number indicates a table; a "b" following a page number indicates a box.